HANDBOOK FOR CLINICAL GYNECOLOGIC ENDOCRINOLOGY AND INFERTILITY

HANDBOOK FOR CLINICAL GYNECOLOGIC ENDOCRINOLOGY AND INFERTILITY

John David Gordon

Co-Director
Dominion Fertility & Endocrinology
Arlington, Virginia;
Clinical Associate Professor
Department of Obstetrics and Gynecology
The George Washington University
Washington, D.C.

Leon Speroff

Professor of Obstetrics and Gynecology
Reproductive Endocrinology
Oregon Health & Science University School of Medicine
Portland, Oregon

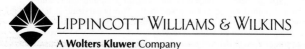

LIPPINCOTT WILLIAMS & WILKINS
A **Wolters Kluwer** Company

Philadelphia · Baltimore · New York · London
Buenos Aires · Hong Kong · Sydney · Tokyo

Acquisitions Editor: Lisa McAllister
Developmental Editor: Denise Martin
Production Editor: Christiana Sahl
Manufacturing Manager: Tim Reynolds
Cover Designer: Patricia Gast
Compositor: Circle Graphics
Printer: Vicks Litho

Library of Congress Cataloging-in-Publication Data

Gordon, John D. (John David)
  Handbook for clinical gynecologic endocrinology and infertility / John David
Gordon, Leon Speroff.
    p. ; cm.
  Companion vol. to: Clinical gynecologic endocrinology and infertility / Leon
Speroff, Robert H. Glass, Nathan G. Kase. 6th ed. c1999.
  Includes index.
  ISBN 0-7817-3164-X
  1. Infertility—Handbooks, manuals, etc. 2. Endocrine gynecology—
Handbooks, manuals, etc. I. Gordon, John David II. Speroff, Leon, 1935-
Clinical gynecologic, endocrinology and infertility. III. Title.
  [DNLM: 1. Genital Diseases, Female—Handbooks. 2. Endocrine Diseases—
Handbooks. 3. Hormones—Handbooks. 4. Infertility—Handbooks. 5.
Reproductive. Medicine—Handbooks. WP 39 G663h 2002]
RC889 .G665 2002
618.1—dc21
                                                                    2001045077

Care has been taken to confirm the accuracy of the information presented
and to describe generally accepted practices. However, the authors and
publisher are not responsible for errors or omissions or for any consequences
from application of the information in this book and make no warranty,
expressed or implied, with respect to the currency, completeness, or accuracy
of the contents of the publication. Application of this information in a
particular situation remains the professional responsibility of the practitioner.
  The authors and publisher have exerted every effort to ensure that drug
selection and dosage set forth in this text are in accordance with current
recommendations and practice at the time of publication. However, in view of
ongoing research, changes in government regulations, and the constant flow of
information relating to drug therapy and drug reactions, the reader is urged to
check the package insert for each drug for any change in indications and
dosage and for added warnings and precautions. This is particularly important
when the recommended agent is a new or infrequently employed drug.
  Some drugs and medical devices presented in this publication have Food and
Drug Administration (FDA) clearance for limited use in restricted research
settings. It is the responsibility of the health care provider to ascertain the
FDA status of each drug or device planned for use in their clinical practice.

10 9 8 7 6 5 4 3 2 1

Contents

Preface

I have had the great privilege to work with Dr. Leon Speroff in bringing the *Handbook for Clinical Gynecologic Endocrinology and Infertility* to press. During my postgraduate training as a house officer at Stanford in Obstetrics and Gynecology and later as a Fellow in Reproductive Endocrinology at the University of California at San Francisco, the earlier editions of *Clinical Gynecologic Endocrinology and Infertility* were essential components of my library. As I prepared for my written and oral board examinations in Reproductive Endocrinology, the sixth edition of the textbook was my constant companion.

For the last 10 years I have actively participated in developing several handbooks for medical professionals in Obstetrics and Gynecology. The concept of a companion handbook to *Clinical Gynecologic Endocrinology and Infertility* was a frequent topic of conversation among two of my fellowship colleagues, Russell Foulk and Collin Smikle, and myself. However, we never found the time to address the project during those years in San Francisco. Five years, two jobs, and one child after completing my fellowship I finally delivered the manuscript for this book to a very patient Lisa McAllister at Lippincott Williams & Wilkins.

The purpose of this handbook is to provide a handy companion to the sixth edition of *Clinical Gynecologic Endocrinology and Infertility*. Its purpose is not to serve in lieu of the textbook; rather, it is a means to distill many of the key points of the textbook into a pocket-sized guide for easy review and reference. The book, written in outline format rather than prose, should help the reader more easily find detailed information on a particular topic in the textbook. My hope is that the book will prove helpful to medical students, house officers, and practicing physicians.

This handbook would not have been possible without the enduring love and patience of my wife, Allison Smith, and our three children, Seth, Aaron, and Leah.

John David Gordon, M.D.

HANDBOOK
FOR CLINICAL
GYNECOLOGIC
ENDOCRINOLOGY
AND INFERTILITY

1

Molecular Biology for Clinicians

I. Historical Perspective
- ♦ Molecular biology—subspecialty of science devoted to understanding the structure and function of the genome (full complement of DNA, the macromolecule containing all the hereditary information).
- ♦ 1860s—Gregor Mendel.
  - • Austrian monk.
  - • First expressed principles of heredity in 1860s through study of his garden peas.
    - ■ Described dominant, recessive traits.
    - ■ Known as "Laws of Transmission."
  - • Theories remained unknown until 1900, 16 years after Mendel's death.
- ♦ 1946—Edward Tatum and Joshua Lederberg demonstrated that DNA carries hereditary information in bacteria.
- ♦ 1953—James Watson and Francis Crick proposed structure of DNA based on x-ray crystallography work of Maurice Wilkins and Rosalind Franklin.
- ♦ 1958—DNA polymerase isolated.
- ♦ 1960—RNA polymerase isolated.
- ♦ 1972—Paul Berg at Stanford produced the first recombinant DNA molecules.
- ♦ 1975—E.M. Southern developed DNA transfer technique to enable DNA to be probed with radiolabeled RNA.

II. The Chromosomes
- ♦ Nomenclature.
  - • Eukaryotes—organisms with true nucleus, bounded by nuclear membrane; multiply by mitosis.
  - • Prokaryotes—organisms without true nucleus; reproduce by cell division.
  - • Chromosomes.
    - ■ Packages of genetic material containing the following:
      - ◇ DNA molecule.
      - ◇ Many proteins.
    - ■ Human somatic cells.
      - ◇ Forty-six chromosomes.
        - o Twenty-two pairs of autosomes.
        - o One pair of sex chromosomes.
      - ◇ Diploid (23 pairs) versus human gametes, which are haploid (22 autosomes, one sex chromosome).
    - ■ Centromere—central portion that divides chromosomes into two arms (p, short; q, long).
    - ■ Autosomes are homologous—paired chromosomes from each parent.
  - • Gene—single unit of DNA within a chromosome, activated to transcribe a specific RNA.

- Gene locus—location on chromosome.
- Homozygous—similar gene between paired chromosomes.
- Heterozygous—dissimilar genes on paired chromosomes.
- Karyotype—arrangement of chromosomes into pairs.
    - Stained with Giemsa to produce banding pattern; bands are numbered from centromere outward.
    - Location specified by chromosome number, arm symbol, region number, and band number (e.g., 7q31.1 is the location of the cystic fibrosis gene).
- Mitosis—process of nuclear division in eukaryotes that occurs in somatic cells.
    - Interphase.
        - All normal cell activity except active division.
        - Inactive X chromosome (Barr body) can be seen in female cells.
    - Prophase.
        - Beginning of cell division.
        - Chromosomes condense.
        - Two chromatids become visible.
        - Nuclear membrane disappears.
        - Centriole forms spindles for cell division.
        - Centriole duplicates itself.
        - Centrioles migrate to opposite poles.
    - Metaphase.
        - Chromosomes migrate to center of cell forming a line designated the equatorial plate.
        - Chromosomes are maximally condensed.
        - Spindles—microtubules of protein that radiate from centrioles to centromeres—form.
    - Anaphase.
        - Division occurs in longitudinal plane.
        - Chromatids move to opposite sides of cell by contraction of spindles.
    - Telophase.
        - Division of cytoplasm results in two complete cell membranes.
        - New nuclei form.
        - DNA serves as template, so DNA content doubles.
- Meiosis.
    - Cell division that forms the gametes (haploid number of chromosomes).
    - Two purposes:
        1. Reduction of chromosome number.
        2. Recombination to transmit genetic information.
    - First meiotic division (meiosis I).
        - Prophase.
            ◇ Lepotene: condensation of chromosomes.
            ◇ Zygotene: pairing of homologous chromosomes (synapsis).
            ◇ Pachytene.

    ○ Each pair thickens to form four strands.
    ○ Crossing over or recombination occurs.
      □ Chiasmata—places of contact where crossing over occurs.
      □ Movement of blocks of DNA creates genetic diversity.
    ○ Insertion of genetic elements can transform host cells.
   ◇ Diplotene: longitudinal separation.
  ■ Metaphase, anaphase, and telophase of meiosis I.
   ◇ Nuclear membrane disappears.
   ◇ Chromosomes move to center of cell.
   ◇ One member of each pair goes to each pole → reduction division.
 • Second meiotic division (meiosis II).
  ■ Follows meiosis I without DNA replication.
  ■ Occurs in oocyte after fertilization.
  ■ End result of meiosis is four haploid cells.

III. The Structure and Function of DNA
  ♦ DNA.
   • Material of the gene responsible for the genetic message.
   • Each DNA molecule has a deoxyribose backbone; nuclear bases, either a purine or a pyrimidine, are attached to each deoxyribose.
    ■ Purine: adenine or guanine.
    ■ Pyrimidine: thymine or cytosine.
   • The nucleotide is the basic building block of DNA; made up of three substances.
    ■ Deoxyribose sugar.
    ■ Phosphate group.
    ■ Nucleic acid base.
   • Phosphate-sugar linkages are asymmetric.
    ■ The five carbon of one sugar links to the three carbon of the next; 5′ end versus 3′ end.
   • By convention, DNA is written from left to right or 5′ to 3′ (direction of transcription).
    ■ 5′ end is the amino end.
    ■ 3′ end is the carboxy end (Fig. 1.1).
   • Double helix.
    ■ Strands are twisted around each other in a clockwise direction.
    ■ Nucleic acids are on the inside with hydrogen bonding of A≡T and C≡G.
    ■ RNA has ribose (not deoxyribose), is single stranded (not double stranded), and has uracil (not thymine).
    ■ The double helix allows DNA to fit into the cell.
    ■ The base pair is the measure of length.
     ◇ We have three billion base pairs of DNA.
     ◇ Only a small portion of these code for protein.
    ■ DNA is not naked within a cell.

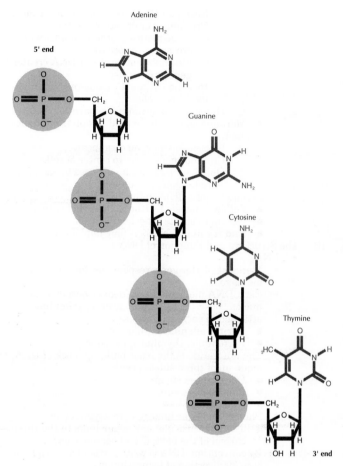

Figure 1.1. The chemical structure of DNA.

- ◇ Winds around a core of protein (histones) to form nucleosome.
- ◇ Nucleosomes condense into bands.
- DNA replication.
  - Replication begins with the separation of strands.
  - DNA polymerase catalyzes synthesis of new duplicate strands.
  - Each daughter molecule contains one parental strand.
  - Original DNA in zygote must be copied 10^{15} times during one's lifetime.
  - Rapidity and accuracy are essential.

- Homeobox.
  - Highly conserved DNA sequence.
  - Encodes 60 amino-acid homeodomain; functions as a transcription factor by binding to DNA.
  - Influences specific tissue functions that are critical for the growth and development of the embryo.
- The human genome.
  - Three billion base pairs.
  - Total of 60,000 to 150,000 genes; accounts for only 3% of all DNA.
  - Nucleotides grouped into three-letter words (codons).
    - Sixty-four possible combinations.
    - Only 20 amino acids (Tables 1.1 and 1.2).
- Gene structure and function.
  - General features.
    - Exon—segment of a gene yielding mRNA product coding for a specific protein.
    - Intron—segment of a gene not represented in mature RNA.
    - Codon.
      - ◇ Sequence of three bases of RNA or DNA coding for a specific amino acid.
      - ◇ Usually one gene codes for one protein.

Table 1.1. The 20 amino acids in proteins

Amino Acid	Three-Letter Abbreviation	Single-Letter Code
Glycine	Gly	G
Alanine	Ala	A
Valine	Val	V
Isoleucine	Ile	I
Leucine	Leu	L
Serine	Ser	S
Threonine	Thr	T
Proline	Pro	P
Aspartic acid	Asp	D
Glutamic acid	Glu	E
Lysine	Lys	K
Arginine	Arg	R
Asparagine	Asn	N
Glutamine	Gln	Q
Cysteine	Cys	C
Methionine	Met	M
Tryptophan	Trp	W
Phenylalanine	Phe	F
Tyrosine	Tyr	Y
Histidine	His	H

Table 1.2. The mRNA genetic code

First Position (5′ end)	Second Position				Third Position (3′ end)
	U	C	A	G	
U	Phe	Ser	Tyr	Cys	U
	Phe	Ser	Tyr	Cys	C
	Leu	Ser	Stop	Stop	A
	Leu	Ser	Stop	Trp	G
C	Leu	Pro	His	Arg	U
	Leu	Pro	His	Arg	C
	Leu	Pro	Gln	Arg	A
	Leu	Pro	Gln	Arg	G
A	Ile	Thr	Asn	Ser	U
	Ile	Thr	Asn	Ser	C
	Ile	Thr	Lys	Arg	A
	Met	Thr	Lys	Arg	G
G	Val	Ala	Asp	Gly	U
	Val	Ala	Asp	Gly	C
	Val	Ala	Glu	Gly	A
	Val	Ala	Glu	Gly	G

Abbreviation: mRNA, messenger RNA.
Reading across the first row of the table, the codon UUU specifies phenylalanine, the codon UCU specifies serine, the codon UAU specifies tyrosine, and the codon UGU specifies cysteine. UAA, UAG, and UGA are stop codons.

◇ Only DNA that is present in exons (parts that exit the nucleus) is transcribed into mRNA and is translated into proteins.
◇ DNA flanking sequences are also important.
  ○ Enhancer region.
    □ Area initiating DNA action.
    □ Enhancer sites are larger than promoter sites.
    □ Can be located anywhere, but are usually in the 5′ flanking end.
    □ Transcription factors are specific proteins that bind to enhancer sites.
  ○ Promoter region.
    □ Sites where transcription actually begins.
      ▲ T–A–T–A–A sequence (TATA box).
      ▲ C–A–A–T sequence (CAT box).
    □ Usually found near start of the coding region.
  ○ Poly A tail.
    □ At 3′ end.
    □ Common for most mRNA molecules.
■ Open reading frame.
  ◇ Long series of base pairs between two stop codons (UAG, UAA, UGA).
  ◇ Usually encountered only in an active gene.

- Gene expression steps.
    1. Transcription of DNA to RNA.
    2. RNA processing to produce functional mRNA by splicing out introns.
    3. Translation of mRNA on a ribosome to create a peptide chain.
    4. Protein structural processing to final functional form.
- Transcription.
    - Synthesis of single stranded mRNA from a gene.
    - RNA polymerase constructs mRNA by reading the DNA strand ("antisense" strand) complementary to the RNA; mRNA is synthesized from the negative template so that it will have the same structure as the positive template (Fig. 1.2).
    - Transcription initiates upstream and continues to the addition of the poly A tail; believed to stabilize mRNA.
    - RNA then moves into cytoplasm where introns are excised; almost all introns begin with GU and end with AG (GT and AG in DNA).
    - 7-Methyl guanosine cap added to 5′ end.
- Transcription factors.
    - Proteins that bind to regulatory elements in DNA (e.g., steroid hormone receptors).
    - Can interact further with other factors (adapter proteins). These interactions explain how similar agents have different actions in different tissues.
- Translation.
    - Amino acids transported by transfer RNA molecules.
    - Amino acids are placed one at a time, beginning at the 5′ end.
    - Process begins at the first AUG triplet and continues until a stop codon.
- Mutations.
    - Any change in the DNA sequence constitutes a mutation.
        - Substitution.
        - Insertion.
        - Deletion.
    - Abnormal mRNA can result from change at coding/noncoding junction.
- Chromosomal abnormalities.
    - Numerical abnormalities.
        - Nondisjunction—failure of separation at anaphase.
        - Aneuploidy—chromosome number not an exact multiple of haploid number.
        - Mosaicism—one or more cell lines with a different karyotype; usually a failure of two paired chromosomes to separate.
        - Polyploidy—multiples of haploid number of chromosomes.

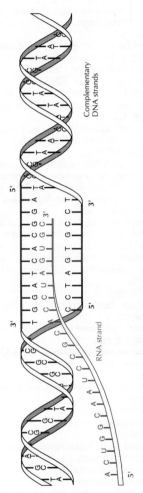

Figure 1.2.   The synthesis of messenger RNA.

- Structural abnormalities.
  - Usually due to breaks induced by radiation, drugs, or viruses.
  - Translocation is an interchange of genetic material between nonhomologous chromosomes.
- Single gene defects.
  - Caused by mutations in specific genes.
  - Follow patterns of Mendelian inheritance.
- Autosomal dominance.
  - Only one allele needs to be abnormal.
  - Two heterozygous parents—75% chance of an affected child.
  - One heterozygous parent—50% chance of an affected child.
  - Subject to variable expression.
    - ◇ Huntington disease.
    - ◇ Neurofibromatosis.
    - ◇ Marfan syndrome.
- Autosomal recessive.
  - Expressed phenotypically only in homozygotes.
  - Heterozygous parents pose 25% risk for each child.
  - Examples include cystic fibrosis, sickle cell anemia, and congenital adrenal hyperplasia.
- X-linked recessive.
  - An affected father can transmit only to daughters.
  - Only homozygous daughters are affected when recessive.
  - Red-green color blindness and hemophilia are examples.
- ◆ Genomic imprinting.
  - Persisting influences on genome function by male and female contributions.
  - Maternal contribution is more important for embryonic development.

IV. Techniques of Molecular Biology
- ◆ Introduction.
  - Restriction enzymes.
    - Will cut DNA only at sites with specific sequences.
    - Discovered in bacteria where they function as defense mechanisms; bacterial DNA is also methylated to prevent digestion.
    - Melding two cut pieces of DNA creates recombinant DNA.
  - DNA polymerase.
    - Enzyme that adds single nucleotides to DNA.
    - Needs DNA template.
  - DNAase.
    - Removes nucleotides.
    - Can be used in conjunction with DNA polymerase to form radiolabeled DNA probe.
  - Reverse transcriptase.

- DNA polymerase that is RNA dependent.
- DNA formed from RNA is called complementary DNA (cDNA).
- Reads only the exons (Fig. 1.3).
- ◆ Southern blot analysis.
  - Allows separation of DNA fragments by size, which is followed by their transfer to nitrocellulose paper.
  - DNA is fixed to paper by baking or exposure to ultraviolet (UV) light.
  - Specific labeled probes can then be introduced.
  - Other types of blotting.
    - Northern blotting.
      - ◇ RNA processing.
      - ◇ Extracted RNA is hybridized with DNA probes.
      - ◇ Useful for determining gene expression.
    - Western blotting.
      - ◇ Electrophoresis is used to separate proteins.
      - ◇ Antibodies are used to hybridize.
    - Dot or slot blotting—hybridization of the probe to DNA without electrophoresis.
- ◆ Hybridization.
  - Reassociation of two complementary strands of DNA.
  - *In situ* hybridization.
    - Placing DNA or RNA probe directly on a slide of tissue or plate of cells.
    - Fluorescence *in situ* hybridization (FISH)—use of a DNA probe with a fluorescent marker.
- ◆ Polymerase chain reaction (PCR).
  - Technique to amplify small fragments or areas of DNA into quantities large enough to analyze.
  - Amplified sequence must be known; can be identified by flanking sequences of DNA called primers.
  - Steps in PCR:
    1. Denature DNA into single strands with heat (92° C).
    2. Lower temperature to 40° C to allow primers to stick.
    3. Raise temperature to 62° C to allow DNA polymerase to synthesize new strands.
    4. Repeat steps 2 and 3 to create exponential increase in DNA formed.
  - Technique works by virtue of heat-resistant DNA polymerase (Taq polymerase); was isolated from a hot water microbe found in the Mushroom Pool in Yellowstone National Park.
- ◆ Cloning DNA.
  - Isolating a gene and making copies.
  - cDNA library is the DNA counterpart of all of the messenger RNA that can be isolated from a particular cell or tissue.
  - Use reverse transcriptase.
  - Insert DNA into appropriate vector.
  - Can also use PCR for cloning.

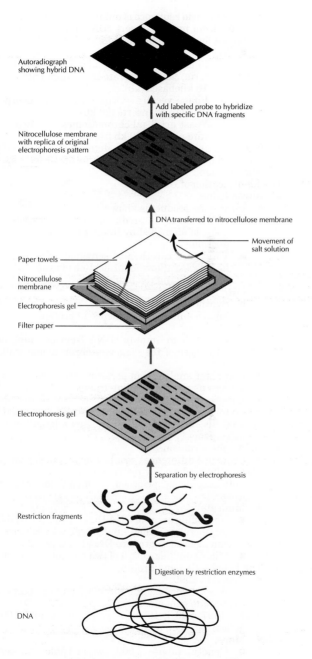

Autoradiograph
showing hybrid DNA

Add labeled probe to hybridize
with specific DNA fragments

Nitrocellulose membrane
with replica of original
electrophoresis pattern

DNA transferred to nitrocellulose membrane

Movement of
salt solution

Paper towels

Nitrocellulose
membrane

Electrophoresis gel

Filter paper

Electrophoresis gel

Separation by electrophoresis

Restriction fragments

Digestion by restriction enzymes

DNA

Figure 1.3. Diagram of Southern blot analysis.

- If amino acid sequence is unknown, can work backward from protein; insert cDNA into vectors and screen for protein production.
  - Vectors.
    - ◊ Plasmid vectors—circular DNA from bacteria; can incorporate DNA fragments up to 10 kilobases (kb).
    - ◊ Phage vectors—viruses that can incorporate larger inserts (20 kb).
    - ◊ Yeast artificial chromosomes can incorporate up to 1,000 kb fragments.
- ◆ Knockout animal models can determine if a specific gene and its protein are essential for life or for a specific function.
- V. The Identification of Genes
  - ◆ Introduction.
    - If the gene product is known:
      - cDNA library is produced, and the DNA fragment is identified by linking it to protein production.
      - Total gene can then be screened using identified cDNA; allows identification of exons, which lead to finding the total gene.
      - **OR**
      - Synthesize oligonucleotide probe based on known amino acid sequence in protein.
      - **OR**
      - Use PCR to amplify cDNA from overlapping sequences of the genome—chromosome walking.
    - Computer analysis can perform entire sequencing process using open reading frames.
    - Localization of gene to specific chromosome when protein product is unknown can be done by linkage analysis; uses restriction fragment length polymorphisms.
  - ◆ DNA polymorphism.
    - Sequence differences result in different fragment lengths produced by restriction enzymes.
    - Polymorphisms governed by mendelian regulations.
    - Minisatellites are a form of polymorphisms.
      - Noncoding areas of DNA that repeat in variable numbers are called tandem repeat sequences; can be used to produce DNA fingerprint.
      - Microsatellites consist of two nucleotide repeats.
  - ◆ The Human Genome Project.
    - Began in 1990.
    - Goal is to sequence the three billion base pairs of the human genome.
    - By 1997, $>60 \times 10^6$ base pairs, or about 50,000 genes, had been analyzed.
    - Maps.
      - Genetic maps—6,000 polymorphic markers have been identified.

- Physical maps—genes localized by comparing overlapping DNA fragments; isolates chromosomal segments for sequencing.
- Sequence maps—most time-intensive mapping process.

VI. Clinical Applications

- ◆ PCR allows molecular diagnosis from even a single blastomere removed from a fertilized embryo.
- ◆ Molecular diagnosis is limited by the prevalence of heterozygote genetic changes (i.e., different mutations in different people).
- ◆ X chromosome is the most studied of all chromosomes.
  - Forty percent of the 160 million base pairs have been cloned.
  - Twenty-six inherited disease genes have been cloned.
  - More than 50 other genes have been localized by linkage analysis.
- ◆ Transgenetic animals and plants result from an embryo injected with foreign DNA; may provide excellent models for disease.
- ◆ Cancer research.
  - Cancer is a genetic disease with malignant cells that are genetically related; oncogenes transform cells from normal to abnormal growth.
  - Tumor suppressor genes also exist.
- ◆ Gene therapy.
  - Can replace missing protein by introducing foreign cells.

  OR
  - Can replace faulty gene (complementary corrected DNA).
  - Could potentially use marker genes to track clones of cells or even to destroy tumor cells.

Hormone Biosynthesis, Metabolism, and Mechanisms of Action

I. Introduction
   - ♦ Hormones are substances that provide a means of communication.
     - Paracrine: intercellular communication involving focal diffusion of regulating substances from a cell to nearby cells.
     - Autocrine: intracellular communication whereby a single cell produces regulating substances that act upon receptors on or within the same cell.
     - Intracrine: intracellular communication occurring when unsecreted substances bind to intracellular receptors.
   - ♦ Estradiol as an example for examining hormone function, formation, and metabolism.
     - Synthesis.
       - Occurs within a special cell (granulosa cell of follicle or corpus luteum).
       - Precursors needed for synthesis.
       - Synthesis occurs in response to a stimulus, which is follicle-stimulating hormone/luteinizing hormone (FSH/LH) secretion.
     - Stimulus.
       - Gonadotropins are too large to enter the cell; second messenger is needed to transduce signal.
       - Gonadotropins activate adenylate cyclase in cell membrane → cyclic adenosine monophosphate (cAMP) (second messenger) is produced.
       - cAMP initiates the process of steroidogenesis.
     - Secretion.
       - Directly follows synthesis.
       - Estradiol exists in two forms: free and bound.
         - ◇ Majority of hormone is bound to protein carriers, such as albumin or sex hormone–binding globulin (SHBG).
         - ◇ Binding may avoid extreme or sudden concentration changes and may limit metabolism.
     - Biologic effects.
       - Determined by a cell's ability to receive and retain hormones.
         - ◇ Free hormone enters cell by diffusion.
         - ◇ Must interact with receptor within the cell.
     - Metabolism.
       - Estradiol is eventually released back into the bloodstream once the mission has been accomplished.

- Unlike testosterone, estradiol is not altered within the target cell.
- Clearance of estradiol depends on conversion (to estrone and estriol) and conjugation (sulfoconjugates and glucuroconjugates).

II. Nomenclature
   ♦ Basic structure is perhydrocyclopentanphenanthrene.
      • Three six-carbon rings.
      • One five-carbon ring.
   ♦ Three main classes of steroids are based on the number of carbon atoms they contain:
      • Twenty-one carbons = pregnane nucleus (progesterones).
      • Nineteen carbons = androstane nucleus (androgens).
      • Eighteen carbons = estrane nucleus (estrogens) (Fig. 2.1).
   ♦ Six centers of asymmetry exist on basic ring structure, so 64 possible isomers.
      • Naturally occurring and active steroids are nearly flat.
      • Alpha substituents are above the plane.
      • Beta substituents are below the plane.
      • Changes in α versus β by one substituent can change its biologic activity.
   ♦ Naming conventions.
      • Basic name depends on number of carbons.
      • Preceded by numbers indicating location of double bonds; name indicates the number of double bonds (e.g., -ene, -diene, -triene).
      • Hydroxy groups are indicated by the number of the carbon to which they are attached; the number of hydroxy residues dictates the name (e.g., -ol, -diol, -triol).
      • Ketone groups are listed last with the number of carbon attachment and designation (e.g., -one, -dione, -trione).
      • Special designations.
         ▪ Dehydro = elimination of two hydrogens.
         ▪ Deoxy = elimination of oxygen.
         ▪ Nor = elimination of carbon.
         ▪ Delta = location of double bond.

III. Lipoproteins and Cholesterol
   ♦ Cholesterol is the basic building block of steroidogenesis; all steroid-producing organs (except the placenta) can synthesize cholesterol from acetate.
   ♦ Major source of cholesterol is the bloodstream; cellular entry is mediated via cell membrane receptors for low-density lipoprotein (LDL).
   ♦ Lipoproteins are large molecules that facilitate transport of nonpolar fats and polar solvents (blood plasma); five major categories exist as follows:
      1. Chylomicrons—large cholesterol (10%) and triglyceride (90%) carrying particles formed in the intestine after a fatty meal.

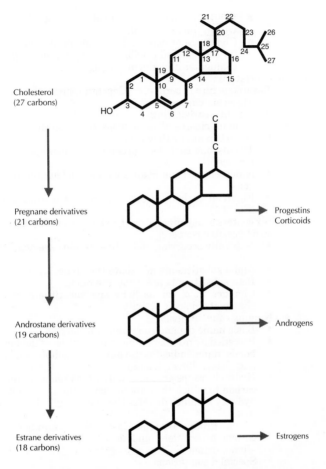

Figure 2.1. The three main groups of sex steroids according to their number of carbon atoms.

2. Very-low-density lipoproteins (VLDLs)—can carry cholesterol but mostly triglycerides; more dense than chylomicrons.
3. Intermediate-density lipoprotein (IDL)—transient formation with removal of some triglycerides from the interior of VLDL.
4. LDL—end product of VLDL catabolism; found after further removal of triglycerides, leaving 50% cholesterol. Carries two-thirds of cholesterol in plasma; related to cardiovascular disease.
5. High-density lipoprotein (HDL)—smallest and most dense, levels are inversely related to athero-

sclerosis. Can be separated into lighter fraction, HDL_2 (strongly associated with cardiovascular disease) and denser fraction (HDL_3).

♦ All lipoproteins contain the following four ingredients:
1. Cholesterol (free on the surface, esterified in the center).
2. Triglycerides in the interior.
3. Phospholipids.
4. Protein (surface proteins called apoprotein).
   - Principal surface proteins:
     ◇ LDL → apoprotein B.
     ◇ HDL → apoprotein A-1.

♦ Lipids for peripheral tissues are provided by secretion of VLDL by the liver.
- Triglycerides (TG) are liberated from VLDL by lipoprotein lipase in capillary endothelial cells and lipase in liver sinusoids.
  - Surface components are transferred to HDL.
  - VLDL is converted to LDL.
- Hepatic lipase enzyme is sensitive to sex steroids.
  - Suppressed by estrogen.
  - Stimulated by androgens.
- LDL is removed from blood by cellular receptors recognizing surface apoproteins.
  - Intracellular levels of cholesterol are partially regulated by number of cell membrane LDL receptors.
  - When receptors are saturated, LDL is taken up by other cells, including arterial intima.
- HDL is secreted by the liver and intestine as a degradation product of VLDL.
  - HDL accepts free cholesterol.
  - Possibly mediated by apoprotein A-1 receptors.
- Particle size increases to HDL_2; HDL_3 remains stable.

♦ Atherosclerotic risk.
- Depends on lipoprotein profiles.
  - HDL is 10 mg/dL higher in women.
  - LDL levels are lower in premenopausal women.
- Protective nature of HDL is due to its ability to pick up free cholesterol; free cholesterol on the surface can be esterified and moved to the center of the lipoprotein.
- LDL receptors alter blood level of LDL; high cholesterol diet → liver-decreased LDL receptor content → increased serum LDL.

IV. Steroidogenesis
♦ Pathways of steroidogenesis are shared by all steroid-producing endocrine organs.
♦ Rules of steroidogenesis (can decrease but never increase number of carbons):
1. Cleavage of side chain (desmolase reaction).
2. Conversion of hydroxyl into ketones or vice versa (dehydrogenase reaction).
3. Addition of hydroxy group (hydroxylation).

4. Creation of double bond (removal of hydrogens).
5. Reduction of double bonds (saturation) by addition of hydrogen.

♦ Steroidogenic enzymes.
- Either dehydrogenases or member of cytochrome P450 (P450) group of oxidases (Table 2.1).
- Structural knowledge of P450 enzymes is derived from amino acid and metabolic sequence studies.
  - Single unique P450scc gene on chromosome 15.
  - Conversion of cholesterol to pregnenolone occurs within mitochondria.
    ◇ One of the principal effects of tropic hormones.
    ◇ Rate-limiting step in steroidogenesis— transfer of cholesterol from outer to inner mitochondrial membrane.
- Acute intracellular cholesterol transfer.
  - Several proposed regulators as follows:
    ◇ Sterol carrier protein 2.
    ◇ Steroidogenesis activator polypeptide.
    ◇ Peripheral benzodiazepine receptor.
    ◇ Steroidogenetic acute regulator (StAR) protein.
- StAR.
  - StAR messenger RNA (mRNA) and protein are induced concomitantly with acute steroidogenesis in response to cAMP.
  - StAR increases steroid production.
  - StAR is imported and localized within mitochondria.
  - StAR gene mutation is found in patients with congenital lipoid adrenal hyperplasia.
    ◇ Failure of adrenal and/or gonadal steroidogenesis.
    ◇ Low level of steroidogenesis is possible (female embryos can feminize), but eventually a loss of all steroidogenic ability is seen.
  - StAR mediates transport in the adrenals and/or gonads but not in the placenta or brain.

Table 2.1. The family of P450 enzymes

Enzyme	Cellular Location	Reactions
P450scc	Mitochondria	Cholesterol side chain cleavage
P450c11	Mitochondria	11-Hydroxylase 18-Hydroxylase 19-Methyloxidase
P450c17	Endoplasmic reticulum	17-Hydroxylase; 17,20-lyase
P450c21	Endoplasmic reticulum	21-Hydroxylase
P450arom	Endoplasmic reticulum	Aromatase

Abbreviation: P450, cytochrome P450.

- StAR synthesized as precursor form with 285 amino acid (aa) precursor; 25 residue sequence cleaved after transport into mitochondria; mutation can prevent this cleavage.
- ◆ Ovarian steroid pathways.
  - Pregnenolone can proceed along two pathways:
    - Δ^4—3-ketone pathway.
    - Δ^5—3β hydroxysteroids.
  - Δ^4 Pathway.
    - Pregnenolone converted to progesterone.
    - 3β Hydroxysteroid dehydrogenase (HSD) enzyme.
      - ◇ Catalyzes both dehydration and isomerization reaction.
      - ◇ Exists in two forms (type I and type II).
      - ◇ Two genes on chromosome 1; type II gene expressed in gonads/adrenals.
    - Once Δ^{4-5} ketone is formed, then progesterone is hydroxylated at C17 (17α hydroxyprogesterone).
    - Side chain is removed to form androstenedione.
    - Reduction to 17β hydroxy forms testosterone.
    - Aromatization results in estradiol.
      - ◇ Loss of C19 carbon.
      - ◇ Ring A aromatization.
  - Alternative pathway takes pregnenolone to dehydroeprandrosterone (DHA) by 17α hydroxylation, followed by cleavage of the side chain.
    - DHA can then be converted into androstenedione.
    - From this point, it proceeds to estrogen as above.
- ◆ P450c17.
  - Mediates all four reactions involved in conversion of progesterones (P_4) and pregnenolone (P_5) to 17-hydroxylase products.
  - Bound to smooth endoplasmic reticulum.
  - Regulated by genes on chromosome 10.
- ◆ P450c21.
  - Only one 21-hydroxylation enzyme in the smooth endoplasmic reticulum (P450c21).
  - Two human genes have been cloned (A and B) on chromosome 6p.
  - Only the B gene is active.
  - P450c21 deficiency can result from gene conversion (B looks like A) or from deletion of the B gene.
- ◆ P450 aromatase.
  - It is found inside the endoplasmic reticulum.
  - Human genome has one gene.
  - Location is on 15q21.1 (denoted CYP19).
  - Gene transcription is regulated by several promotor sites responding to the following:
    - Cytokines.
    - Cyclic nucleotides.
    - Gonadotropins.
    - Glucocorticoids.
    - Growth factors.

- Highly regulated expression in the ovary; non-regulated expression in the placenta and adipose tissue.
- Specific inhibitors have been developed.

◆ 17β Hydroxysteroid dehydrogenase and 5α-reductase reactions.
  - Non-P450 enzymes.
  - 17β HSD bound to endoplasmic reticulum.
  - 5α-Reductase bound to nuclear membrane.
  - 17β HSD represents the following four isoenzymes:
    - Type I (placenta): estrone → estradiol.
    - Type II: testosterone → androstenedione.
    - Type III (testes): androstenedione → testosterone.
    - Type IV: estradiol → estrone.

V. The Two-Cell System

◆ Logical explanation of ovarian follicular steroidogenesis.

◆ First proposed by Falck in 1959.

◆ Important facts are as follows:
  1. FSH receptors are present on granulosa cells.
  2. FSH receptors are induced by FSH.
  3. LH receptors are present on theca cells but initially absent on granulosa cells. However, FSH induces appearance of LH receptors on granulosa.
  4. FSH induces aromatase in granulosa.
  5. The above actions are modulated by autocrine and paracrine factors secreted by theca and granulosa cells.

◆ Follicular development.
  - Primordial → preantral conversion occurs independent of hormones.
    - Stimulus is unknown.
    - Continued growth is dependent on FSH.
    - FSH receptors increase in numbers.
    - FSH activates aromatase in granulosa.

◆ Autocrine/paracrine factors.
  - Insulin-like growth factor (IGF) is secreted by theca cells.
    - Enhances LH stimulation of androgen production.
    - Enhances FSH-mediated aromatization.
  - Other factors include epidermal growth factor (EGF), fibroblast growth factor (FGF), inhibin, and activin.
  - Paracrine regulation of inhibin and/or activin is mediated via modification of the expression of steroidogenic enzymes (especially P450c17).
  - Luteal phase.
    - Dominance of luteinized granulosa layer is dependent on the preovulatory induction of an adequate number of LH receptors; depends on preovulatory adequate exposure to FSH.
    - Conversion of granulosa layer from FSH-mediated activity to LH-mediated activity.

- Granulosa cells lack P450c17, so they are dependent on androgen substrate from theca; in the corpus luteum, theca luteal cells continue to produce androgens that are used by granulosa luteal cells to produce estrogens.

VI. Blood Transport of Steroids (Table 2.2)
   - Majority of sex steroids are bound to SHBG.
   - Level of SHBG is inversely related to weight, insulin levels, and distribution of fat.
   - SHBG contains a simple binding site for androgens and estrogens.
     - Homodimer (two monomers).
     - Gene localized to 17 p12-13; also codes for androgen-binding protein present in seminiferous tubules.
   - Transcortin (corticosteroid-binding globulin [CBG]).
     - Binds cortisol, progesterone, deoxycorticosterone, and corticosterone.
     - Seventy-five percent of circulating cortisol is bound to CBGs.
       - Fifteen percent is attached to albumin.
       - Ten percent is free.
   - Hormone action is determined by unbound hormone (free hormone); concept is controversial.
     - Hormone protein complex may be involved at target cell plasma membrane.
     - Albumin-bound fraction may be available because of low affinity; concentration of albumin-bound fraction may be significant.

VII. Estrogen Metabolism
   - Androgens are the common precursors of estrogens; 17β HSD converts androstenedione to testosterone, which is aromatized to estradiol.
   - Estradiol also arises from estrone.
   - Estriol is the peripheral metabolite of estrone and estradiol, not a secretory product of the ovary.
   - Peripheral conversion in adipose and skin can generate significant amounts of estrogens; adrenal gland is major source of circulating androgen (androstenedione).

Table 2.2.   Circulation of principal sex steroids

	Free (Unbound)	Albumin-Bound	SHBG-Bound
Estrogen	1%	30%	69%
Testosterone	1%	30%	69%
DHA	4%	88%	8%
Androstenedione	7%	85%	8%
Dihydrotestosterone	1%	71%	28%

Abbreviations: DHA, dehydroepiandrosterone; SHBG, sex hormone–binding globulin.

- ♦ Pattern of circulating steroids is influenced by the following:
    - • Secretion rate: direct organ secretion.
    - • Production rate: secretion plus peripheral conversion.
    - • Metabolic clearance rate (MCR): volume of blood cleared of hormone/unit of time.
    - • Blood production rate (PR) = MCR × [concentration].
- ♦ Normal estrogen production.
    - • Estradiol = 100 to 300 µg/day.
    - • Androstenedione = 3 mg/day → 1% conversion; accounts for 20% to 30% of estrone.
    - • Testosterone = 250 µg/day → 0.15% conversion to estradiol (0.375 µg/day).

VIII. Progesterone Metabolism
- ♦ Peripheral conversion to progesterone not seen in nonpregnant female; progesterone production is a combination of adrenal and ovarian secretion.
- ♦ Blood production rate <1 mg/day in preovulatory phase.
- ♦ Approximately 10% to 20% is excreted as pregnanediol.
    - • Preovulation urine excretion <1 mg/day.
    - • Postovulation urine excretion peaks between 3 to 6 mg/day.
- ♦ Blood levels in preovulatory or prepubertal females <100 ng/dL.
    - • Luteal phase: 500 to 2,000 ng/dL.
    - • Congenital adrenal hyperplasia patients can have 50 times the normal levels.
- ♦ Pregnanetriol is the chief urinary metabolite of 17α-hydroxyprogesterone.
    - • Clinically significant in adrenogenital syndrome.
    - • Now replaced clinically by measurement of 17α-hydroxyprogesterone in blood.

IX. Androgen Metabolism
- ♦ Major androgen products of the ovary.
    - • DHA and androstenedione.
    - • Testosterone secretion—significant in androgen secreting tumors.
- ♦ Adrenal steroid hormones.
    - • Three groups of hormones: glucocorticoids, mineralocorticoids, sex steroids; adrenal sex steroids are intermediate byproducts—synthesis of glucocorticoids and mineralocorticoids.
    - • Androstenedione—50% ovary, 50% adrenal.
    - • DHA.
        - ■ Fifty percent adrenal.
        - ■ Twenty-five percent ovary.
        - ■ Twenty-five percent peripheral.
    - • Testosterone (0.2 mg/day).
        - ■ Fifty percent peripheral conversion of androstenedione.
        - ■ Twenty-five percent ovary.
        - ■ Twenty-five percent adrenal.
    - • Testosterone binding ↓ by androgens.

- Total concentration can be normal, but free protein portion is elevated; presence of hirsutism or virilism indicates increased androgen effect.
- If both total and unbound testosterone are normal in patient with hirsutism or virilism, these can be explained by excessive intracellular androgen effect (testosterone → dihydrotestosterone [DHT]).
- Reduction of Δ^4 unsaturation of testosterone.
  - Irreversible pathway.
  - 5β-Derivatives are not androgenic.
  - 5α-Derivative is very potent (DHT).
    ◇ In men, circulating DHT is derived from testosterone.
    ◇ In women, blood DHT is primarily derived from androstenedione and DHA; skin production of DHT is predominantly influenced by androstenedione.
- 5α-Reductase exists in two forms as follows:
  - Type I—skin.
  - Type II—reproductive tissue.
- DHT metabolized intracellularly.
  - Blood DHT is one-tenth of circulating testosterone.
  - DHT enters nucleus.
  - DHT can initiate androgenic actions, even in cells without 5α-reductase.
- DHT is further reduced to 3α-androstanediol.
- Male development.
  - Testosterone dependent for development of wolffian duct structures—epididymis, vas deferens, seminal vesicle.
  - DHT dependent for development of urogenital sinus, tubercule—external genitalia, urethra, and prostate.

X. Excretion of Steroids
  ♦ Steroids are excreted as sulfoconjugates and glucuroconjugates.
  ♦ Conjugation usually reduces or eliminates biologic activity.
  ♦ Hydrolysis can restore active form.

XI. Cellular Mechanism of Action
  ♦ Two major types of hormone action at target tissue as follows:
    • Tropic hormones (peptide and glycoprotein hormones) have receptors at cell membrane level.
    • Steroid hormones enter cells and interact with intracellular receptors.
  ♦ Receptors in the nucleus lead to transcription activation (e.g., estrogen receptor [ER]).
  ♦ G protein receptors—single polypeptide chain spanning the cell membrane.
    • Binding of hormone leads to interaction with G protein and second messenger.
    • Examples include tropic hormones, prostaglandins.

♦ Ion gate channels—component of multiple cell surface units.
  • Ion channels open after binding.
  • Example is acetylcholine receptor.
♦ Receptors with intrinsic enzyme activity.
  • Transmembrane with intracellular tyrosine or serine kinase component.
  • Examples: insulin, activin, inhibin receptors.
♦ Other receptors—receptors not fitting in the above categories include LDL, prolactin, and growth hormone.

XII. Mechanism of Action for Steroid Hormones
♦ Introduction.
  • Specificity to sex steroids due to intracellular receptor proteins.
  • Mechanism of action:
    1. Diffusion of hormone across cell membrane.
    2. Binding of hormone to receptor protein.
    3. Interaction of hormone-receptor complex with DNA.
    4. Synthesis of mRNA.
    5. Transport of mRNA to ribosomes.
    6. Protein synthesis.
  • Other mechanisms exist that allow steroid receptors to regulate gene transcription (e.g., posttranscription events and nongenomic events) (Fig. 2.2).
  • Localization of receptors differs among classes of steroids.
    ■ Glucocorticoid, mineralocorticoid, probably androgen receptors; unbound receptors present in cytoplasm.
    ■ Estrogen, progesterone receptors; unbound receptors within nucleus.
  • Free hormone rapidly transfuses across the cell membrane.
  • Following receptor binding, the receptor undergoes a conformational change: transformation or activation of receptor.
    ■ Exposes DNA-binding region.
    ■ Heat shock protein complex dissociates.
  • Hormone receptor complex binds to specific DNA sites—hormone response elements.
    ■ Located upstream of gene.
    ■ Results in RNA polymerase initiation of transcription.
    ■ Biologic activity maintained only while nuclear site is occupied.
      ◊ Duration of exposure to hormone is as important as dose.
      ◊ ER complex has a long half-life compared with cortisol or progesterone complexes.
  • Estrogen increases concentration of its own receptor and also progesterone and androgen receptors—replenishment.
  • Progesterone and clomiphene block receptor replenishment mechanism.

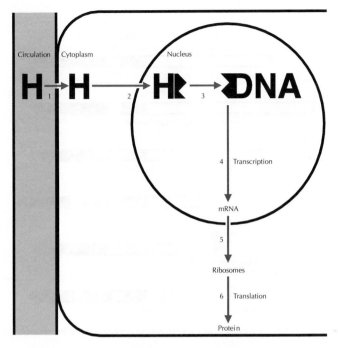

Figure 2.2. The mechanism of action for steroid hormones.

- Estrogen and progesterone receptors must move into nucleus quickly.
  - Nuclear membrane has 3,000 to 4,000 pores.
  - 1×10^6 histone molecules enter the nucleus every 3 minutes.
  - Proteins have localization signals in hinge region.
  - Some diseases may be due to "poor traffic control."
- Receptor processing—conversion of high affinity receptor sites to a rapidly dissociating form with loss of binding activity; completed in 6 hours for ER.
- Estriol has only 20% to 30% affinity for ER when compared with estradiol; in pregnancy, the high concentration of estriol makes it an important hormone.
- ERs and progestins.
  - Progestins accelerate turnover of preexisting receptors and inhibit estrogen-induced receptor synthesis; interrupt transcription of estrogen-regulated genes.
  - Androgens do not deplete ERs but do decrease estrogen-induced RNA activity in cytoplasm.
- The receptor superfamily.

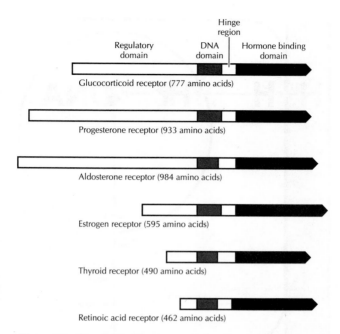

Figure 2.3. Structures of various receptors for steroid hormones.

- Steroid receptors share a common structure with the following:
    - Thyroid hormone receptor.
    - 1,25-Dihydroxy vitamin D_3 receptor.
    - Retinoic acid receptor.
- This "superfamily" contains about 150 proteins in a wide variety of species; many are "orphan" receptors, as no ligands have been identified (Fig. 2.3).
- The estrogen receptor.
    - Two ERs have been identified: ER-α, ER-β.
        - ER-α.
            - Discovered in 1960.
            - Amino acid sequence determined in 1986.
            - Translated from 6.8 kilobase mRNA; eight exons, chromosome 6q.
            - Molecular weight: 66,000; 595 amino acids.
            - Half-life: 4 to 7 hours.
        - ER-β.
            - More recently discovered.
            - Localized to chromosome 14,q22-q24; close proximity to Alzheimer disease genes (Fig. 2.4 and Table 2.3).
    - Comparison of ER-α, ER-β.
        - Phytoestrogens have greater affinity for ER-β.
        - Regulatory domains differ; ER-β may not work via transcription-activation function 1 (TAF-1).

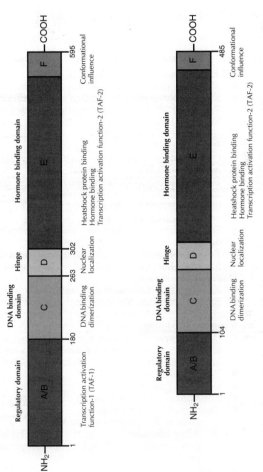

Figure 2.4. The structures of the estrogen receptor-α (top) and the estrogen receptor-β (bottom).

**Table 2.3.   Homology of
estrogen receptor domains and regions**

	ER-α and ER-β Homology
The regulatory domain	17.5%
The DNA-binding domain	97%
The hinge	30%
The hormone-binding domain	59.1%
The F region	17.9%

- AB region, the regulatory domain.
  - Most variable region in the superfamily.
  - ER-α contains phosphorylation sites and TAF-1; TAF-1 can stimulate transcription in absence of hormone binding.
- C region, DNA-binding domain.
  - Binds to DNA.
  - One hundred amino acids with nine cysteines in fixed portions—zinc fingers.
  - Domain essential for activation of transcription.
  - This domain controls which gene will be regulated; specificity is determined by zinc fingers, especially the first finger.
  - Substitution can lead to "loss of function" mutation.
  - Functional specificity localized to second zinc finger (D box).
- D region, the hinge.
  - Important for movement of receptor into nucleus.
  - Site of rotation for inducing conformational change.
- E region, the hormone-binding domain.
  - Carboxy end of ER-α is hormone-binding domain for estrogens and antiestrogens; 251 amino acids.
  - Responsible for dimerization.
  - Contains TAF-2.
  - Site of heat shock protein–binding (hsp90).
  - Characteristic structure.
    - ◇ Helices form a pocket (sandwich fold).
    - ◇ After hormone binding, this region creates new sites for coactivation and corepressor proteins.
- F region.
  - C-terminal segment made up of 42 amino acids in ER.
  - Modulates gene transcription by estrogens and antiestrogens.
    - ◇ Conformation of receptor-ligand complex differs between estrogens and antiestrogens
    - ◇ Conformation also differs with or without F region.

- Not required for transcription response to estrogen.
  ◇ Does affect the magnitude of activity.
  ◇ Alters activity of both TAF-1 and TAF-2.
♦ Mechanism of action.
  • ER undergoes nucleocytoplasmic shuttling—receptors are more rapidly degraded in cytoplasm; agents that inhibit dimerization impair shuttling (pure estrogen antagonist).
  • hsp90 is the critical protein for maintaining the inactive state and proper folding for membrane transport; "activation" or "transformation" refers to the dissociation of hsp90.
  • Hormone binding results in hsp dissociation and allows dimerization—hormone-binding domain pocket (sandwich fold) undergoes conformational change.
    - Different with each ligand.
    - Determines exact message transmitted to gene.
  • Cavity in estrogen-receptor, hormone-binding domain is large; allows acceptance of various ligands.
  • Thyroid and retinoic acid–receptor subfamily members do not exist as inactive complexes with hsp; can form dimers and bind to DNA response elements but do act as repressors in the absence of ligands.
  • Mutant ERs that do not bind estradiol can be created.
    - Can form dimers with wild type.
    - Can bind to estrogen response element (ERE).
    - Cannot activate transcription; transcription is dependent on the structural change following estradiol binding.
  • Receptor dimerization.
    - True for estrogen, progesterone, androgen, and glucocorticoid receptors.
    - ER-α can form homodimer or heterodimer.
      ◇ Same for ER-β.
      ◇ Allows for variation in response.
  • Hormone response elements (HRE).
    - DNA-binding domain is specific for an enhancer site in the gene promoter (5′ flanking region).
    - Activity of HRE requires hormone-receptor complex.
  • At least four different HREs as follows:
    - Glucocorticoids/progestins/androgen.
    - Estrogen.
    - Vitamin D.
    - Thyroid/retinoic acid.
  • Binding to HRE induces many changes, including conformational change in DNA.
  • Transcription factors.
    - Polypeptides complexed with one of three different RNA polymerases (I, II, III).
    - Modulate transcription either at promoter site or at a segment further upstream.

- Steroid hormone receptors are transcription factors.
- Effect can be either activation or repression.

- Steroid hormone receptor activates transcription in partnership with several groups of proteins as follows:
  1. Other transcription factors—peptides that interact with polymerase enzymes and DNA.
  2. Coactivators/corepressors—peptides that interact with the TAF areas of the receptor (adapter protein).
  3. Chromatin factors—structural organizational changes that allow an architecture appropriate for transcription response.

- Estrogen action.
  - Binding to EREs allows efficient RNA transcription, which is regulated by coactivator/corepressor action on TAF areas.
  - Most genes regulated by estrogen respond within 1 to 2 hours; a few respond within minutes (depends on the need to synthesize regulatory proteins).
  - Binding of estradiol increases affinity of receptor for estradiol (positive cooperativity); clomiphene induces negative cooperativity.

- Ligand binding induces conformational changes, allowing TAFs to function.
  - TAF-1 can stimulate transcription in absence of hormone when fixed to DNA; also promotes DNA binding in intact receptor.
  - TAF-2 consists of dispersed elements united after estrogen binding.

- Activity of the TAFs depends on cellular context; same hormone can have different responses in different cells.

- Phosphorylation.
  - Can regulate receptor function.
  - Can transmit signal from cell membrane receptors.
  - cAMP and protein kinase A increase transcription of ERs.
  - Epidermal growth factor (EGF), IGF-I, transforming growth factor-α (TGF-α) can activate ERs in the absence of estrogen.
    - $\diamond$ Can be blocked by pure antiestrogens.
    - $\diamond$ Exact mechanism of action unknown.
  - Can also explain positive feedback relationship between estrogen and growth factors.

- Summary of steps in the steroid hormone-receptor mechanism.
  1. Binding of the hormone to the hormone-binding domain that has been kept in an inactive state by various heat shock proteins.
  2. Activation of the hormone-receptor complex, by *conformational* change, follows the dissociation of the heat shock proteins.

  3. Dimerization of the complex.
  4. Binding of the dimer to the hormone-responsive element on DNA by the zinc finger area of the DNA-binding domain.
  5. Stimulation of transcription, mediated by TAFs, and influenced by the protein (other transcription factors and coactivators/corepressors) *context of the cell* and by *phosphorylation*.
- Summary of factors that determine biologic activity.
  1. Affinity of hormone for the hormone-binding domain of the receptor.
  2. Target tissue differential expression of the receptor subtypes (e.g., ER-α and ER-β).
  3. Conformational shape of the ligand-receptor complex, with effects on two important activities: dimerization and modulation of adapter proteins.
  4. Differential expression of target tissue adapter proteins and phosphorylation.
- Different roles for ER-α, ER-β.
  - ER-α mouse knockout studies.
    - Both sexes infertile.
    - Male mice demonstrate reduced spermatogenesis, progressive testicular atrophy; mounting activity was unchanged, but intromission, ejaculation, and aggression were reduced.
    - Female mice do not ovulate.
      ◇ Ovaries do not respond to gonadotropins.
      ◇ High levels of estrogen, testosterone, LH, FSH-β; FSH is at normal levels.
      ◇ Uterine development normal, but growth impaired.
      ◇ No mammary gland, duct, or alveolar development.
      ◇ No sexually receptive behavior.
  - Implies differential expression of ERs.
    - ER-β in brain, cardiovascular system, and human granulosa cells.
    - Human breast has both.
    - Rat brain exhibits differential localization.
  - Differential functions also exist.
    - Estradiol can stimulate gene transcription with ER-α but can inhibit with ER-β in same system.
    - May be explained by TAF-1, TAF-2 differences.
- Progesterone receptor.
  - Induced by estrogens at the transcriptional level and decreased by progestins at both transcription and translation.
  - Two major forms (A and B).
    - Expressed by a single gene.
    - Consequence of transcription from different promoters.

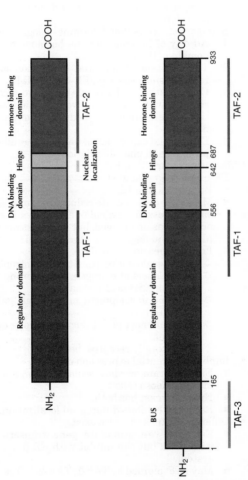

Figure 2.5. The structures of the progesterone receptor-A (top) and the progesterone receptor-B (bottom).

- ■ Each form is associated with additional proteins.
- ■ B has unique upstream 164 amino acid segment called B upstream segment (BUS) (Fig. 2.5).
- • TAF-1 located in 91-aa segment upstream of DNA-binding domain.
- • TAF-2 located within hormone-binding domain.
- • TAF-3 located in BUS; can autonomously activate transcription or can synergize with other TAFs.
- • In absence of hormone binding, the C-terminal region exerts inhibitory effect on transcription.
  - ■ Agonist induces a conformational change that overcomes this inhibitory function.
  - ■ Antagonist allows inhibitory actions to be maintained.
- • Variety of responses based on homodimer or heterodimer formation.
- • Both receptors expressed in breast and endometrial cancer cell lines.
- • Relative levels differ during menstrual cycle.
- • In most cells, B is positive regulator.
  - ■ A inhibits B activity.
  - ■ A inhibits estrogen, glucocorticoid, mineralocorticoids, and androgen-receptor activity.
  - ■ Either A competes with ER for a critical protein, or the target is a critical protein (an essential transcription activator).
- ◆ Androgen receptor.
  - • Cellular mechanism is more complex for androgens.
  - • Androgens can work in one of three ways:
    1. Intracellular conversion of testosterone to DHT (testosterone → DHT)—intracrine activity.
    2. Via testosterone itself (endocrine activity).
    3. Via intracellular conversion of testosterone to estradiol (aromatization)—intracrine activity.
  - • Wolffian duct derivatives respond via testosterone pathways.
  - • Hair follicles, urogenital sinus, and urogenital tubercle derivatives respond via DHT.
  - • Hypothalamus converts androgens to estrogens; suggests role of aromatization in the brain.
  - • DHT system allows for amplification of signal secondary to increased receptor affinity; antiandrogens bind with 20% of the affinity of testosterone → fails to activate biologic response.
  - • A and B forms.
    - ■ Full-length B form, truncated A form; probably represent functional differences.
    - ■ DNA-binding domain most similar to progesterone receptor; they cross react at pharmacologic doses.
    - ■ Progestins also compete for 5-α reductase; dihydroprogesterone further competes with testosterone and DHT for receptor.
    - ■ Estrogen can modify androgen responsive gene expression.

- Androgen insensitivity syndrome (testicular feminization).
  - Congenital abnormality in androgen intracellular receptor (200 unique mutations identified).
  - Androgen receptor gene is at Xq11-12; only steroid receptor gene on X chromosome.
  - X-linked disorder.
  - Molecular studies reveal deletions in steroid-binding domain with a spectrum of clinical presentations.
    ◇ Complete absence of binding—complete testicular feminization.
    ◇ Intermediate forms—clinically mixed picture.
    ◇ Minimal changes in 25% of infertile men who have normal genitalia but present with azoospermia.
  - Androgen receptor also involved in motor neuron physiology: specific mutation results in Kennedy disease; X-linked spinobulbar muscular atrophy.
- Nongenomic actions of steroid hormones.
  - Genomic actions require greater than 1 hour.
  - Some steroid hormone effects are immediate.
    - Calcium/sodium transport.
    - Neural effects.
    - Oocyte/sperm reactions.
  - Estrogen-induced vasodilation of coronary arteries is probably a nongenomic calcium flux mechanism.
XIII. Agonists/Antagonists
- Introduction.
  - Agonists.
    - Substance that stimulates a response.
    - Activity follows receptor binding; message stimulated by receptor association.
  - Antagonists.
    - Completely inhibit actions of agonists.
    - Activity follows receptor binding; blockage of receptor message or nontransmission.
    - Most hormone nuclear receptor antagonists have mixed agonist/antagonist responses (e.g., tamoxifen, RU486).
  - Short-acting antagonists (e.g., estriol).
    - Mixed combinations of agonistic and antagonistic depending on tissue.
      ◇ Short-term estrogen response elicited because estriol binds to receptor.
      ◇ Long-term response eliminated because binding is short-lived.
    - Antagonism results when estriol competes with estradiol; a potent estrogen response is possible in the constant presence of weak hormones.
  - Long-acting antagonists (e.g., clomiphene, tamoxifen).

- Endometrium very sensitive to agonistic response.
- Breast more sensitive to antagonistic response.
- Antagonistic action results from alteration in receptor and DNA processing → failure of hormone replenishment.

- Gonadotropin-releasing hormone (GnRH) agonists/antagonists.
  - Action depends on location of substitution in this decapeptide hormone.
    ◇ Multiple positions → antagonist.
    ◇ Position 6 or 10 → agonist.
  - Agonists initially stimulate the pituitary, but down-regulation and desensitization then occur.
  - Antagonists bind to receptor but fail to transmit message.
  - Agonists have many uses.

- Physiologic antagonists.
  - A progestin is not, strictly speaking, an estrogen antagonist; it modifies estrogen action.
  - Androgens do block estrogen action.
    ◇ Mechanism unclear; gene activity subsequent to ER binding.
    ◇ High levels can produce binding to both estrogen and progesterone receptors.

- ◆ Antiestrogens.
  - Currently two groups: pure and mixed.
    - Mixed includes triphenylethylene derivatives (clomiphene and tamoxifen) and nonsteroidal benzothiophene (raloxifene).
    - Ideal antiestrogen has the following characteristics:
      1. Pure antagonistic activity on proliferating breast cancer cells.
      2. Resistance rare or requiring long exposure.
      3. High affinity for the ER.
      4. No interference with beneficial action.
      5. No toxic or carcinogenic effects.
  - Tamoxifen.
    - Very similar to clomiphene.
    - Competitively inhibits estrogen binding; 100 to 1,000 times lower binding affinity when compared with estrogen.
    - Action is hydrostatic.
    - Tamoxifen–ER complex binds with DNA; agonistic versus antagonistic response depends on presence of other promoter elements.
    - Prolonged disease-free survival of breast cancer patients (20% increase in 5 years).
      ◇ Response rates in advanced cancer are 30% to 35%.
      ◇ They are 75% in tumors highly positive for ER.
    - Serum protein changes reflect agonistic action.

    ◊ Decrease antithrombin III, cholesterol, and LDL cholesterol.

    ◊ Increase HDL, SHBG.

- Nearly as potent as 2 mg estradiol in lowering FSH levels in postmenopausal women (26% versus 34%).
- Stimulates progesterone-receptor synthesis; maintains bones and estrogenic effects on vaginal mucosa and endometrium.
- No significant increase in cardiac or vascular mortality.
- Can induce endometrial hyperplasia, polyps, or cancer, as well as a flare-up of endometriosis.

- Mechanism of action.
  - TAF-1 and TAF-2 can both activate transcription.
    - ◊ TAF-2 activates transcription only when bound by estrogen.
    - ◊ Tamoxifen can activate TAF-1 (agonistic activity) but competitively inhibits TAF-2 (antagonistic activity).
  - Estrogen-associated protein binds to right-hand side of TAF-2.
    - ◊ Estrogen induces binding of this protein.
    - ◊ Protein recognizes only activated conformation, not the tamoxifen conformation.
    - ◊ In some cells, TAF-1 is dominant.
    - ◊ In some cells, both are necessary.
    - ◊ No cells have yet been identified as TAF-2 dominant.
    - ◊ In most cells, TAF-1 is too weak to initiate transcription (except in endometrium, bone, liver); antiestrogens have no effect on TAF-1–dependent transcription in breast cells.
  - Raloxifene—may activate an estrogen response chain via response elements separate from ERE; requires specific activating peptides.
  - Summary: response of cells to estrogens and antiestrogens depends on the following:
    1. Nature of the ER.
    2. Estrogen response elements and nearby promoters.
    3. Cellular context of protein coactivators and corepressors.
    4. Properties of the ligand.
    5. Modulation by growth factor and agents that affect protein kinases and phosphorylation.

- Tamoxifen-negative and ER-negative tumors and/or tamoxifen resistance.
  - Other actions of tamoxifen may explain responses:
    1. Tamoxifen and clomiphene inhibit protein kinase C activity (phosphorylation).

2. Tamoxifen inhibits calmodulin-dependent cAMP phosphorylation by calmodulin binding.
3. Tamoxifen has effects on other growth factors, opposing the estrogen effect (e.g., increased TGF-β, decreased IGF-I and IGF-II) (Fig. 2.6).

- Tamoxifen resistance.
  - Treatment of breast cancer patients beyond 5 years may worsen survival/recurrence rates.
  - Possible explanations:
    ◇ Loss of ER—no good supporting evidence.
    ◇ Variant and mutant ER—unlikely.
    ◇ Changes in coactivators—agonistic actions of tamoxifen could occur in cells that previously were demonstrating antagonistic response.
    ◇ Crosstalk between signaling pathways.
      ○ Synergy exists between ER and protein hormone pathways.
      ○ ER phosphorylation, other protein phosphorylation.
        □ Agonistic activity if tamoxifen induced.
        □ Not true for pure antiestrogens.
    ◇ Binding to other proteins—remote possibility.
    ◇ Differential cellular transport—overexpression of efflux pump could decrease intracellular tamoxifen.
    ◇ Differential metabolism—little evidence seen.
- ♦ Pure antiestrogens.
  - Derivatives of estradiol with long hydrophobic side chains at position 7.
  - Binding with pure antiestrogens prevents DNA binding; sterically interferes with dimerization.
  - Also increases cellular turnover of ERs; receptors degraded in cytoplasm.
    - Half-life of ER with estrogen is approximately 5 hours.
    - Half-life of ER with antiestrogen is less than 1 hour.
  - May also increase insulin-like growth factor–binding protein 3 (IGFBP-3) production.
- ♦ Selective estrogen receptor modulators.
  - Raloxifene and droloxifene have antiestrogenic activity in uterus and breast.
  - They have agonistic activity on bone, lipids (but no effect on HDL).
- ♦ RU486.
  - Forms HRE-ER complex similar to progesterone; slightly different conformational change in hormone-binding domain prevents full gene activation.
  - Some agonistic activity.

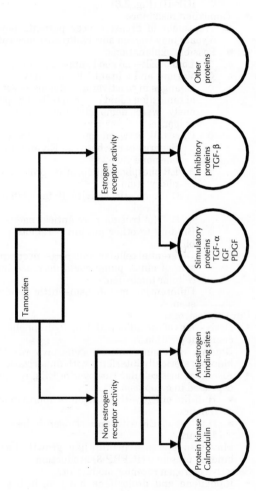

Figure 2.6. Receptor and nonreceptor-mediated actions of tamoxifen.

- 19-Nortestosterone derivative; dimethylaminophenyl side chain at carbon 11.
    - Long half-life.
    - High affinity for PR.
    - Active metabolites.
- Progesterone receptor affinity of RU486 is 5 times greater than progesterone.
- Low affinity binding to androgen receptor.
- High affinity binding to glucocorticoid receptor but need high dose to produce effect secondary to high circulating cortisol concentration.
- Changes transcription activity of progesterone receptor B.
- Stimulates A receptor inhibition of transcription activity for all steroid hormone receptors.
- ◆ Androgen antagonists.
    - Cyproterone acetate and spironolactone.
        - Bind to androgen receptor.
        - Mixed agonist and antagonist functions; in presence of high androgen levels, antagonism predominates.
    - Flutamide.
        - Nonsteroidal pure antiandrogen.
        - Blocks androgenic action at target sites by competitive inhibition.

XIV. Mechanism of Action for Tropic Hormones
- ◆ Introduction.
    - Includes hypothalamic-releasing hormones and a variety of anterior pituitary and placental peptides and glycoproteins.
    - Specificity dependent on presence of cell membrane receptors.
    - Functions of receptor proteins.
        - Ion channel.
        - Enzyme function.
        - Coupled to intracellular messenger systems.
            - ◇ cAMP.
            - ◇ Inositol 1,4,5-triphosphate (IP_3).
            - ◇ 1,2-Diacylglycerol (DG).
            - ◇ Calcium.
            - ◇ Cyclic guanosine 3′,5′-monophosphate (cGMP).
- ◆ cAMP mechanism.
    - Intracellular messenger for FSH, LH, human chorionic gonadotropin (hCG), thyrotropin (TSH), adrenocorticotropin (ACTH).
    - Tropic hormone binding activates adenylate cyclase; adenosine triphosphate (ATP) → cAMP.
    - Sensitivity imparted by large number of receptors, but only 1% need to be occupied.
        - Protein kinase activated by cAMP-receptor protein complex.
        - Tetramer with two regulatory/two catalytic subunits.

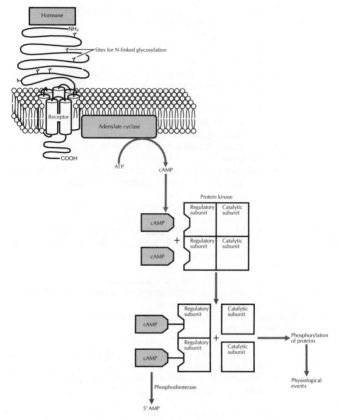

Figure 2.7. The mechanism of cyclic AMP action (cAMP).

- ■ cAMP binding to regulatory units releases catalytic subunits.
- ■ Serine and threonine residues are phosphorylated (Fig. 2.7).
- • DNA contains response elements that bind proteins phosphorylated by catalytic units.
  - ■ cAMP-response element functions as an enhancer element.
  - ■ cAMP regulatory element–binding protein activates many genes.
- • Other pathways may also exist.
- • Specificity depends on differential gene expression; adenylate cyclase also exists in several isoforms.
- • Amplification of the faint hormone signal is important.
- • Prostaglandins (PG) stimulate adenylate cyclase, but PGs are synthesized after cAMP in signaling pathway.

- Probably cell wall effect of PGs facilitates tropic hormone response.
- Specificity depends on differential gene expression.
- PGs and cGMP may participate in an intracellular negative feedback mechanism.
- Hormones not using adenylate cyclase mechanisms include the following:
  - Oxytocin, insulin, growth hormone, prolactin, cytokines; single transmembrane domain–receptor family.
  - Prolactin operates via several mechanisms, including ion channels and nuclear kinase activation.
  - Gonadotropin-releasing hormone (GnRH) is calcium dependent; uses IP_3 and 1,2-DG as second messengers.
    - ◇ Requires G protein.
    - ◇ Associated with cyclic release of calcium ions and opening of cell membrane channels.
- ♦ Calcium messenger system.
  - Intracellular calcium is regulator of both cAMP and cGMP; activation of cell surface receptors either opens cell membrane channel or releases calcium from internal stores.
  - Linked to hormone-receptor function by phospholipase C.
    - Catalyzes hydrolysis of phosphatidylinositol.
    - Two intracellular messengers.
      - ◇ IP_3, DG.
      - ◇ Initiate function of two parts of calcium system:
        - ○ Protein kinase—sustained response.
        - ○ Calmodulin—acute response.
  - Calmodulin identified in all animal/plant cells.
    - Very ancient protein.
    - One hundred forty-eight amino acids.
    - Four calcium-binding sites.
    - One percent of total cell protein (10×10^6 molecules).
- ♦ Kinase receptors.
  - Tyrosine kinase receptors.
    - Insulin.
    - IGF.
    - EGF.
    - Platelet-derived growth factor (PDGF).
    - FGF.
  - All have similar structures.
    - Extracellular ligand-binding domain.
    - Single transmembrane domain.
    - Cytoplasmic domain—undergoes conformational change with ligand binding and autophosphorylation.
  - Insulin receptor is more complex.
    - 2α, 2β subunits.

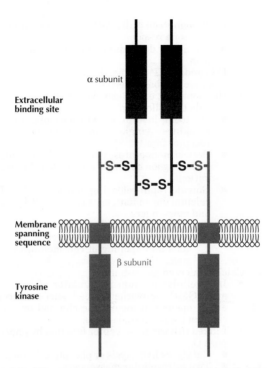

Figure 2.8.   The receptor structure for insulin and insulin-like growth factor.

- ■ Transmembrane domains connected extracellularly by disulfide bridges.
- • Serine-specific protein hormones; activin, inhibin receptors.
- • Significant homology among kinase receptors in cytoplasmic domain; many substrates are enzymes/proteins in other messenger systems that allow crosstalk (Fig. 2.8).
- XV. Regulation of Tropic Hormones
  - ◆ Introduction.
    - • Regulation can be divided into four major components as follows:
      1. Autocrine/paracrine regulation factors.
      2. Heterogeneity of the hormone.
      3. Up-regulation or down-regulation of receptors.
      4. Regulation of adenylate cyclase.
  - ◆ Autocrine/Paracrine.
    - • Growth factors are polypeptides that modulate activity in either the cells in which they are produced (autocrine) or nearby cells (paracrine).

- Produced by local gene expression; bind to cell-membrane receptors.
  - Intracellular component with tyrosine kinase activity.
  - Others work via second messengers (cAMP, IP_3).
- Growth factors important for embryonic/fetal growth.
  - Can operate in cooperative, competitive, or synergistic fashion with other hormones.
  - For instance, IGF-I plus FSH, but not IGF-I alone, increases LH receptors, P_4 synthesis, and aromatization in granulosa cells.
- Activin/inhibin.
  - Disulfide-linked dimers; 1α, 2β subunits.
  - Three forms of activin:
    - ◇ Activin A: $beta_A$–$beta_A$.
    - ◇ Activin AB: $beta_A$–$beta_B$.
    - ◇ Activin B: $beta_B$–$beta_B$.
  - Two forms of inhibin:
    - ◇ Inhibin A: $alpha$–$beta_A$.
    - ◇ Inhibin B: $alpha$–$beta_B$.
  - Each subunit is encoded by separate genes.
    - ◇ Precursor proteins cleave to form subunits.
    - ◇ Free subunits, related monomeric products can be secreted.
  - Function as antagonists in some systems; belong to same gene family as TGF-β, antimüllerian hormone (AMH).
  - Activin activity is regulated by protein binding (follistatin).
  - Receptors are transmembrane serum kinases.
- TGF-β and others.
  - Activity depends on target cell and/or presence or absence of other growth factors.
  - In granulosa cell, they enhance actions of FSH and antagonize down-regulation of FSH receptors.
  - EGF is structural analog of TGF-α; 1α, 2β subunits.
  - FGF is a potent mitogen.
    - ◇ Enzyme activity.
    - ◇ Angiogenesis.
- IGFs.
  - Also called somatomedins.
  - Single-chain polypeptide.
  - Involved in growth and differentiation in response to growth hormone.
  - IGF-II prominent during embryogenesis.
  - IGF-I more active postnatally.
    - ◇ Only the liver makes more IGF-I than the ovary.
    - ◇ Amplifies action of gonadotropins.
    - ◇ Coordinates theca/granulosa.
      - ○ IGF-I action on granulosa cells increases the following:

- □ FSH.
- □ LH receptors.
- □ Steroidogenesis.
- □ Secretion of inhibin.
- □ Oocyte maturation.
    - ○ IGF-I action on theca cells increases steroidogenesis.
  - ■ Granulosa cells also contain insulin receptors; insulin can bind to an IGF-I receptor.
  - ■ IGF-I receptor.
    - ◇ Heterotetramer (2α, 2β).
    - ◇ Insulin can bind to an α subunit ligand-binding domain and can activate the β subunit (protein kinase).
- • IGFBPs.
  - ■ Modulate biologic potency and/or availability.
    - ◇ Six IGFBPs have been identified.
    - ◇ Nearly all IGFs are bound to IGFBPs.
  - ■ Differ in actions and individual expression.
  - ■ Tissue-specific regulation can change bioavailability at specific sites.
  - ■ Direct IGFBP effects also exist.
  - ■ A complex system with endocrine, autocrine, and paracrine functions.
- ◆ Orphan receptors involved in steroidogenesis.
  - • Nuclear receptors for which no specific ligands have been identified.
  - • They include the following:
    - ■ Steroidogenic factor 1 (SF-1).
      - ◇ Influences expression of genes encoding steroidogenic enzymes.
      - ◇ Animal knockout models—gonads and/or adrenals fail to develop.
      - ◇ Regulates transcription of StAR gene.
      - ◇ Regulates genes encoding gonadotropin subunits and GnRH receptors.
    - ■ Dosage-sensitive sex reversal adrenal hypoplasia congenita region on X chromosome.
      - ◇ Mutations result in adrenal hypoplasia.
      - ◇ Believed to work with SF-1 to regulate development/function of steroid-producing tissue.
- ◆ Heterogeneity.
  - • FSH/LH are not single proteins but a family of heterogeneous forms.
    - ■ Isoforms arise via the following ways:
      - ◇ Different DNA promoter action.
      - ◇ Alternative RNA splicing.
      - ◇ Point mutations.
      - ◇ Posttranslational carbohydrate changes.
    - ■ Isoforms differ in clearance, binding, and activity.
    - ■ At least 20 to 30 isoforms present during the menstrual cycle.
  - • Synthesis.

- Nonglycosylated subunits are synthesized in the endoplasmic reticulum.
- Glycosylation occurs.
- Glycosylated subunits combine and travel to the Golgi for carbohydrate processing.
- Protein moiety binds to target receptors.
- Carbohydrate component couples hormone-receptor complex to adenylate cyclase.
- Chemical makeup of glycoproteins.
  - Essential in determining receptor-binding activity.
  - Heterodimers of α and β subunits; tightly bound noncovalent association.
  - Alpha-chain shared; made up of 92 amino acids.
  - Beta-chains differ.
- β hCG.
  - Largest β subunit; 145 amino acid residues.
  - Unique carboxy terminal tail piece of 24 amino acids.
    - ◊ Allows formation of highly specific antibodies for immunoassays.
    - ◊ Four glycosylation sites → longer half-life.
  - These unique structural features are associated with different promoter and transcriptional sites upstream in hCG β subunit gene.
  - No hormone response element; thus, no sex steroid feedback regulation.
  - Rate-limiting step in synthesis of all the glycopeptides is the availability of β subunits.
    - ◊ Excess α found in blood and tissue.
    - ◊ Half-life of α hCG: 6 to 8 minutes.
    - ◊ Half-life of placental whole hCG: 24 hours, which is longer than hCG from all other tissues.
  - Glycosylation—sialic acid is key sugar moiety for increased half-life.
- Comparison of FSH and LH.

FSH:	LH:
Alpha chain: 92 aa	Alpha chain: 92 aa
Beta chain: 118 aa	Beta chain: 121 aa
Four carbohydrate side chains	Three carbohydrate side chains
Half-life: 3 to 4 hours	Half-life: 20 minutes

- Gene regulation.
  - Promoter (enhancer) inhibitor regions in 5′ flanking region upstream.
  - Respond to second messengers (cAMP), as well as to steroids.
  - Single human gene present for α subunit.
    - ◊ Located on chromosome 6p21.1-23.
    - ◊ Single promoter site in both the placenta and pituitary.

- ■ β Subunits are more restricted in cell type.
  - ◇ TSH β—thyrotrope, regulated by thyroid hormone.
  - ◇ FSH β—gonadotropes; regulated by GnRH, activin, inhibin, and steroids.
  - ◇ LH β—gonadotropes; regulated by GnRH, unaffected by inhibin/activin.
- ■ α Subunit gene activation.
  - ◇ Requires activation of distinct regulatory elements in thyrotrope, gonadotrope, and placenta.
  - ◇ In gonadotropes → GnRH signaling pathway via DG, IP_3, and calcium to activate protein kinase C; growth factor and/or steroid influence in the pituitary versus cAMP in placenta.
- ■ FSH-β gene.
  - ◇ Chromosome 11p13.
  - ◇ Activin markedly influences pituitary expression.
    - ○ Unique to FSH-β.
    - ○ Follistatin/inhibin antagonize expression.
- ■ LH, hCG, and TSH-β subunit genes.
  - ◇ Located in cluster on 19q13.3.
    - ○ Six genes for β hCG (96% identical with LH).
      - □ Each has different promoters.
      - □ Recent evolution; possible read-through mutation of LH.
      - □ Present only in primates and horses.
    - ○ One gene for β LH; not expressed in placenta.
    - ○ One LH variant relatively common.
      - □ Two point mutations.
      - □ Northern Europeans.
      - □ May provide abnormal immunoassay readings.
  - ◇ β Subunit specifies biologic activity, but both α and β are necessary for full hormonal activation.
- • Variations in carbohydrate content (CHO).
  - ■ Isoform mixture influenced by GnRH and sex steroid feedback.
  - ■ Certain clinical conditions may arise.
    - ◇ Low estrogen environment results in production of increased carbohydrate content and decreased biologic activity.
    - ◇ Greater FSH bioactivity is found at midcycle with increased production in a less sialated form.
  - ■ CHO modifications affect target tissue response in the following two ways:
    - ◇ Metabolic clearance.
      - ○ Increased sialic acid, decreased clearance.

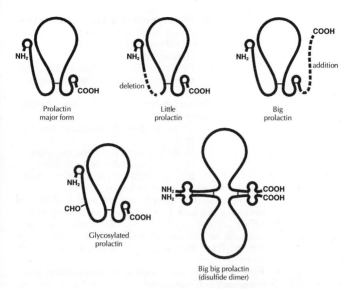

Figure 2.9.   Various forms and structures of prolactin resulting from structural modifications.

- ○ Other factors also contribute.
- ◇ Biologic activity.
- ○ Binding and/or activation.
- ○ Carbohydrate component does not alter binding but lowers activity.
- • Prolactin—most common prolactin in mammals is 190 amino acids.
    - ■ Forty percent homology with growth hormone and human placental lactogen; probably all three arise from the same ancestral protein.
    - ■ Bioassays and immunoassays reveal discrepancies (Fig. 2.9).
        - ◇ Differences originally based on size.
        - ○ Other aspects also differ among isoforms.
            - □ Glycosylation.
            - □ Phosphorylation.
            - □ Variations in binding and charge.
        - ◇ Prolactin encoded on a single gene on chromosome 6.
            - ○ Major form exists as three loops with disulfide bonds.
            - ○ Most variants are posttranslational modifications.
                - □ Little prolactin from a splicing variant.
                - □ Big prolactin from a failure to remove introns.

□ Big-big prolactin from separate molecules binding together.

○ Other differences also exist.
  □ Glycosylation.
  □ Different CHO moities, although major circulating form is nonglycosylated.

○ Prolactin-receptor gene on chromosome 5.
  □ Close to growth hormone receptor gene.
  □ Probably more than one receptor.
  □ May also function as a cytokine.
  □ Signal mediated via tyrosine kinase.

♦ Up-regulation and down-regulation.
  • Up-regulation is poorly understood; GnRH and prolactin can both increase their own receptors.
  • Down-regulation could result from dissociation of complex or the loss of receptors; internalization results from excess concentration of tropic hormone.
  • Episodic secretion avoids down-regulation; pulse frequency is a key factor.
  • Receptors inserted randomly in the cell membrane.
  • Receptor hormone complex migrates to coated pit in the presence of a high tropic hormone concentration.
    ■ Each cell contains 500 to 1,500 coated pits.
    ■ Clustering allows increased internalization via endocytosis.
  • Coated pit.
    ■ Lipid vesicle hanging on a basket of specific proteins (clathrins).
    ■ Internal margin has brush border.
    ■ Clathrin network binds internal binding receptor.
    ■ When it is fully occupied, the coated pit pinches off → receptosome.
      ◊ Delivered to lysosome.
      ◊ Undergoes degradation.
      ◊ Internalized hormones may mediate biologic response.
  • Potocytosis: internalization of small molecules/ions.
    ■ Uses cholesterol rich invaginations called caveolae; G proteins, kinases, and growth-factor receptors have all been detected.
    ■ Fewer in number than clathrin-coated pits.
    ■ Nitric oxide resides in caveolae.
    ■ Caveolae facilitate endocytosis and exocytosis.
    ■ Cell membrane receptors are usually internalized and then degraded in lysosomes.
      ◊ Coated pit may immobilize hormone-receptor complexes.
      ◊ hCG is degraded in some tissues but is potentially recycled back to the cell surface

in the placenta as a means of transport into circulation.

- ■ Cell membrane receptors are found within pits.
  - ◇ They are internalized and then recycled.
  - ◇ Examples include LDL, cobalamin (vitamin B_{12}), transferrin (iron), and IgG transferred across the placenta.
- • LDL receptor.
  - ■ LDL is a sphere.
    - ◇ Approximately 1,500 cholesterol molecules in center.
    - ◇ Core contained by lipid bilayer.
    - ◇ Apoproteins project on the surface; recognized by receptors.
    - ◇ Critical for steroid-producing cells; some cells (e.g., granulosa) can extract cholesterol from HDL.
  - ■ LDL receptor is a mosaic protein; it is derived from exons of different gene families (EGF, complement) (Fig. 2.10).
  - ■ Precursor of 860 aa.
    - ◇ 21 aa hydrophobic signal sequence.
    - ◇ 839 aa protein with five domains as follows:
      1. NH_2-terminal 292 aa (40 aa repeat with variation seven times); LDL-binding site.
      2. 400 aa segment, 35% homologous to EGF precursor.
      3. Sugar-linked site.
      4. 22 aa hydrophobic cell membrane–spanning region; deletion results in failure of receptor insertion into membrane.
      5. 50 aa cytoplasmic tail; clusters LDL receptor into pits.
    - ◇ Endocytosis occurs when the coated pit is fully occupied.
      - ○ Pit moves to Golgi.
      - ○ It is routed to lysosome.
    - ◇ Intracellular level of free cholesterol influences the following:
      - ○ Cholesterol synthesis.
      - ○ Reesterification of excess cholesterol.
      - ○ Synthesis of LDL receptors.
    - ◇ Cholesterol fate is variable.
      - ○ Internalized in mitochondria for steroidogenesis.
      - ○ Reesterification for storage.
      - ○ Used in membranes.
      - ○ Excreted; involves cell surface caveolae.
    - ◇ Synthesis and/or insertion of LDL receptors.
      - ○ Function of LH in gonads, ACTH in adrenal.
      - ○ Very fast process—LDL receptor makes one round trip every 10 minutes during its 20-hour life span.

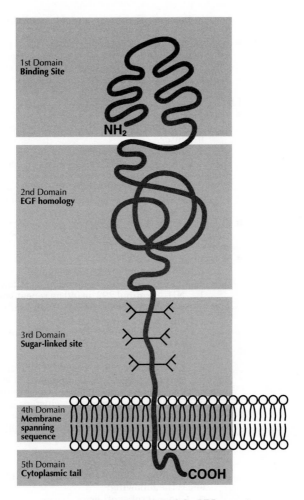

Figure 2.10.   The domains of the LDL receptor.

- Regulation of adenylate cyclase LDL receptor—another means by which biologic activity of polypeptide/glycoprotein hormones can be altered.
- G protein system.
  - Nobel Prize–winning (1994) description by Gilman and Rodbell.
  - Three protein units.
    - ◇ Receptor.
    - ◇ Guanyl nucleotide regulatory unit.

- ◇ Coupling protein; regulated by guanosine triphosphate (GTP).
- ◇ Catalytic unit—converts ATP to cAMP.
- ◇ Receptor and regulatory unit are structurally linked but are inactive prior to binding.
- ◇ With receptor binding, GTP is taken up by the regulatory unit; this activates catalytic unit ATP → cAMP.
- ◇ Enzyme activity is terminated by hydrolysis of GTP → guanosine diphosphate (GDP).
- ■ G protein has been purified.
  - ◇ Family of G proteins.
  - ◇ Stimulatory and inhibitory nucleotides regulates the G proteins: α, β, γ (Fig. 2.11).
  - ◇ β and γ are not all alike; have selectivity for specific receptors.
  - ◇ Each G protein has unique α.
  - ◇ Four subfamilies.
    - ○ $G_s\alpha$, $G_q\alpha$, $G_i\alpha$, G_{i2}.
    - ○ G_i is inhibitory.
  - ◇ α Subunit binds GDP in inactive state.
    - ○ Hormone binding changes α conformation.
    - ○ β and γ freed.
    - ○ GTP-α binds to catalytic unit; can also activate ion channels.
  - ◇ Intrinsic GTPase activity changes GTP-α to GDP-α.
- ■ G protein receptors.
  - ◇ More than 200 receptors linked to the G protein.
    - ○ Inserted in membranes.
    - ○ Long 7 helix polypeptide chain.
    - ○ Amino extracellular and carboxy intercellular.
    - ○ Can be activated by hormones, neurotransmitters, growth factors, odorants, and light.
  - ◇ LH/hCG receptor.
    - ○ Highly conserved in mammals—expression is especially regulated by FSH.
    - ○ Activates G protein and calcium pathways.
    - ○ Gene on chromosome 2.
  - ◇ FSH receptor.
    - ○ Similar to LH/hCG receptor but structurally distinct.
    - ○ Major sequence divergence in extracellular domain.
    - ○ Gene on chromosome 2p21.
    - ○ Regulated by FSH, estradiol.
- ■ Mutations in G protein system.
  - ◇ Loss of function mutations.
    - ○ TSH receptor → hypothyroidism.

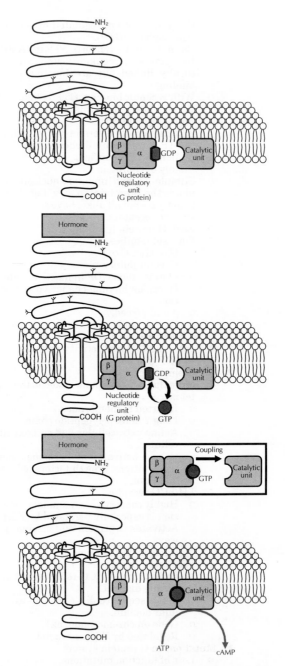

Figure 2.11.   The G protein in its inactive state (top and middle) and in its active state (bottom).

Table 2.4. Some genetic diseases due to specific G protein system mutations

Mutation	Disorder
Activating LH receptor	Precocious puberty in boys
Inactivating LH receptor	Male pseudohermaphroditism
Inactivating FSH receptor	Premature ovarian failure
$G_s\alpha$ (stimulatory)	McCune–Albright syndrome
$G_i\alpha$ (inhibitory)	Hypothyroidism
Rhodopsin	Retinitis pigmentosa
Vasopressin	Diabetes insipidus

Abbreviations: FSH, follicle-stimulating hormone; LH, luteinizing hormone.

- ○ LH receptor → male pseudohermaphroditism.
- ○ $G_s\alpha$ receptor → pseudohypoparathyroidism.
- ◇ Gain of function mutations.
  - ○ $G_s\alpha$ mutation leading to unregulated activity.
  - ○ Example is McCune–Albright syndrome.
    - □ Sexual precocity.
    - □ Café-au-lait spots.
    - □ Polyostotic fibrous dysplasia.
    - □ Endocrine gland autonomy (Table 2.4).
- • Coupling, uncoupling, and/or desensitization.
  - ■ LH stimulates steroidogenesis through coupling of stimulatory regulatory units to catalytic units.
  - ■ Prostaglandin F $(PGF)_{2\alpha}$ is directly luteolytic; may uncouple catalytic unit via inhibitory subunit.
  - ■ Desensitization is rapid, acute change without loss of receptors; LH/hCG receptor undergoes this process in response to LH or hCG via C terminal.
  - ■ Phosphorylation; true for GnRH stimulation as well.
- • Summary of down-regulation.
  - ■ Down-regulation is a decrease in response in the presence of continuous stimulation.
  - ■ It involves the following three mechanisms:
    1. Desensitization by autophosphorylation of the cytoplasmic segment of the receptor.
    2. Loss of receptors by internalization, a relatively slow mechanism.
    3. Uncoupling of the regulatory and catalytic subunits of the adenylate cyclase enzyme.

The Ovary: Embryology and Development

I. Historical Perspective
   - Soranus of Ephesus (A.D. 98–138) provided the first accurate description of the ovary; the great text was lost for centuries but was eventually published in 1838.
   - Galen (A.D. 138–200) was felt to be the ultimate authority on anatomy.
   - da Vinci (1452–1511) accurately drew the ovary and uterus.
   - Vesalius (1514–64) was the first to describe ovarian follicles and the corpus luteum.
   - Fallopius (1534–62) described oviducts (fallopian tubes).
   - William Harvey maintained the Aristotelian belief that the egg was a product of conception (corrected by Niles Stensen [1667]).
   - Regnier DeGraaf (1672) thought the whole follicle was the egg.
   - Leeuwenhoek (1677) discovered spermatozoa (mammalian).
   - von Baer (1827) described the egg residing within the follicle.
   - Newport (1853) described the process of fertilization.

II. The Human Ovary
   - Responsible for the release of gametes (eggs) and the production of steroid hormones.
   - The ovary is a heterogeneous cyclic tissue.
   - It consists of the following three major portions:
     - Outer cortex.
       - Outermost portion is tunica albuginea.
       - It is topped by a single layer of cuboidal epithelium.
       - Oocytes are present within the follicles.
     - Hilum.
       - Point of attachment to mesovarium.
       - Contains nerves, blood vessels, and hilus cells.
     - Stromal tissue.
       - Derived from mesenchymal cells.
       - Forms connective tissue and interstitial cells.
       - Central medullary region contains mesonephric cells.

III. The Fetal Ovary
   - Four stages of development as follows:
     1. Indifferent gonad stage.
     2. Stage of differentiation.
     3. Oogonial multiplication and oocyte formation.
     4. Follicular formation.
   - Indifferent gonad stage.

- At 5 weeks of gestation, gonads are structurally consolidated coelomic prominences.
  - Form gonadal ridges.
  - Morphologically identical in ovaries and testes.
- This stage lasts 7 to 10 days.
- Mesonephros and genital ridge are the urogenital ridge.
- Origin of gonadal somatic cells is uncertain.
  - Possibly from the invasion of germinal epithelium into underlying mesenchyme.
  - Possibly arising from the mesonephros (not coelomic epithelium).
- Primordial germ cells originate within the primitive ectoderm.
  - Specific cells of origin cannot be distinguished.
  - First identified at end of third week after fertilization; located in primitive endoderm and yolk sac.
  - Gonadal ridge is the only place germ cells can survive.
    - ◇ Germ cells "migrate" along dorsal mesentery of genital ridges; in rodents, this involves stem cell factor and its receptor c-kit.
  - Germ cells begin proliferation during migration; by the sixth gestational week → 10,000 germ cells.
- ◆ Stage of differentiation.
  - If the gonad is destined to become a testis, differentiation occurs at 6 to 9 weeks.
  - If the fetus is female, internal and external genitalia differentiation precedes gonadal maturation.
  - The testes.
    - Testis-determining factor is a product of a gene on Y chromosome.
      - ◇ Best candidate is within the sex-determining region on Y chromosome (SRY).
      - ◇ The protein product of the gene contains a DNA-binding domain.
    - Normal testes also require other genes; SOX genes (similarity with SRY b*ox* region) possess DNA-binding sequence.
    - SRY expression confined to the genital ridge in fetal life but it is also active in adult germ cells.
    - Male phenotype is dependent on antimüllerian hormone (AMH) and testosterone; female phenotype occurs in the absence of these fetal gonadal products.
    - AMH inhibits formation of müllerian ducts.
      - ◇ Begins at 7 weeks.
      - ◇ Regression dependent on adequate number of Sertoli cells and regulation of AMH receptor.
      - ◇ Secreted after regression of müllerian system but has no known function.

- o Produced in granulosa cells.
- o Possible relationship to autocrine/paracrine actions in oocyte maturation/follicular development.
- Testis begins differentiation in week 6 to 7.
  - ◇ Sertoli cells appear; aggregate to form testicular cords.
  - ◇ Primordial germ cells embedded in testicular cords that will form Sertoli cells (spermatogonia).
  - ◇ Mature Sertoli cells make androgen-binding protein and inhibin.
- By week 8, Leydig cells differentiate.
  - ◇ They form mesenchymal cells of interstitial components.
  - ◇ Secretion of AMH by Sertoli cells precedes steroidogenesis in the Leydig cells.
  - ◇ Peak androgen secretion at 15 to 18 weeks.
    - o Leydig cells then begin to regress.
    - o Only a few left at birth.
- Cycle of fetal Leydig cells follows rise and decline of human chorionic gonadotropin (hCG) (peak at 10 weeks; nadir at 20 weeks).
  - ◇ Presence of hCG receptor in fetal testes also suggests a regulatory role—fetal hCG levels are 5% of maternal levels.
  - ◇ Testosterone production peaks at 15 to 18 weeks, similar to androgen, and then declines.
    - o Initially responds to fetal levels of hCG.
    - o Further maintained by fetal pituitary.
- Fetal Leydig cells avoid down-regulation; eventually, these cells are replaced by adult generation of Leydig cells.
  - ◇ Functional at puberty.
  - ◇ Respond to high levels of hCG and luteinizing hormone (LH) with down-regulation.
- Fetal spermatogonia.
  - ◇ Derived from primordial germ cells.
  - ◇ Located in testicular cords; surrounded by Sertoli cells.
  - ◇ Do not start meiotic division until puberty (Fig 3.1).
- Differentiation of wolffian system begins with increase in testicular testosterone.
  - ◇ Classic experiments by Jost—effect of testosterone due to local action.
- Not all androgen-sensitive tissue is dependent on dihydrotestosterone (DHT).
  - ◇ Wolffian duct structure dependent on testosterone as the intracellular mediator.
  - ◇ Urogenital sinus and tubercles require DHT.
- In female fetus, loss of wolffian system is due to the lack of testosterone locally.

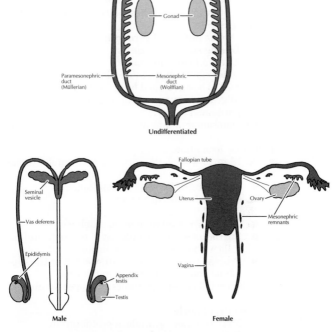

Figure 3.1. Differentiation of the internal duct systems in male and female fetuses.

- ◆ Oogonal multiplication and oocyte formation.
    - • First signs of ovarian differentiation reflected in rapid mitotic multiplication—6 to 7 million by week 16 to 20; maximal oogonial content of the gonad.
    - • Oogonia formed by mitosis; become oocytes as they enter the first meiotic division.
        - ■ Arrest in diplotene stage of prophase.
        - ■ Possibly in response to a product from the rete ovarii.
        - ■ Arrest maintained by granulosa cell–inhibiting substances in prophase.
    - • Single ovum formed by two meiotic divisions of oocytes.
        - ■ One division prior to ovulation.
        - ■ Second division at time of sperm penetration.
        - ■ Excess genetic information extruded as the polar body.
    - • Gonadotropin and growth factors can induce resumption of meiosis.
        - ■ Only true in oocytes with cumulus–granulosa cells.

- ■ Family of sterols present in follicular fluid; activates meiosis (Figs. 3.2 and 3.3).
- • Loss of germ cells takes place throughout all of these events.
  - ■ During mitosis of germ cells.
  - ■ During stages of meiosis.
  - ■ After follicular formation.
- • Oocytes regress during meiosis.
  - ■ Fail to be enveloped by granulosa cells.
  - ■ Migrate to surface and are eliminated in the peritoneal cavity.
- • Chromosomal anomalies can accelerate germ cell loss.
- ♦ Follicular formation.
  - • At 18 to 20 weeks, the cortex is perforated by vascular channels.
    - ■ Beginning of follicular formation.
    - ■ Other cells also drawn in.
  - • Primordial follicle.
    - ■ Oocyte arrested in meiotic prophase.
    - ■ Surrounded by a single layer of pregranulosa cells with a basement membrane.
    - ■ Process continues until all oocytes in the diplotene stage can be found in follicles.
  - • Primary follicle—pregranulosa changes to cuboidal layer.
  - • Preantral follicle.
    - ■ More complete granulosa proliferation.
    - ■ Call–Exner body formation.
    - ■ Found in the sixth month of gestation.
  - • Antral follicles.
    - ■ Present by the end of pregnancy.
    - ■ Not seen in large numbers.
    - ■ Theca cells found only in third trimester.
    - ■ No estrogen production until late in pregnancy; gonadal steroids not needed for phenotype development.
  - • Ovary at birth can contain cystic follicles.
- ♦ Anterior pituitary.
  - • Begins development between 4 and 5 weeks of fetal life.
  - • Median eminence apparent by week 9.
  - • Hypothalamic–pituitary portal circulation functional by the fourth week.
    - ■ Pituitary levels of follicle-stimulating hormone (FSH) peak between 20 to 23 weeks;
    - ■ Levels are higher in the female fetus until last 6 weeks.
      - ◊ Ovaries in the anencephalic fetus are smaller at term (no gonadotropin-releasing hormone [GnRH], no gonadotropin).
      - ◊ However, progression through meiosis to primordial follicles occurs.

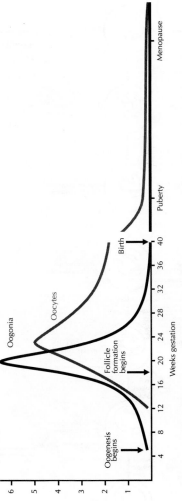

Figure 3.2.   Production of oogonia and oocytes prior to birth and during the lifetime of the female.

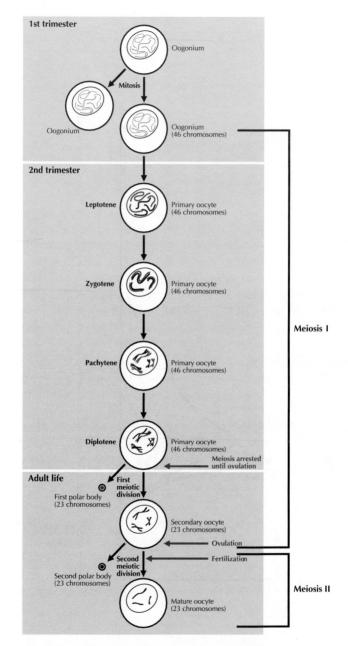

Figure 3.3. Development of an oocyte from oogonium (prenatal) to mature oocyte (adulthood).

- Gonadotropin receptors present only in second half of pregnancy.
  - ◇ Loss of oocytes cannot be explained solely by decline in gonadotropins.
  - ◇ Follicular growth and/or development in second half of pregnancy is gonadotropin-dependent.

IV. Neonatal Ovary
  - ◆ Four to five million oocytes lost over 20 weeks; newborn has lost approximately 80% of her oocytes.
  - ◆ Ovary is 1 cm in diameter.
    - Weighs 250 to 350 mg at birth.
    - Right gonad is larger.
  - ◆ Higher pituitary and circulating FSH/LH levels in female fetuses, as well as a more sustained postnatal FSH rise.
    - Decreases by 1 year of age.
    - Follicular growth relatively common in the first 6 months of life.
    - Postnatal rise important for normal hypothalamic–pituitary function.
    - Levels reach nadir by 1 to 2 years in girls; rise slightly between 4 and 10 years of age.

V. Ovary in Childhood
  - ◆ Low levels of gonadotropins in the pituitary.
  - ◆ Ovary is not quiescent.
    - Follicles grow at all times.
    - Some reach antral stage.
  - ◆ Oocytes are active; monkey experiments suggest prepubertal suppression of GnRH and gonadotropin is partially dependent on presence of ovaries, thus suggesting some functional activity of ovary in childhood (Fig 3.4).

VI. Adult Ovary
  - ◆ Overview.
    - At onset of puberty, germ cell mass is 300,000 to 500,000 gametes. Over 30 years, 400 to 500 oocytes will ovulate.
    - Loss is accelerated in the last 10 to 15 years before menopause.
      - Decreased levels of inhibin and insulin-like growth factor I (IGF-I).
      - Elevations in FSH.
      - Cycles become shorter, probably resulting from the increase in FSH with earlier recruitment.
    - Follicles and oocytes are lost through atresia.
      - Apoptosis = programmed cell death.
      - Its precise function is not known.
    - Sympathetic and sensory neurons are present in primate ovaries.
  - ◆ Follicular growth.
    - Stages of development are observed even during prenatal period.
      - Granulosa proliferation.
      - Theca interna formation.
      - Zona pellucida formation.

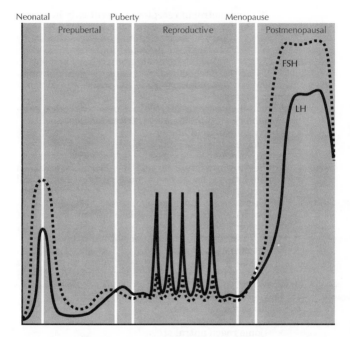

Figure 3.4.   Pituitary hormone activity during different periods of female growth and development.

- From development of primary follicle to ovulation to ovulatory oocytes = 85 days.
- Growth is independent of gonadotropins for the majority of time.
- FSH-dependent stage is seen later; FSH receptors are found on granulosa cells.
  - Formation of Call–Exner bodies.
  - Transudate forms.
  - Granulosa remain avascular.
- Some follicles arrest and regress (Fig. 3.5).
- Ovulation.
  - If a follicle has adequate gonadotropin stimulation, it will advance to ovulation.
    - Antrum distends.
    - Granulosa compress.
    - Capsule weakens.
    - Oocyte is extruded.
  - Physical expulsion is dependent on surge in prostaglandin (PG) synthesis; inhibition results in trapped oocytes.
- Corpus luteum.
  - Profound alterations occur in the ruptured follicle.
    - Granulosa cells hypertrophy.

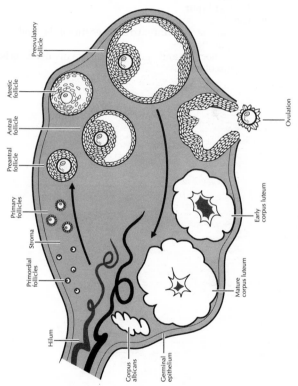

Preovulatory follicle

Atretic follicle

Antral follicle

Preantral follicle

Primary follicles

Primordial follicles

Stroma

Hilum

Corpus albicans

Germinal epithelium

Ovulation

Early corpus luteum

Mature corpus luteum

Figure 3.5. The cycle of maturation of a follicle up to ovulation.

- ■ Granulosa cells become luteinized.
- ■ Theca becomes less prominent.
- • Formation of corpus luteum.
  - ■ Dependent on low levels of LH.
  - ■ Without new emerging source of LH (i.e., hCG), the corpus luteum rapidly ages.
- ◆ Modulators of function—complex sequence of events, which includes the following systems:
  - • Endocrine.
  - • Paracrine/intracrine.
  - • Autocrine.
  - • Neural input.
  - • Cytokines.
    - ■ Corpus luteum attracts eosinophils and T-lymphocytes.
    - ■ Monocytes and macrophages are involved, as is luteolysis.

The Uterus

I. Introduction
   ♦ Anatomic knowledge slow to accumulate regarding the uterus.
     • Soranus (A.D. 98–138) accurately described the uterus; treated prolapse with pessaries.
     • Galen's (A.D. 138–200) descriptions were of animal uteri only.
     • Fallopius (1561) described uteri tuba (tubes).
     • Vesalius (1514–1564) revealed the presence of the endometrial cavity.
II. Development of the müllerian system
   ♦ Wolffian (mesonephric) and müllerian (paramesonephric) ducts coexist for up to 8 weeks.
   ♦ Hormonal control of duct differentiation was established by Alfred Jost; testicular secretions clearly play an important role in differentiation.
     • AMH (antimüllerian hormone; müllerian inhibiting factor).
     • Testosterone.
   ♦ Antimüllerian hormone.
     • Member of the transforming growth factor (TGF)-β family.
     • Gene has been mapped to chromosome 19.
     • It is synthesized by Sertoli cells.
     • It induces ipsilateral regression by 8 weeks of gestation; lack of regression is found in mutations.
     • Normal müllerian development requires the prior appearance of mesonephric ducts; müllerian anomalies are often associated with renal anomalies (Fig. 4.1).
   ♦ Internal genitalia possess an intrinsic tendency to feminize.
     • Lack of AMH allows retention of müllerian structures.
     • Wolffian duct regresses in the absence of testosterone.
     • In the presence of the ovary or the absence of any gonad, müllerian duct development occurs.
   ♦ Paramesonephric ducts connect in the midline to form Y-shaped primordium.
     • Uterus, tubes, upper one-third of vagina.
     • Occurs by tenth week of gestation.
     • Canalization of uterus, cervix, vagina occurs by 22 weeks.
   ♦ Endometrium is derived from mucosal lining of fused müllerian ducts; it is one of the most complex tissues in the body (Fig. 4.2).
III. Histologic Changes in the Endometrium During the Ovulatory Cycle
   ♦ Overview.
     • Carefully studied by Noyes.

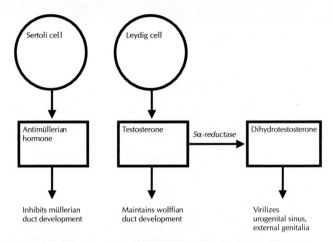

Figure 4.1. The regulation of differentiation for internal duct structures of the fetus.

- Five phases are as follows: (a) menstrual; (b) proliferative; (c) secretory; (d) implantation; (e) breakdown.
- Endometrium is divided morphologically.
  - Upper two-thirds called "functionalis"; prepares for the implantation of blastocyst.
  - Lower one-third known as "basalis"; provides regenerative endometrium following menstrual loss.
- Uterine vasculature.

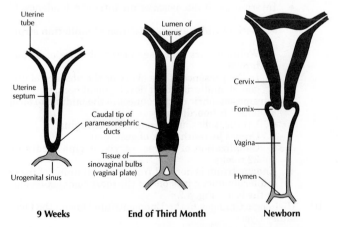

Figure 4.2. The chronology of müllerian duct development in the female fetus.

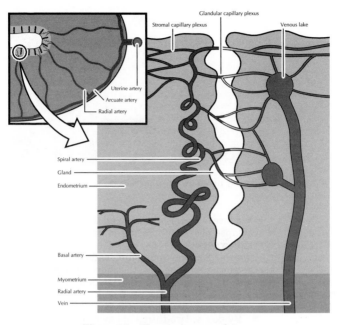

Figure 4.3.   The uterine vasculature.

- Paired uterine arteries are branches of the internal iliac.
- Uterine artery separates.
  - Vaginal branch.
  - Ascending branch.
    - ◇ Divides into arcuate arteries.
    - ◇ Run parallel to uterine cavity.
    - ◇ Form a vascular ring.
      - ○ Small centrifugal branches—radial arteries.
        - □ Supply myometrium.
        - □ Enter endometrium as basal arteries or continue into functionalis as spiral arteries.
      - ○ Spiral arteries.
        - □ Hormonal responses.
        - □ End arteries (Fig. 4.3).
- Menstrual endometrium.
  - Thin but dense.
  - Stable, nonfunctioning basalis; small amount of residual stratum spongiosum.
    - Disarray and breakage of glands.
    - Fragmented vessels.
    - Necrosis.
    - White cell infiltrate.
    - Red cell interstitial diapedesis.

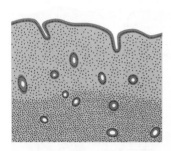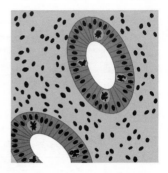

Figure 4.4.   The early proliferative phase. Right is a magnified view.

- Evidence of repair present in all tissue components.
- Collapse of the supporting matrix contributes to shallowness.
- Two-thirds of the functioning endometrium is lost; the more rapid the loss, the shorter the flow is.
- New surface emanates from flanks of gland stumps.
  - Isthmic area of corpus and cornual recesses remain intact.
  - By day 4, two-thirds of cavity is covered with new epithelium.
  - By day 5 to 6, entire cavity is reepithelialized; stromal growth begins.
- ◆ Proliferative phase.
  - Associated with ovarian follicle growth, increased estradiol secretion.
  - Glands are narrow and tubular at first.
  - Epithelium extends peripherally.
  - Stromal component evolves.
    - Dense → edematous → loose syncytial-like status.
    - Spiral arteries extend immediately below the epithelial-binding membrane.
    - Proliferation peaks by day 8 to 10 (Figs. 4.4 and 4.5).
    - Endometrium grows from 0.5 mm up to 3.5 mm to 5.0 mm.
      - ◇ Mainly in functionalis.
      - ◇ The increase in height is secondary to the "reinflation" of the stroma.
    - Increased presence of ciliated/microvillus cells is seen.
    - Population of marrow-derived lymphocytes and macrophages is always present.
- ◆ Secretory phase.
  - After ovulation, a combined reaction to estrogen and progesterone occurs.
  - Endometrial height is fixed.

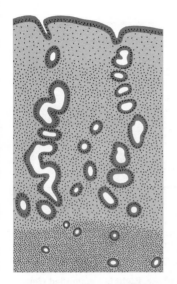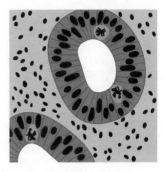

Figure 4.5.   The late proliferative phase. Right is a magnified view.

- Epithelial proliferation ceases 3 days postovulation; probably effect of progesterone.
  - Interference with estradiol receptor expression.
  - 17β-Hydroxysteroid dehydrogenase and sulfotransferase expression increased.
  - Suppresses estrogen-mediated enzyme expression.
- Confinement of growth to fixed structure leads to tortuous glands.
- Granulosa cells are vacuolated (Fig. 4.6).
- Stroma increases in edema.
- First histologic sign of ovulation is found.
  - Appearance of subnuclear intracytoplasmic glycogen vacuoles (day 17 to 18).
  - Giant mitochondria and "nucleolar channel system" appear.
- Tortuous glands begin secreting glycoproteins and peptides; transudate of plasma contributes.
- Immunoglobulins are delivered to the endometrial cavity.
- Implantation.
  - Significant changes occur by day 21 to 27; 13 days postovulation, the following three distinct zones are observed:
    - ¼ = Unchanged basalis.
    - ½ = Lace-like stratum spongiosum, loose edematous stroma.
    - ¼ = Stratum compactum.

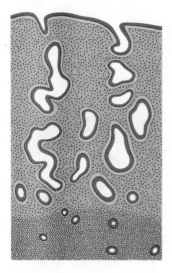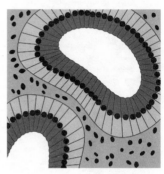

Figure 4.6.   The early secretory phase. Right is a magnified view.

- ◇ Superficial layer of endometrium.
- ◇ Stromal cells.
- ◇ Cytoplasmic expansion of one cell abuts the other.
- ◇ Necks of glands are compressed and less prominent.
- At the time of implantation, the predominant morphological feature is edema of the endometrial stroma; may be prostaglandin (PG)-related–estrogen-mediated and/or progesterone-mediated.
- Mitosis seen in vascular cells by day 22; results in the coiling of the spiral arteries.
- K cells (Körnchenzellen) appear.
  - ▪ Granulocytes have immunoprotective role in implantation; they are located perivascularly.
  - ▪ By day 26 to 27, stroma are infiltrated by polymorphonucleocytes.
  - ▪ Stromal cells respond to hormonal signals.
    - ◇ Decidual cells produce wide array of substances, including prolactin, relaxin, renin, insulin-like growth factors (IGFs).
    - ◇ They emanate from the primitive uterine mesenchymal stem cells.
- Decidualization.
  - ▪ Begins in luteal phase under the influence of progesterone; mediated by autocrine/paracrine factors.
  - ▪ Predecidual cells identified by day 22 to 23.
    - ◇ Perivascular.

◇ Cytonuclear enlargements.
- Plays key role in menstrual cycle and implantation/placentation.
- Inhibition of endometrial hemorrhage is attributed to the following:
  ◇ Lower plasminogen activator level.
  ◇ Reduced expression of stromal degradative enzymes (metalloproteinase).

♦ Endometrial breakdown.
- Predecidual transformation forms "compacta" layer by day 25.
- In absence of pregnancy, estrogen and progesterone levels drop.
- Withdrawal of estrogen and progesterone support initiates the following important events:
  1. Vasomotor reaction.
  2. Apoptosis.
  3. Tissue loss.
  4. Menstruation.
- Vasomotor reactions.
  - Spiral arteries undergo rhythmic vasoconstriction and relaxation; successive spasms are prolonged and profound; endometrial ischemia and stasis result.
  - White and red blood cells permeate the stratum.
  - Thrombin plugs appear in the vessels.
  - Prostaglandin $F_{2\alpha}$ ($PGF_{2\alpha}$) concentration increases; followed by vasoconstriction and myometrial contraction.
  - Endothelin-1 (potent vasoconstrictor) is produced by stromal cells.
- Apoptosis (programmed cell death).
  - Lysosomal membranes lose their integrity; enzymes are released into cytoplasm.
  - Cell-to-cell adhesion breakdown; cadherins, catenins.
- Enzyme activity.
  - Matrix metalloproteinase degrades components.
    ◇ Collagenases—degrade interstitial/basement membrane.
    ◇ Gelatinases—result in further degradation of collagens.
    ◇ Stromelysins—degrade fibronectin, laminin, and glycoproteins.
  - Metalloproteinase expression correlates with menstrual cycle; it is sex steroid–response related.
  - Expression is suppressed in early pregnancy; it is mediated by TGF-β (Fig. 4.7).
  - Progesterone withdrawal can lead to an endometrial breakdown via a mechanism that is independent of vascular events.
  - Tumor necrosis factor–α (TNF-α) probably plays a major role in menstruation.
    ◇ Induces apoptotic signal.

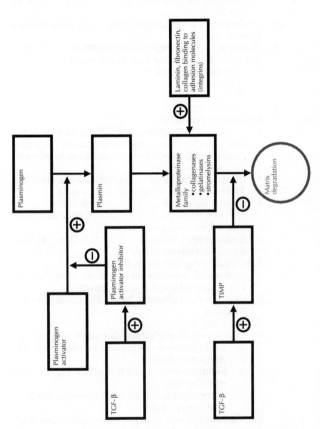

Figure 4.7. Components of endometrial tissue breakdown. Abbreviation: TGF, transforming growth factor; TIMP, tissue inhibitors.

◇ Peaks at menstruation.
◇ Causes loss of adhesion proteins as well.
- Eventually interstitial hemorrhage occurs.
- Menstrual bleeding is influenced by activation of clotting and fibrinolysis; plasmin is formed from plasminogen.
- Endometrial cell tissue factor and plasminogen activator inhibitor 1 (PAI-1) govern the amount of bleeding.
- Cleavage point develops between the basalis and spongiosum.
  ◇ It is initiated in the fundus.
  ◇ Within 13 hours, endometrium shrinks from 4 to 1.25 mm.
- Bleeding stops as a result of prolonged vasoconstriction, tissue collapse, vascular stasis, and estrogen-induced healing; myometrial contractions are not important.

♦ Normal menses.
- Fifty percent of menstrual detritus in first 24 hours.
- Ninety percent of women cycle every 24 to 35 days.
  - Menarche is followed by 5 to 7 years of increasingly regular cycles.
  - By the age of 40 years and older, cycles lengthen again.
- Usual flow lasts between 4 and 6 days.
- Usual volume is 30 mL.
- A volume greater than 80 mL is considered abnormal.

♦ Dating the endometrium.
- Described by Noyes et al. in 1950.
- Biopsy obtained 2 to 3 days prior to menses.
- Most accepted method for diagnosing a luteal phase defect (Fig. 4.8).

IV. Teleologic Theory of Endometrial Menstrual Events
♦ Menstruation is a very recent phenomenon in evolution.
♦ Goal of every cycle is conception.
♦ Ovum must be fertilized within 12 to 24 hours after ovulation.
- Remains unattached in tube for 2 days.
- Enters uterus for 2 to 3 more days.
- By day 6, the embryo is ready to implant.

V. The Uterus as an Endocrine Organ
♦ Endometrial products.
- Endometrium produces a nourishing, supportive environment for the early embryo.
- Suppresses immune response (Table 4.1).
- Cytokines.
  - Interleukins stimulate PG production and other cytokines.
  - Colony-stimulating factor–1: influences cellular proliferation of macrophages.
  - Interferon: T-lymphocyte product inhibits endometrial and epithelial proliferation.

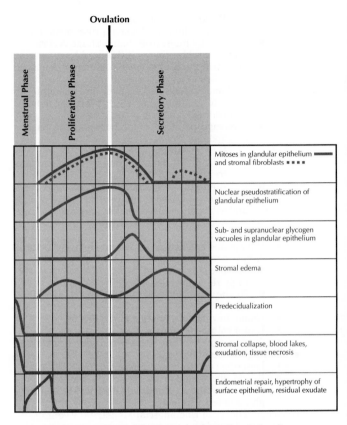

Figure 4.8.   Timetable for the menstrual cycle by phases.

- Leukocyte inhibitory factor: most abundant during secretory phase; possible role in implantation.
- TNF-α: increased in proliferative, midsecretory phases.
- Growth factors.
  - Epidermal growth factor (EGF): present in endometrial stromal and epithelial cells during follicular phase and in stromal cells in luteal phase.
  - TGF-α: uses same receptor as EGF; peaks at midcycle.
  - IGFs: promote cellular mitosis and differentiation.
    - ◊ IGF-I: predominant in proliferative and early secretory phases.

Table 4.1.   Endometrium-produced substances

Lipids	Cytokines	Peptides
Prostaglandins	Interleukin-1α	Prolactin
Thromboxanes	Interleukin-1β	Relaxin
Leukotrienes	Interleukin-6	Prorenin and renin
	Interferon-γ	Endorphin
	Colony-stimulating factor-1	Endothelin-1
	Tumor necrosis factor-α	Corticotropin-releasing hormone
	Leukemia-inhibiting factor	Fibronectin
		Uteroglobin
		Lipocortin-1
		Parathyroid hormone–like protein
		Integrins
		EGF family
		EGF
		Heparin-binding EGF
		TGF-α
		IGF family
		IGF-I
		IGF-II
		IGFBPs 1–6
		Platelet-derived growth factor
		TGF-β
		Fibroblast growth factor
		Vascular endothelial growth factor

Abbreviations: EGF, epidermal growth factor; IGF, insulin-like growth factor; IGFBP, insulin-like growth factor–binding protein; TGF, transforming growth factor.

- ◇ IGF-II: mid-to-late secretory phase.
- ◇ Dependent on insulin-like growth factor–binding proteins (IGFBPs).
  - ■ TGF-β: greatest in secretory phase, may increase IGFBP-3 synthesis.
- PGs.
  - ■ Reach peak levels in late secretory phase.
  - ■ $PGF_{2\alpha}$ is predominant PG.
  - ■ Decreased production following implantation.
  - ■ Endometrial stromal cells produce PGs and thromboxane in estradiol-responsive fashion.
  - ■ Alterations in PG production can affect menstrual bleeding; this explains the efficacy of non-steroidal antiinflammatory drugs (NSAIDs).
- Other proteins.
  - ■ Fibronectin.

- Laminin.
- Integrins.
- Uteroglobin.
- Endothelins: endothelin-1 is involved in vaso-constriction to stem menstrual bleeding.
    - ◇ Can also produce contractions.
    - ◇ Can promote healing and reepithelialization of endometrium.
- Vascular endothelial growth factor and other angiogenic factors.
  - Steroid receptors.
    - Estradiol-receptor changes reflect estradiol and progesterone concentration.
        - ◇ Reaches maximum in late follicular phase; greatest in glandular epithelium.
        - ◇ Decreases in early luteal phase.
        - ◇ Increases again in mid to late luteal phase.
    - Progesterone receptor reaches maximum in late follicular or early luteal phase.
        - ◇ Nearly undetectable at midpoint of secretory phase.
        - ◇ High concentration in decidualizing stromal cells.
        - ◇ In general, progesterone antagonizes estrogen stimulation.
            - ○ Decrease in estradiol receptor.
            - ○ Suppression of estradiol-mediated transcription of oncogenes.
            - ○ Modulation of estradiol secretion via enzyme effects.
  - Androgen receptor.
    - Constant throughout the cycle.
    - Present in all stages of the menstrual cycle.
- The decidua.
  - Specialized endometrium of pregnancy; consists of vigorous active tissue.
  - Possible role for alpha substrate in decidualization and prolactin secretion.
  - Derived from stromal cells of endometrium.
    - Appears in luteal phase.
    - Secretes a host of substances, including the following:
        - ◇ Prolactin (same as pituitary prolactin but not responsive to drug therapy); decidual prolactin-releasing factor identified.
        - ◇ Relaxin.
        - ◇ Renin.
        - ◇ IGFs.
        - ◇ IGFBPs.
  - Lipocortin 1.
    - Calcium-binding and phospholipid-binding protein; inhibits prolactin release.
        - ◇ Independent of glucocorticoids and phospholipase action.
        - ◇ Appears in luteal phase.

- ■ Amniotic fluid prolactin is most likely derived from the decidua.
  - ◇ Unaffected by bromocriptine.
  - ◇ Regulates amniotic fluid volume and electrolytes.
  - ◇ Involved in surfactant synthesis.
  - ◇ Inhibits uterine contractility.
  - ◇ Suppresses immune response.
- • Other proteins.
  - ■ Fibroblast growth factor (FGF).
  - ■ Corticotropin-releasing hormone.
  - ■ Prorenin.
  - ■ Relaxin.
  - ■ IGFs, IGFBPs: IGFBP-1.
    - ◇ Appears in midluteal phase.
    - ◇ Major production through first trimester.
    - ◇ Previously known as placental protein 12 or pregnancy-associated α-globulin.
    - ◇ High levels continue until a drop in the third trimester.
    - ◇ May limit trophoblast invasion and endometrial growth; possible mechanism of action of progesterone-producing IUDs.
  - ■ TGF-β.
    - ◇ Can be a messenger from the fetus to the decidua.
    - ◇ May also limit trophoblast invasion.
- ♦ Summary: the uterus is an endocrine organ.

  One cannot dispute the fact that the uterus is an endocrine organ, but the vast array of active substances can be bewildering and overwhelming. Keeping in mind a fundamental and relatively simple description can help: the endometrium is necessary for reproduction, and the synchronous, complex cycle of events is dependent on the endocrine guidance of estradiol and progesterone, which are modulated and mediated by a plethora of locally produced biochemical agents. Each and every signaling substance utilizes one of the pathways discussed in Chapter 2 and makes a contribution to the dynamic sequence of morphologic and biochemical events repeatedly dedicated to nourishing and supporting an early embryo.

VI. Anatomic Abnormalities of the Uterus
- ♦ Introduction.
  - • Relatively common findings.
  - • Can contribute to infertility, recurrent pregnancy loss, and poor pregnancy outcome (25% of women with abnormalities).
  - • Cervical cerclage often indicated.
  - • Can also result in dysmenorrhea and dyspareunia.
  - • Can be present even with normal ovaries and ovarian function (Tables 4.2 and 4.3).
  - • Can originate in fusion failure, connection failure, or luminal formation failure.
  - • Vaginal outflow obstruction can be minimal or complete.

Table 4.2. Incidence of müllerian defects

Overall	5%
Fertile women	2% to 3%
Infertile women	3%
Women with recurrent miscarriages	5% to 10%
Women with late miscarriages and preterm deliveries	>25%

- ◆ Unicornuate uterus.
  - Failure of development of one müllerian duct.
  - Increased obstetrical complications.
  - Rudimentary horn may be present; prophylactic removal recommended.
  - Forty percent of cases associated with urinary tract anomalies.
- ◆ Uterus didelphys.
  - Obstruction is variable.
  - Increased risk for malpresentation and/or preterm labor.
- ◆ Bicornuate.
  - Partial lack of duct fusion.
  - Relatively common finding.
  - Pregnancy outcome may be normal.
- ◆ Septate uterus.
  - Partial lack of resorption.
  - Not associated with infertility but potentially a cause of miscarriage.
    - Ninety percent rate of pregnancy loss before hysteroscopy treatment.
    - Ten percent rate of pregnancy loss after hysteroscopic treatment.
  - Arcuate uterus likely has no adverse impact on pregnancy.
- ◆ Rare anomaly: cervical agenesis—best treated by hysterectomy.
- ◆ Diethylstilbestrol.
  - Exposure to high levels of estrogen in uterus leads to multiple anomalies, both uterine and cervical.
  - Poor pregnancy outcomes.
  - Cerclage is the only treatment option.
- ◆ Diagnosis—ultrasound and magnetic resonance imaging (MRI) are very helpful.

Table 4.3. Distribution of specific uterine anomalies

Bicornuate uterus	37%
Arcuate uterus	15%
Incomplete septum	13%
Uterus didelphys	11%
Complete septum	9%
Unicornuate uterus	4.4%

VII. Leiomyomata
- ◆ Benign neoplasms arising from uterine smooth muscle.
- ◆ Monoclonal; multiple myomas are not clonally related.
- ◆ Sarcomas arise either independently or from existing myomata; incidence is very low.
- ◆ Seventy-seven percent of hysterectomy specimens have myomata.
  - • Seventeen percent of hysterectomies are performed for leiomyomata.
  - • Approximately 10% to 11% of all women require hysterectomies for leiomyomata.
- ◆ Rate is 2 to 3 times higher in black women.
- ◆ They are encountered in 1% of pregnant women.
  - • Pregnancy reduces the risk of myomata.
  - • Smoking decreases the risk of myomata.
  - • Obesity increases the risk of myomata.
  - • Oral contraceptives are associated with no increased risk.
- ◆ Local hyperestrogenic environment.
  - • Estradiol and progesterone receptors increased.
  - • Increased levels of aromatase.
  - • Endometrial hyperplasia may be seen at the margins.
- ◆ Progesterone may stimulate growth.
  - • RU486 treatment may be helpful.
  - • Bcl-2 protein expression prevents apoptosis.
- ◆ Other growth factors.
  - • EGF, IGF-I, IGF-II, decreased IGFBP-3.
  - • Prolactin.
  - • Angiogenic factors.
- ◆ Reproductive function and leiomyomata.
  - • Infrequent cause of infertility; mechanical obstruction and distortion effect on implantation.
  - • Hysteroscopic resection very helpful if greater than 50% protrusion into the cavity.
  - • MRI may help to map out fibroids.
  - • Recurrence rate is 15%; hysterectomy is needed for 1% to 5% of cases.
  - • Long-term recurrence rate is 27%.
  - • Medical therapy is not recommended for infertile patients; most myomata do not grow in pregnancy.
- ◆ Medical therapy of leiomyomata.
  - • Goal of medical therapy: temporarily reduce symptoms with gonadotropin-releasing hormone (GnRH) agonist.
  - • Native GnRH.
    - ■ Short half-life due to rapid cleavage of bonds between amino acids 5-6, 6-7, and 9-10.
    - ■ Substitution at position 6 or replacement of C-terminal glycine amide produces agonist.
      - ◇ Long-acting.
      - ◇ Initial response is a flare effect.
      - ◇ After 1 to 3 weeks, desensitization and/or down-regulation; also postreceptor mechanisms lead to secretion of biologically inactive gonadotropins (still immunoactive).

- Treatment.
  - Mean uterine volume decreases 30% to 64% after 3 to 6 months.
  - Decrease in operative blood loss in cases of fibroid uterus after it reaches size of a 16-week pregnancy.
  - Return to preterm uterine size in 3 to 4 months.
  - May also be useful in treatment of leiomyomatosis peritonealis disseminata and adenomyosis.
- Side effects.
  - Hot flashes in 75% of patients.
  - Vaginal dryness, headaches, joint stiffness, and depression in 15%.
  - Local allergic reaction in 10%.
  - Delayed vaginal hemorrhage in 2%.
  - Fetal exposure has not resulted in adverse effects.
- GnRH agonists and steroid add-back.
  - May permit long-term use without bone loss.
  - Progestin is the only add-back that reduces hot flashes, but it has a decreased effect on reduction in uterine size.
  - Traditional hormone-replacement therapy add-back is very effective.
  - GnRH antagonist therapy may be even better as a future treatment option.

Neuroendocrinology

I. The hypothalamic–Hypophyseal Portal Circulation
   ♦ The hypothalamus is at the base of the brain above the junction of optic nerves; a direct neural connection to pituitary does not exist.
      • Blood supply connects hypothalamus to pituitary; superior hypophyseal arteries form capillary network in median eminence.
         ▪ Drain into portal vessels.
         ▪ Portal vessels descend along pituitary stalk to anterior pituitary.
      • Retrograde flow delivers pituitary hormones back to the hypothalamus.
II. The Neurohormone Concept
   ♦ Pituitary function is dependent on hypothalamic signals transported via the portal system.
      • A section of the pituitary stalk affects gonadal, adrenal, and thyroid activity.
      • Pituitary transplantation results in gonadal failure; function resumes if pituitary is retransplanted under median eminence.
      • Stalk section and transplantation induces increased prolactin; implies negative hypothalamic control of prolactin secretion.
   ♦ Neuroendocrine agents
      • Exist in the hypothalamus.
      • Stimulatory effects on growth hormone (GH), thyrotropin (TSH), adrenocorticotropin (ACTH), follicle-stimulating hormone (FSH), and luteinizing hormone (LH).
   ♦ Corticotropin-releasing hormone (CRH).
      • Forty-one–amino acid polypeptide.
      • Principal regulator of ACTH secretion.
      • Also activates sympathetic nervous system.
      • Can suppress gonadotropins via endorphin inhibition of gonadotropin-releasing hormone (GnRH).
   ♦ GnRH.
      • Ten–amino acid peptide; some variation among various mammals.
      • Stimulates both FSH and LH; divergent response patterns depend on feedback effect of steroids and other autocrine and/or paracrine agents.
      • Ninety-two–amino acid precursor protein.
         ▪ Gene found on short arm of chromosome 8.
         ▪ Twenty-three–amino acid signal sequence.
         ▪ Ten–amino acid true peptide (GnRH).
         ▪ Three–amino acid proteolytic-processing site.
         ▪ Fifty-six–amino acid GnRH-associated peptide.
            ◊ Inhibits prolactin, stimulates FSH and LH.
            ◊ Physiologic role not well-established.

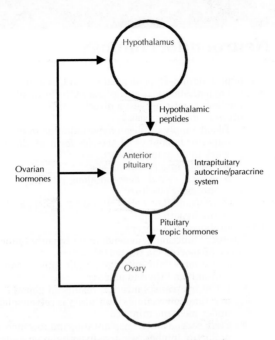

Figure 5.1.   The hypothalamic–pituitary–ovarian axis.

- Present in neural and nonneural tissue.
- Identical in all mammals; has existed for 500 million years.
- GnRH-II exists in other species, as well as in humans.
    - Gene is located on chromosome 20p13.
    - Gene produces similar precursor protein.
    - Expression is highest outside the brain and in the midbrain nucleus.
- GnRH-III is present in fish.

♦ Pituitary as the master gland.
  - Function is essential for sustaining life.
  - Development and control are under hypothalamic regulation.
  - Responses are modulated by hormonal messages from target tissues (Fig. 5.1).

♦ Prolactin secretion.
  - Gene expression in the lactotrophs of the anterior pituitary and in decidualized endometrium and myometrium; prolactin from different tissues is identical, but differences in messenger RNA (mRNA) exist.
  - Gene transcription is regulated by transcription factor (Pit-1).

- Binds to the 5′ promoter region.
- Also necessary for GH and TSH.
- Prolactin secretion is also regulated by estrogen and glucocorticoid receptors with 5′ flanking sequences.
- Pit-1 is also involved in differentiation and growth of anterior pituitary cells; mutations can lead to absent GH, prolactin, and TSH and to the absence of their trophic cells in the pituitary.
- Pit-1 is not involved in pituitary tumor formation.
- Main function of prolactin is lactogenesis (osmoregulation in fish).
- Further regulation of prolactin gene expression is accomplished via the following:
  - Estrogen.
  - Other peptide hormones.
  - Agents controlling cyclic adenosine monophosphate and calcium channels.
- Inhibitory control of prolactin results from hypothalamic dopamine release.
  - Mediated by receptors coupled to inhibition of adenylate cyclase.
  - Five forms of dopamine receptor.
    - ◊ The 2 functional groups are D_1 and D_2; D_2 is predominant in the pituitary.
    - ◊ G protein receptor.
    - ◊ Dopamine binding suppresses adenylate cyclase and intracellular levels of calcium.
    - ◊ Pit-1 binding sites are involved.
    - ◊ D_2 receptor binding also inhibits lactotroph growth and development.
- Prolactin-releasing factors.
  - Thyrotropin-releasing hormone (TRH).
  - Vasoactive intestinal polypeptide.
  - Epidermal growth factor (EGF).
  - Possibly GnRH.
- ♦ Hypothalamus and GnRH secretion.
  - Hypothalamus represents part of the diencephalon at the base of the brain; it forms the floor of the third ventricle.
  - Contains peptidergic neural cells that secrete hormones.
    - These neural cells have characteristics of both neurons and endocrine gland cells.
    - They respond to bloodstream signals and neurotransmitters within the brain; neurosecretion—neurohormone or neurotransmitter are synthesized in cytoplasm and transported by active axonal flow.
  - GnRH-producing cells originate in the olfactory area.
    - Migrate along cranial nerves from the nose towards the forebrain; eventually, 1,000 to 3,000 GnRH-producing cells are found in the arcuate nucleus.

- Failure of olfactory axonal and GnRH neuronal migration from the olfactory placode leads to Kallmann syndrome.
  ◇ Anosmia and absence of GnRH.
  ◇ Failure of secondary sexual development; three modes of transmission of Kallmann syndrome.
    ○ X-linked; the most common, based on a 5 to 7 times ↑ frequency in boys.
    ○ Autosomal dominant.
    ○ Autosomal recessive.
  ◇ Absence of fibronectin-like protein is necessary for neuronal migration.
- Olfactory and GnRH neurons have cilia.
  ◇ Evolutionary link via pheromones—airborne chemicals released by one individual that can affect another of the same species.
  ◇ Clinical evidence supports pheromone effects in humans.
- GnRH neuroanatomy.
  - Primary network of cell bodies is found within medial basal hypothalamus; most are within the arcuate nucleus.
  - Neurons exist in a complex network; allows for multiple interactions with neurotransmitters, hormones, and growth factors.
  - GnRH is delivered to portal circulation via the tuberoinfundibular tract.
  - GnRH fibers are also identified in the posterior hypothalamus descending into the posterior pituitary and in the anterior hypothalamic area projecting to sites within limbic regions.
    ◇ Only the arcuate nucleus is critical for GnRH secretion into portal system.
    ◇ Other sites may be involved in behavioral responses.
- GnRH secretion.
  - The half-life of GnRH is only 2 to 4 minutes; biologically effective amounts do not escape the portal system.
  - Biologic action is dependent upon interplay between neurohormones, pituitary gonadotropins, and gonadal steroids; both positive and negative feedback effects exist.
  - Long feedback loop—action of target gland hormones on the hypothalamus and pituitary.
  - Short feedback loop—negative feedback of pituitary hormones on their own secretion via effects on the hypothalamus.
  - Ultrashort feedback—inhibition by the releasing hormone on its own synthesis.
  - These signals, as well as those from higher centers, modify GnRH secretion.
    ◇ GnRH neurons lack estradiol receptors.
    ◇ Steroid hormone regulation is mediated via neurotransmitters.

- Pulsatile release.
  - Classic experiments by Knobil revealed critical range of GnRH pulse frequency and amplitude; in monkeys; 1 mg GnRH × 6 minutes with 1 pulse/hour yields peak gonadotropin secretion.
    - ◊ Increased frequency or ↑ dose extinguishes secretion.
    - ◊ Decreased frequency leads to ↓ LH but ↑ FSH.
  - Gonadotropins are secreted in pulsatile fashion and, thus, gonadal steroid release is also.
  - Pubertal changes in GnRH pulsatility eventually mature into the adult pattern.
- Timing of GnRH pulses.
  - Measured by determining LH pulses; the long half-life of FSH limits its utility.
  - Characteristic pulse frequency and amplitude of LH are as follows:

Phase	LH pulse mean amplitude:
Early follicular phase	6.5 IU/L
Midfollicular phase	5.0 IU/L
Late follicular phase	7.2 IU/L
Early luteal phase	15.0 IU/L
Midluteal phase	12.2 IU/L
Late luteal phase	8.0 IU/L

Phase	LH pulse mean frequency:
Early follicular phase	90 min
Late follicular phase	60 to 70 min
Early luteal phase	100 min
Late luteal phase	200 min

- Control of GnRH pulses.
  - Critical range of frequency and amplitude is needed for normal function.
  - Dopamine tract.
    - ◊ Cell bodies for dopamine synthesis are found in arcuate and periventricular nucleus; they arise within the medial basal hypothalamus and project to the median eminence.
    - ◊ Administration of dopamine suppresses circulation of prolactin and gonadotropins; the effect is mediated via GnRH release in the hypothalamus.
    - ◊ Dopamine may directly suppress both arcuate GnRH activity and pituitary prolactin via the portal system transport.
- The norepinephrine tract.
  - Cell bodies are located in mesencephalon and lower brain stem; these cell bodies also synthesize serotonin.

- Axons ascend into medial forebrain bundle and terminate in various brain structures.
- Neuropeptide Y.
  - Secretion and gene expression in hypothalamic neurons are regulated by gonadal steroids.
  - Stimulates pulsatile release of GnRH.
  - Potentiates pituitary response to GnRH.
  - Inhibits gonadotropin secretion in the absence of estrogen; the proposed mediator of a link between nutrition and reproductive function.
- Current concept.
  - Biogenic catecholamines modulate GnRH pulsatile release.
  - Norepinephrine has stimulatory effects on GnRH discharge ($\uparrow$ frequency, possibly $\uparrow$ amplitude).
  - Dopamine and serotonin have inhibitory effects (Fig. 5.2).
- Pituitary gonadotropin secretion.
  - Gene for α subunit is expressed in both the pituitary gland and the placenta.
    - β-Human chorionic gonadotropin (hCG) gene is expressed in the placenta but only minimally in the pituitary.
    - LH β subunit is expressed in the pituitary gland but not the placenta.
  - Sex steroids interact at level of gonadotropin gene transcription, as well as at membrane level, to affect GnRH/receptor interactions.
  - Both LH and FSH are secreted by gonadotroph.
    - Localized in the lateral pituitary.
    - Responsive to GnRH pulsatility.
    - GnRH action is calcium-dependent; 1,4,5-triphosphate (IP$_3$) and 1,2-diacylglycerol (1,2-DG) serve as second messengers.
    - Functions via the G protein receptor.
    - Gene for GnRH receptor is found on chromosome 4q13. to 14q21.1.
    - Regulation of GnRH receptor.
      - ◇ GnRH.
      - ◇ Inhibin and/or activin.
      - ◇ Sex steroids.
    - Gonadotropin synthesis.
      - ◇ Occurs on the rough endoplasmic reticulum.
      - ◇ Packaged into secretory granules by Golgi.
      - ◇ Secretion requires migration.
      - ◇ Rate-limiting step is the availability of β subunits.
    - Response to GnRH.
      - ◇ Immediate secretory release of granules.
      - ◇ Delayed response.
        - ○ Self-priming action of GnRH; greater release in response to subsequent pulses.
          - □ Important for midcycle surge.
          - □ Requires estrogen.

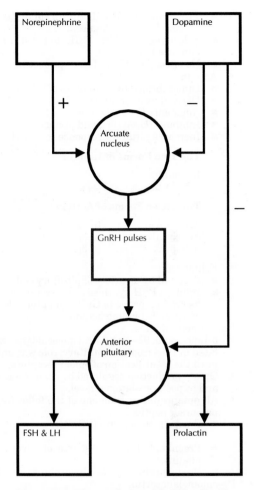

Figure 5.2.   The regulation of GnRH pulsatility.

- ○ Augmented by progesterone and requires the following:
  - ▲ Estrogen exposure for ↑ in progesterone receptors.
  - ▲ Progesterone receptor activation by GnRH.
- ◆ Intrapituitary, autocrine, and paracrine system.
  - • Activin, inhibin, and follistatin: activin and inhibin are members of the transforming growth factor-β family.
  - • Inhibin.
    - ■ Dimer of α and β subunits that are linked by disulfide bonds.

- Two forms purified (distinct β subunits).
- Secreted by granulosa cells.
- Selectively inhibits FSH, but not LH; may enhance LH activity.
- No effect on GH, ACTH, or prolactin.
- Activin.
  - Dimer formed by β subunits of inhibin.
  - Derived from granulosa cells.
  - Augments FSH secretion.
  - Inhibits GH, ACTH, and prolactin.
  - Increases pituitary response to GnRH.

The Two Forms of Inhibin

Inhibin-A: α-β_A
Inhibin-B: α-β_B

The Three Forms of Activin

Activin-A: β_A-β_A
Activin-AB: β_A-β_B
Activin-B: β_B-β_B

- Follistatin.
  - Secreted by a variety of pituitary cells.
  - Inhibits FSH synthesis and secretion, as well as FSH response to GnRH; its probable means of action is binding activin.
- Endogenous opiates.
  - β-Lipotropin: 91–amino acid molecule that was isolated in 1964 from the pituitary; role was unknown until the identification of opioid receptors.
  - Opiate production regulated by gene transcription and at posttranslational level.
  - All opiates derive from one of the following three precursor peptides:
    - Proopiomelanocortin (POMC)—source of endorphins.
    - Proenkephalin A/B—source of several enkephalins.
    - Prodynorphin—yields dynorphins (Fig. 5.3).
- Proopiomelanocortin.
  - First precursor peptide identified.
  - Produced in anterior/intermediate lobe of pituitary, hypothalamus, sympathetic nervous system, gonads, placenta, gastrointestinal (GI) tract, and lungs.
  - Split into two fragments (see Fig. 5.3); no role for β–melanocyte-stimulating hormone (MSH) in humans.
  - In adults, major products in pituitary are ACTH and β-lipoprotein, as well as small amounts of endorphin; regulated via CRH and glucocorticoids.
  - During fetal life, in the intermediate lobe, ACTH → corticotropin-like intermediate lobe peptide and β-MSH.

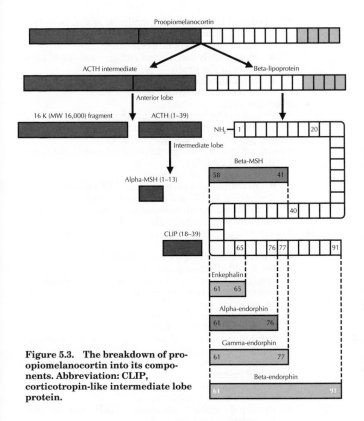

Figure 5.3.   The breakdown of pro-opiomelanocortin into its components. Abbreviation: CLIP, corticotropin-like intermediate lobe protein.

- In the placenta, POMC → α-MSH and β-endorphins.
- In the brain, major products are the opiates; in the hypothalamus, they are mainly β-endorphins and α-MSH, which are regulated via sex steroids.
- High concentrations of the POMC family are found in follicular fluid; only β-endorphin shows significant changes during the menstrual cycle.
- β-Endorphin.
  - A neurotransmitter, neurohormone, and neuromodulator.
  - Influences a variety of hypothalamic functions, such as the following:
    - Reproduction.
    - Temperature.
    - Cardiovascular and respiratory.
  - Influences extrahypothalamic functions: pain and mood.
- Proenkephalin A.

- Produced in the adrenal medulla, brain, posterior pituitary, spinal cord, and GI tract.
- Yields several enkephalins.
  - Most widely distributed endogenous opioid peptides in the brain.
  - Inhibitory neurotransmitters that modulate the autonomic nervous system.
- Prodynorphin.
  - Found in the hypothalamus and GI tract.
  - Has similar functions to endorphins.
- Opioid peptides and the menstrual cycle.
  - Opioid tone is an important part of menstrual functions and cyclicity.
    - Estradiol ↑ endorphins.
    - Estradiol and progesterone ↑↑↑ endorphins.
  - Reduction in LH pulse frequency is linked to increased endorphin release; naloxone increases the frequency and amplitude of LH pulses.
- Endogenous opioids suppress hypothalamic GnRH release.
  - No effect on pituitary response to GnRH.
  - No opioid effect on postmenopausal and/or ovariectomized levels of gonadotropins; the response is restored with sex steroid administration.
  - In pubertal boys/girls, naloxone could not prevent the suppression of LH by estradiol; possibly, a direct estradiol effect on GnRH.
  - Inhibitory tone is reduced at the time of the ovulatory surge; probably a response due to the estrogen-induced decrease in opioid receptor binding and/or opioid release.
  - Suppression of gonadotropins in pregnancy also reflects opioid inhibition.
  - Principal opioids affecting GnRH release are β-endorphin and dynorphin.
    - Probably function via modulation of catecholamine pathways.
    - α-MSH counteracts β-endorphin; a potential site for neuroendocrine regulation.
- Clinical implications.
  - Changes in opioid tone may affect various aspects of reproduction as follows:

Not Important	**Important**
Puberty	Hypogonadotropic state
Delayed puberty	Elevated prolactin
Kallmann syndrome	Exercise
Other hypothalamic causes of amenorrhea	

  - Naltrexone can restore normal function in hypothalamic amenorrhea patients.
- Corticotropin-releasing hormone (CRH) directly inhibits GnRH secretion.
  - Via direct effect and by augmenting opioid secretion.

- Women with hypothalamic amenorrhea demonstrate hypercortisolism; link between stress and reproductive function exists.
- Evidence for coupling between neuroregulatory system of adrenal and gonad.
- CRH gene contains two segments similar to estrogen-response elements; allows estrogen enhancement of CRH activity.

♦ Prolactin release.
  - Morphine, enkephalin analogs, and β-endorphin all cause prolactin release.
  - Effect is mediated by inhibition of dopamine secretion in tuberoinfundibular tract neurons in median eminence.
  - No effect of naloxone on prolactin; physiologic role for endogenous opioid regulation of prolactin is elusive.
  - GnRH suppression associated with ↑ prolactin may be mediated by endogenous opiates.

♦ Catecholestrogens.
  - Enzyme that converts estrogens to catecholestrogens (2-hydroxylase) is richly concentrated in the hypothalamus.
  - Higher concentrations of catecholestrogens than of estrone or estradiol.
  - May serve as possible interaction between catecholamines and GnRH secretion (Fig. 5.4).

♦ GnRH agonists and antagonists.
  - GnRH has a short half-life (minutes).
    - Rapid cleavage of bonds between amino acids 5-6, 6-7, and 9-10 occurs.
    - Analogues have altered amino acids at these positions—substitution at position 6 or replacement of C-terminal glycine amide.
  - Agonists can be delivered either intramuscularly, subcutaneously, or intranasally.
    - Initial agonist effect ("flare"), which is greatest in the early follicular phase.
    - After 1 to 3 weeks, desensitization and down-regulation produce hypogonadotropic hypogonad state.
      ◇ Initial response is desensitization.
      ◇ Later response is due to receptor loss and uncoupling.
  - Clinical entities treated with GnRH include the following:
    - Endometriosis.
    - Uterine leiomyomata.
    - Precocious puberty.
    - Prevention of menstrual bleeding.
    - Cancer therapy: breast, pancreatic, prostate, testicular, and ovarian.
  - GnRH antagonists.
    - Synthesized by multiple amino acid substitutions.

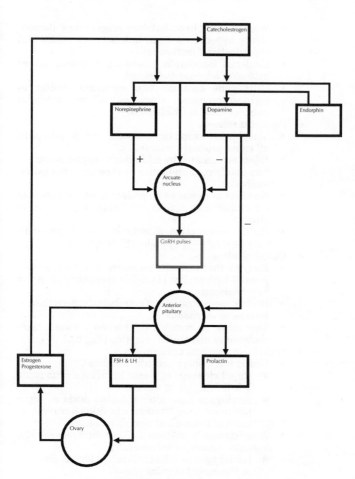

Figure 5.4. Catecholestrogens and reproductive function.

- Bind the GnRH receptor.
  - ◇ Provide competitive inhibition.
  - ◇ Produce immediate decline in gonadotropins.
- Early products lacked potency or had significant histamine release–related side effects (Fig. 5.5 and Table 5.1).
- Tanycytes.
  - Specialized ependymal cells whose ciliated cell bodies line the third ventricle over the median eminence.
  - Cells terminate on portal vessels; can transport materials from cerebrospinal fluid (CSF) to the portal system—pineal gland.

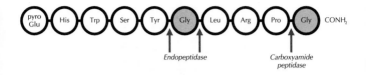

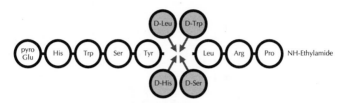

**Figure 5.5.   Top: Gonadotropin-releasing hormone (GnRH).
Bottom: GnRH agonists.**

- Posterior pituitary pathways.
  - Posterior pituitary is a direct prolongation of the hypothalamus.
  - Neurosecretory cells in superoptic and paraventricular nuclei make vasopressin and oxytocin (both are nine–amino acid proteins, which include two half cystines forming a bridge from positions 1 to 6); human vasopressin contains arginine (animal vasopressin contains lysine).
  - Oxytocin and vasopressin are carried by large transport proteins called neurophysins.
    ◇ Neurophysin I (stimulated by estrogen).
    ◇ Neurophysin II (stimulated by nicotine).
  - Genes for oxytocin and vasopressin.
    ◇ Found on chromosome 20.
    ◇ Common ancestor gene is approximately 400×10^6 years old.
  - Transcription is regulated by sex steroids and thyroid hormone; hormone response elements are found upstream.
  - Two large protein molecule precursors.
    ◇ Propressophysin = neurophysin II + vasopressin.
    ◇ Prooxyphysin = neurophysin I + oxytocin (Fig. 5.6).
  - Posterior pituitary pathway is complex; secretion into CSF also occurs.
    ◇ Influence extends into the anterior pituitary.
      ○ Vasopressin cooperates with CRH.
      ○ Oxytocin increases gonadotropin release.
    ◇ Secretion exhibits a circadian rhythm.
  - Peak levels of oxytocin are present at the time of LH surge.
    ◇ Oxytocin may inhibit GnRH metabolism.

Table 5.1. GnRH agonists in clinical use

Position	1	2	3	4	5	6	7	8	9	10
Native GnRH	pGlu	His	Trp	Ser	Tyr	Gly	Leu	Arg	Pro	Gly-NH$_2$
Leuprolide						D-Leu				NH-Ethylamide
Buserelin						D-Ser (tertiary butanol)				NH-Ethylamide
Nafarelin						D-Naphthylalanine (2)				
Histrelin						D-His (tertiary benzyl)				NH-Ethylamide
Goserelin						D-Ser (tertiary butanol)				Aza-Gly
Deslorelin						D-Trp				NH-Ethylamide
Tryptorelin						D-Trp				

Abbreviation: GnRH, gonadotropin-releasing hormone.

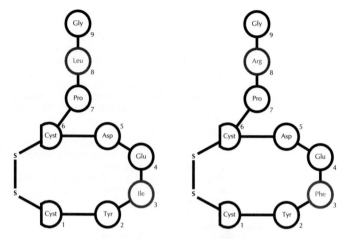

Figure 5.6.   Structures of oxytocin (left) and arginine-vasopressin (right).

- ◇ Vasopressin may be involved in learning and memory.
- ◇ Both circulate as free peptides; they have a rapid half-life (1 minute for the first component; 2 to 3 minutes for the second component).
- Vasopressin.
  - Sources of stimulation for release.
    - ◇ Changes in blood osmolality are detected by hypothalamic osmoreceptors.
    - ◇ Changes in blood volume are detected by volume receptors in the left atrium, aortic arch, and carotid sinus.
    - ◇ Psychogenic stimuli include pain and/or fear.
  - Major function is the regulation of osmolality and blood volume; a powerful vasoconstrictor and antidiuretic hormone.
    - ◇ Defective action results in diabetes insipidus.
    - ◇ Excessive action results in the syndrome of inappropriate secretion of antidiuretic hormone (SIADH).
- Oxytocin.
  - Stimulates muscular contractions in the uterus and myoepithelial contractions in the breast.
  - Episodic release.
    - ◇ Three spurts every 10 minutes.
    - ◇ Released during coitus (Ferguson reflex), as well as from olfactory, visual, and auditory stimuli.

- Increase in nocturnal release prior to parturition.
  - ◊ Oxytocin levels rise significantly during labor, especially during the second stage.
  - ◊ They may also be released by the fetal pituitary (controversial concept).
  - ◊ Stimulates prostaglandin release in the decidua and myometrium; local oxytocin production is found in the amnion, chorion, and decidua.
  - ◊ Oxytocin receptor.
    - ○ Low concentration in nonpregnant state.
    - ○ Increases 80-fold throughout gestation.
    - ○ Doubles during labor.
  - ◊ Suckling response is mediated by the third, fourth, and fifth thoracic nerves.
  - ◊ Opioids inhibit release.
- ♦ The brain and ovulation.
  - • Classic rodent studies.
    - ■ Tonic center and cyclic center.
    - ■ LH feedback from estrogen is dependent on concentration.
      - ◊ Low concentration of estrogen = negative feedback.
      - ◊ High concentration of estrogen = positive feedback.
    - ■ Mechanism not inaccurate BUT is different in primates.
  - • Primates—midcycle surge center located in the pituitary, not the hypothalamus.
    - ■ Feedback responses are dependent on ovarian steroid feedback to the anterior pituitary; proven in the classic experiment by Knobil, in which medial basal hypothalamic lesions were produced.
    - ■ Administration of GnRH produces a biphasic response.
    - ■ The three principal positive actions of GnRH are as follows:
      1. Synthesis and storage of gonadotropin.
      2. Activation (self-priming).
      3. Direct secretion.
  - • Functions change during cycle.
    - ■ Low estradiol (E_2) → low secretion and storage.
    - ■ Rising E_2 → increased storage; premature release is prevented by the inhibitory release of estradiol.
    - ■ Midcycle → increase in GnRH receptor results in increased priming.
    - ■ Surge → when estradiol levels exceed critical concentration and duration, then LH surge is initiated.
  - • GnRH.
    - ■ Gene contains hormone response elements, but no estrogen receptors have been detected on GnRH neurons; possibly an estrogen receptor β.

- GnRH surge probably helps to fine-tune the response.
  - ◇ Role must be essential for LH surge as GnRH antagonists block LH surge.
  - ◇ Pulse frequency and pituitary receptor concentration are affected.
  - ◇ Bioactivity of LH is also modulated by GnRH pulsatility.
- FSH surge.
  - Needed to induce granulosa LH receptors.
  - Also accomplishes intrafollicular changes.
- Progesterone.
  - At low levels and in the presence of estrogen, pituitary LH secretion is augmented; progesterone is also responsible for FSH surge.
  - Full luteinization after ovulation followed by a marked rise in progesterone.
    - ◇ Decreased GnRH centrally at hypothalamus.
    - ◇ Decreased estrogen-induced response of pituitary GnRH (Figs. 5.7A and 5.7B).
- Summary of the section's key points:
  1. Pulsatile GnRH secretion must be within a critical range for frequency and concentration (amplitude). This is absolutely necessary for normal reproductive function.
  2. GnRH has only positive actions on the anterior pituitary: synthesis and storage, activation, and secretion of gonadotropins. The gonadotropins are secreted in a pulsatile fashion in response to the similar pulsatile release of GnRH.
  3. Low levels of estrogen enhance FSH and LH synthesis and storage, have little effect on LH secretion, and inhibit FSH secretion.
  4. High levels of estrogen induce the LH surge at midcycle, and high steady levels of estrogen lead to sustained elevated LH secretion.
  5. Low levels of progesterone acting at the level of the pituitary gland enhance the LH response to GnRH and are responsible for the FSH surge at midcycle.
  6. High levels of progesterone inhibit pituitary secretion of gonadotropins by inhibiting GnRH pulses at the level of the hypothalamus. In addition, high levels of progesterone antagonize pituitary response to GnRH by interfering with estrogen action.
- ◆ The pineal gland.
  - No physiologic role has been firmly established in humans; may exert inhibitory control over the hypothalamus.
  - Pineal arises as an outgrowth of the roof of the third ventricle.

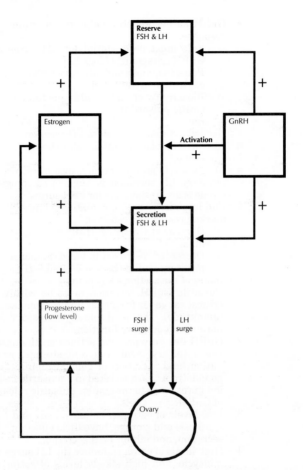

**Figure 5.7A. Effects of progesterone levels on LH, GnRH, and FSH.
A: Low levels of progesterone. B: High levels of progesterone.**

- ■ After birth, it loses all afferent and efferent neural connections.
- ■ New sympathetic neural connections arise—photic and hormonal stimuli.
- Hydroxyindole-O-methyltransferase (HIOMT) is found in pineal parenchymal cells—essential enzyme for melatonin.
- Melatonin synthesis is controlled by the following:
  - ■ Norepinephrine stimulation of adenylate cyclase.
  - ■ Norepinephrine that is initially liberated due to the absence of light.

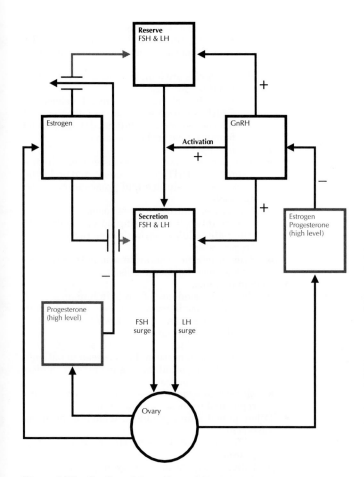

Figure 5.7B. Continued from the previous page.

- Excision of pineal gland → no melatonin.
- Relationship of pineal gland to reproduction.
  - Probable source of gonadal inhibitory substances.
  - Rat experiments with constant light versus dark; darkness → ↑ melatonin → ↓ GnRH.
- The pineal is involved in circadian rhythms; desynchronization may result in jet lag.
- The pineal rhythm requires a suprachiasmatic nucleus; possibly the site where pineal and light changes are coordinated.
- Melatonin.
  - It circulates like a classic hormone.

◇ Affects distal target organs.
◇ Mainly circulates in the blood (versus CSF).
- Gonadal changes are mediated via the hypothalamus.
- Highest levels are found in the first year of life.
  ◇ Gradual decrease.
  ◇ Possibly relates to eventual release of GnRH suppression prior to puberty; does not correspond with human data that blind females have earlier menarche.
- Pineal activity.
  - Receptors for estradiol, testosterone, dihydrotestosterone (DHT), progesterone, and prolactin.
  - Converts testosterone and progesterone to 5α metabolites.
  - Aromatizes androgens to estrogens.
  - Unique interaction causing norepinephrine to stimulate cellular synthesis of estrogen and androgen receptors.
  - Sympathetic nervous system activity takes precedence over hormonal effects.
- Role in humans.
  - No definite evidence of a role in humans.
  - Seasonal distribution with regard to human conception is seen; ↓ in dark winter months.
  - Can disrupt normal gonadal function.
    ◇ Increased levels → delayed puberty.
    ◇ Increased nocturnal levels seen in patients with hypothalamic amenorrhea and/or anorexia nervosa.
  - Menstrual synchrony—results are not always replicated in these clinical studies.
- Other pineal gland products, including arginine vasotocin.
  - Differs from oxytocin by single amino acid in position 8.
  - Differs from vasopressin by single amino acid in position 3.
  - Inhibitory action on gonads and on pituitary secretion of prolactin and LH.
♦ Gonadotropin secretion through fetal life, childhood, and puberty.
- Puberty is not an awakening but just another stage in development.
  - Development of anterior pituitary begins at 4 to 5 weeks of life.
    ◇ By the twelfth week, the vascular connection between the hypothalamus and pituitary is functional.
    ◇ High fetal levels of FSH/LH.
    ◇ GnRH is detectable by 10 weeks; FSH/LH are produced by 10 to 13 weeks.
    ◇ Peak pituitary levels at 20 to 23 weeks.
    ◇ Peak circulatory levels at 28 weeks.

- ■ Increasing sensitivity to steroids by midgestation; decrease in gonadotropins.
- ■ Gonadotropins rise after birth secondary to the loss of placental steroid inhibition.
- ■ Testicular function is correlated with hormone patterns.
  - ◇ Initially dependent on hCG.
  - ◇ Later switches to pituitary control.
  - ◇ Fetal Leydig cells avoid down-regulation; they are replaced by an adult generation, which becomes functional at puberty and responds with down-regulation and ↓ steroid production.
- • Sexual differences in fetal circulation.
  - ■ Higher pituitary and circulatory FSH and LH in female fetuses.
  - ■ Lower male levels, possibly secondary to testicular testosterone and inhibin.
  - ■ Postnatal rise is more marked in female infants, but LH level is not as high as in males; low inhibin levels.
  - ■ Nadir is reached at age 6 months in boys and at age 1 to 2 years in girls.
    - ◇ Low levels of LH and FSH in the pituitary and in the blood.
    - ◇ Little response of the pituitary to GnRH; maximal hypothalamic suppression.
- • Pubertal initiation.
  - ■ The precise signal is unknown.
  - ■ In girls, the following occurs:
    - ◇ First steroids to ↑ are dehydroepiandrosterone and dehydroepiandrosterone sulfate at 6 to 8 years of age; occurs just prior to FSH ↑.
    - ◇ Estrogen and LH do not rise until the age of 10 to 12 years.
    - ◇ Adrenarche is an independent stage of development.
    - ◇ Prepubertal gonadotropins are still associated with irregular pulses; puberty is preceded by ↑ in pulse frequency, amplitude, and regularity (especially at night).
    - ◇ At the appearance of secondary sexual characteristics, the mean LH level is 2 to 4 times higher during sleep.
    - ◇ FSH levels plateau in midpuberty.
      - ○ LH and estradiol levels continue to rise until late puberty.
      - ○ Biologically active LH also rises proportionally more than immunoreactive LH.
    - ◇ Rise of gonadotropins occurs independent of gonads; the same pattern is seen in gonadal dysgenesis patients (Fig. 5.8).

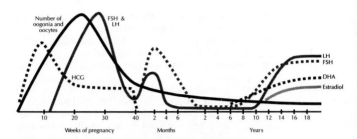

Figure 5.8.   Levels of gonadotropins at various stages of development.

- Maturational changes in the hypothalamus.
  - Orderly and predictable sequence of events.
  - Increased GnRH secretion leads to ↑ pituitary response to GnRH.
    - ◇ Increasing production and secretion of gonadotropins; increased gonadotropins are responsible for follicular growth.
    - ◇ Rising estrogen concentration contributes to adult pattern of GnRH secretion; cyclic menstrual patterns are established.
- Pituitary demographics.
  - Trend toward lowering of menarchal age and period of accelerated growth has now halted.
  - Mean age of menarche is 12.83 years (range, 9.14 to 17.7).
  - Age of onset is variable.
    - ◇ Genetic factors.
    - ◇ Socioeconomic conditions.
    - ◇ General health.
  - Has a relationship with body weight (<48 kg) and percentage of body fat (17%); concept is helpful, *but* extreme variability is present.
  - Pubertal sequence.
    - ◇ Begins at 8 to 14 years.
    - ◇ Usually occurs over 2 to 4 years.
    - ◇ Growth spurt → thelarche → pubarche → menarche.
    - ◇ Great variation of sequence order.
- Pubertal suppression.
  - Puberty is reactivation of hypothalamic–pituitary axis that previously was fully active in fetal life.
  - Decrease in sensitivity of hypothalamic centers due to negative-inhibitory action of gonadal steroids.
    - ◇ Slowly rising set point; GnRH pulsatility.
      - ○ FSH rises first; low frequency GnRH pulses.
      - ○ Ovarian stimulation; gonadal steroids.

- Cannot be solely reliant on negative effect of steroids.
  - ◇ Agonadal children also demonstrate some decline in gonadotropins.
  - ◇ CNS mechanism must exist.
    - ○ Must represent the dominant mechanism.
    - ○ Search for this mechanism continues.

Regulation of the Menstrual Cycle

I. The Follicular Phase
- ♦ The primordial follicle.
  - • Introduction.
    - ■ Primordial germ cells originate in endoderm of the yolk sac, allantois, and hindgut.
    - ■ They migrate to the genital ridge by 5 to 6 weeks.
    - ■ Mitotic multiplication causes them to reach quantities of 6 to 7×10^6 by 16 to 20 weeks.
    - ■ Growth and atresia are not interrupted by pregnancy, anovulation, or ovulation.
    - ■ Four hundred follicles will ovulate over a lifetime.
    - ■ The mechanism that selects follicles for growth is unknown; the number of follicles that start growing is dependent on the size of the residual pool.
  - • Rescue from atresia (apoptosis).
    - ■ The follicle destined for ovulation is recruited in the first few days of the cycle.
    - ■ Early growth of follicles occurs over timespan of several cycles.
      - ◊ The ovulatory follicle is a member of the cohort recruited at luteal–follicular transition.
      - ◊ The total duration to ovulatory status = 85 days.
    - ■ Once follicles reach the follicle-stimulating hormone (FSH)-dependent stage of growth, they must either be selected or undergo apoptosis.
  - • Follicular development.
    - ■ The first physical signs are an increase in oocyte size and a change in granulosa cell appearance (become cuboidal).
    - ■ Small gap junctions are formed between granulosa cells and oocytes; these allow the exchange of nutrients, ions, and regulatory molecules.
    - ■ The granulosa cell development is influenced by oocyte-derived factors, such as growth differentiation factor 9 in mice.
  - • Primary follicles.
    - ■ The primordial follicle is surrounded by approximately 15 granulosa cells.
    - ■ The granulosa cells are separated from stromal cells by the basement membrane (basal lamina).

- ■ The stromal cells differentiate into concentric layers as follows:
  - ◇ Theca interna versus theca externa.
  - ◇ Theca appears when granulosa cells reach three to six layers.
- ■ Gonadotropin-independent growth is rapidly followed by atresia of most follicles, except in those responsive to increased FSH levels of bioactivity in the mid- to late luteal phase.
- ■ Follicles become gonadotropin-responsive after approximately 60 days of development (Fig. 6.1).
  - ◇ Usually three to 11 follicles in the ovary initiate growth.
  - ◇ Decreased luteal phase steroids and inhibin A induce increases in FSH secretion.
- ■ Follicular growth in nonprimates versus primates.
  - ◇ A classic description of events places estradiol as the key local and feedback hormone.
  - ◇ This role has been replaced by local, autocrine, and/or paracrine peptide hormones in the primate.
- ♦ The preantral follicle.
  - • The granulosa undergoes proliferation.
    - ■ Dependent on gonadotropins.
    - ■ Correlated with increasing estrogen production.

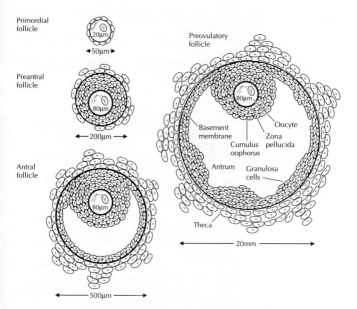

Figure 6.1. Stages of development of the follicle.

- Follicle can synthesize all three classes of steroids; significantly more estrogens than androgens are produced.
- FSH initiates steroidogenesis (aromatization) and stimulates cell growth.
- FSH receptors appear at this stage.
  - Estrogen concentration is limited by the FSH-receptor content; FSH induces its own receptor.
  - This phenomenon is mediated by growth factors.
  - FSH receptors quickly reach 1,500 receptors per granulosa cell.
- FSH operates via G proteins and the adenylate cyclase system; multiple signaling pathways regulate steroidogenesis, including the following:
  - Adenylate cyclase.
  - Ion gate channels.
  - Tyrosine kinase receptors.
  - Phospholipase system of second messengers.
- FSH and estrogens promote rapid accumulation of FSH receptors; this allows follicles to respond to a relatively low concentration of FSH.
- Intrafollicular communication means that not every cell has to contain gonadotropin receptors.
  - Signals can transfer by gap junctions.
  - Promotes coordinated cellular response.
- Role of androgens.
  - Very complex.
  - Androgen receptors are present in granulosa cells.
  - Androgens serve as substrate for estrogen production.
  - Androgen enhance aromatization at low concentrations.
  - At high concentrations, androgens are converted to 5α-reduced forms.
    - ◇ The 5α-reduced forms cannot be converted to estrogen.
    - ◇ Aromatase is inhibited.
    - ◇ FSH induction of luteinizing hormone (LH) receptors is inhibited (Fig. 6.2).
- Balancing act.
  - Androgen concentration can swing the follicle into the atretic pathway.
  - The follicle will progress only if FSH is elevated and LH is low.
- Summary of events.
  1. Initial follicular development occurs independently of hormone influence.
  2. FSH stimulation propels follicles to the pre-antral stage.
  3. FSH-induced aromatization of androgen in granulosa results in estradiol production.
  4. FSH and estradiol together increase FSH-receptor content of follicles.
- The antral follicle.
  - Introduction.

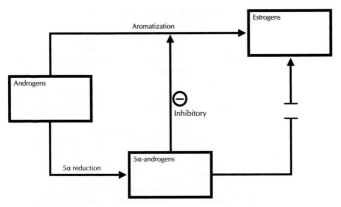

Figure 6.2. The role of androgens in early follicular development.

- Under the influence of FSH and estrogen, follicular fluid increases and a cavity forms; cumulus oophorus develops.
- In the presence of FSH, estrogen becomes dominant; in absence of FSH, androgen is predominant.
- A premature increase in LH results in decreased granulosa cell mitotic activity, increased androgens, and degenerative changes.
- Two-cell, two-gonadotropin system.
  - The granulosa cell possess much greater aromatase activity than theca.
  - LH receptors are present only on theca cells, FSH receptors are only on granulosa cells; theca interstitial cells possess 20,000 LH receptors in their membranes.
  - Conversion of androgen microenvironment to estrogen microenvironment is dependent on a growing sensitivity to FSH.
  - Theca cells begin to express genes for the LH receptors, P450scc, and 3β-hydroxysteroid dehydrogenase (HSD); LH-regulated entry of low-density lipoprotein (LDL) cholesterol into the mitochondria is essential.
  - After luteinization, granulosa cells can use high-density lipoprotein (HDL) cholesterol in a novel fashion.
    ◇ Lipoproteins are not internalized.
    ◇ Cholesterol esters are extracted from lipoprotein at the cell surface.
  - As the follicle grows, theca cells express P450c17 (c21 → androgens); this is not expressed by the granulosa.
  - P450 aromatase is expressed only in the granulosa.
- Two-cell, two-gonadotropin in primates.

- Treatment of gonadotropin-deficient women with recombinant FSH.
    - ◇ Follicular development occurs.
    - ◇ Estradiol production is limited.
- Similar response is found in gonadotropin-releasing hormone (GnRH) antagonist–treated monkeys.
- Only FSH is required for folliculogenesis; autocrine and paracrine peptides have replaced estrogen.
- Selection of the dominant follicle.
    - Selection is mediated by estradiol as follows:
        - ◇ Local interaction between estradiol and FSH within the follicle (nonprimate model).
        - ◇ Effect of estrogen on pituitary FSH.
    - Gonadotropin support is withdrawn from less-developed follicles.
    - Factors governing the loss of follicles and/or oocytes via atresia.
        - ◇ Gonadotropin withdrawal.
        - ◇ Ovarian steroids.
        - ◇ Autocrine and paracrine factors.
    - Apoptosis.
        - ◇ Natural programmed cell death.
        - ◇ Heralded by specific messenger RNA (mRNA) changes in contrast with pathologic cell death (necrosis).
        - ◇ Once cells enter apoptosis, their response to FSH is modulated by local growth factors; tumor necrosis factor (TNF) inhibits FSH stimulation of estradiol secretion.
    - Estrogen and follicular selection.
        - ◇ Asymmetry in ovarian steroid production can be detected by day 5.
            - ○ Critical time in the cycle.
            - ○ Exogenous estrogens can disrupt the recruitment of dominant follicles.
        - ◇ Estrogen feedback inhibits development of all but the dominant follicle.
            - ○ The dominant one has increased FSH receptors.
            - ○ Enhancement of FSH action occurs.
                - □ Due to estrogen (nonprimate).
                - □ Due to peptides (primate).
        - ◇ Thecal vasculature develops.
            - ○ By day 9, dominant follicle has increased its vascularity by 2×.
            - ○ Allows the preferential delivery of gonadotropins to the dominant follicle.
            - ○ Synthesis of vascular endothelial growth factor (VEGF) may play an important role in this process.
    - LH receptors must be induced to prepare for ovulation; in the nonprimate model, this occurs as follows:

      ◊   Increased estrogen switches FSH from up-regulation of its own receptor to increased LH-receptor formation; LH can also up-regulate its own receptor in FSH-primed cells.

      ◊   Obligatory role for estrogen—inhibition prevents FSH-stimulated increase in LH receptor.

- The feedback system.
  - The dominant follicle optimizes its own environment to the detriment of the lesser follicles.
  - Pattern of GnRH and gonadotropin secretion is the result of the feedback from steroids and peptides.
    - ◊ Increase in GnRH accompanies LH surge so that estrogen feedback occurs at both pituitary and hypothalamic levels; negative estrogen feedback also is seen at these levels.
    - ◊ Progesterone has inhibitory action at the hypothalamus and positive action at the pituitary.
  - FSH secretion is inhibited by estrogen at low levels.
  - LH secretion is inhibited by estrogen at low levels but is stimulated at high levels.
    - ◊ Two critical features are as follows:
      - Concentration greater than 200 pg/mL.
      - Length of exposure greater than 50 hours.
    - ◊ This occurs only when the follicle is greater than 15 mm.
  - Pulsatile release of gonadotropins.
    - ◊ Pattern is a direct result of GnRH.
    - ◊ Amplitude and frequency are modulated by steroid feedback (Table 6.1).
  - In the luteal phase, gonadotropin secretion is still characterized by infrequent LH pulses and a low FSH level.
  - As transition to the follicular phase occurs, estradiol and progesterone levels decrease, and decreases in inhibin lead to increased GnRH pulse secretion.
    - ◊ The following general changes occur:
      - Frequency increases 4.5×.
      - FSH concentration increases 3.5×.
      - LH concentration increases 2×.
    - ◊ Changes in pulse frequency correlate with the duration of exposure to progesterone.
    - ◊ Changes in pulse amplitude are influenced by the progesterone concentration.
    - ◊ Steroids affect pulse frequency (hypothalamus) and amplitude (pituitary).
      - Possibly mediated by hypothalamic endogenous opioid peptides; estrogen en-

Table 6.1. Pulsatile pattern for gonadotropin secretion

Phase	Time
LH Pulse Frequency:	
Early follicular phase	90 min
Late follicular phase	60–70 min
Early luteal phase	100 min
Late luteal phase	200 min
LH Pulse Amplitude:	
Early follicular phase	6.5 IU/L
Midfollicular phase	5.0 IU/L
Late follicular phase	7.2 IU/L
Early luteal phase	15.0 IU/L
Midluteal phase	12.2 IU/L
Late luteal phase	8.0 IU/L

Abbreviation: LH, luteinizing hormone.

hances the stimulatory action of luteal phase progesterone on the endogenous opioids.
- ○ Plasma endorphin rises 2 days before LH peak.
  - □ Maximal at LH surge.
  - □ Nadir during menses.
- ■ Estrogen also modulates the biologic activity of gonadotropins.
  - ◇ Modulation of sialylation, size, and activity of gonadotropins.
  - ◇ Augments release of gonadotropins.
- ■ FSH and LH exhibit a nocturnal decline during the follicular phase; diurnal rhythm of LH found only in the early follicular phase.
- • Inhibin, activin, and follistatin.
  - ■ Introduction.
    - ◇ Synthesized by granulosa cells.
    - ◇ Expression present in many tissues.
    - ◇ Inhibin—inhibits FSH secretions.
    - ◇ Activin—stimulates FSH release in the pituitary and augments FSH action in the ovary.
    - ◇ Follistatin—suppresses FSH by binding activin.
  - ■ Inhibin.
    - ◇ Two subunits (α and β) are linked by disulfide bonds.
    - ◇ Two forms are purified.
      - ○ Identical α subunits.
      - ○ Two distinct β subunits as follows:
        - □ Inhibin A, α-β$_A$.
        - □ Inhibin B, α-β$_B$.
    - ◇ FSH stimulates inhibin and is suppressed by it; inhibin B form is predominantly secreted in the follicular phase.

◇ Inhibin secretion is decreased by GnRH and epidermal growth factor (EGF) and is increased by insulin-like growth factor-I (IGF-I) (Table 6.1).

◇ Secretion of inhibin B further augments the withdrawal of FSH from other follicles.

◇ Secretion is pulsatile (60 to 70 minutes).
  ○ Peaks in early/midfollicular phases.
  ○ Decreases with approaching ovulation.
  ○ Reaches its nadir in midluteal phase.

◇ Inhibin B level is lower and FSH levels are higher in the follicular phase of women from 45 to 49 years of age.

◇ As follicle changes into corpus luteum, inhibin comes under LH control.
  ○ Expression changes to inhibin A.
  ○ Peaks at midluteal phase.
  ○ Contributes to suppression of FSH to nadir levels.

◇ Multiple inhibitory effects on gonadotropin secretion are found.
  ○ Blocks synthesis and secretion of FSH.
  ○ Prevents up-regulation of GnRH receptors by GnRH.
  ○ Reduces the number of GnRH receptors.
  ○ Promotes (at high concentrations) intracellular degradations of gonadotropins.

◇ Enhances stimulatory action of LH and/or IGF-I on thecal cells.

■ Activin.
  ◇ Related to inhibin, but with the opposite action.
  ◇ Contains two subunits identical to β subunits of inhibin.
  ◇ Each subunit encoded by a distinct gene.
  ◇ Structure homologous to transforming growth factor-β (TGF-β); antimüllerian hormone (AMH) is also a member of this family.
  ◇ Three forms of activin:
    ○ Activin A, $\beta_A\beta_A$.
    ○ Activin B, $\beta_B\beta_B$.
    ○ Activin AB, $\beta_A\beta_B$.
  ◇ Activin is present in many cell types:
    ○ In ovarian follicles.
      □ Increases FSH binding in granulosa cells; regulates receptor number.
      □ Augments FSH stimulation of aromatization and inhibin production.
      □ Suppresses action of LH and IGF-I on theca; suppresses granulosa progesterone production to prevent premature luteinization.

○ In boys.
  □ Inhibits LH stimulation of andro-gen; inhibin facilitates androgen production.
  □ Stimulates spermatogonial prolifer-ation; inhibin decreases spermato-gonial proliferation.
○ In the anterior pituitary.
  □ Locally produced activin B aug-ments FSH secretion.
  □ Activin A directly stimulates GnRH receptors in pituitary cells.
- Follistatin.
  ◇ Secreted by a variety of pituitary cells, including gonadotropes.
  ◇ Also called FSH-suppressing protein.
  ◇ Main action: inhibits FSH synthesis and secretion and FSH response to GnRH.
  ◇ Mode of action: binds activin and thus decreases its activity.
  ◇ Feedback regulation.
    ○ It is stimulated by activin.
    ○ Inhibin prevents this response.
    ○ It is stimulated by FSH action on gran-ulosa cells.
- Summary.
  ◇ Pituitary secretion of FSH can be regulated by the balance of activin, inhibin, and fol-listatin.
  ◇ Within the follicle, activin and inhibin influence growth and development by mod-ulating the theca and granulosa response.
  ◇ This family of peptides can be considered a class of tumor-suppressor proteins.
    ○ Mice deficient in inhibin α subunit form gonadal stromal tumors.
    ○ Questionable contribution of increased FSH levels on tumor development.
- Growth factors.
  - Insulin-like growth factor–binding protein (IGFBP)—polypeptides that modulate cell proliferation and differentiation.
    ◇ Bind to specific cell membrane receptors.
    ◇ *Not* classic endocrine substances; they act locally in paracrine and autocrine mode.
  - IGFs.
    ◇ Also called somatomedins.
    ◇ Structurally and functionally similar to insulin.
    ◇ Single-chain polypeptides with three disulfide bonds.
    ◇ IGF-I is encoded on 12q; IGF-II, on 11p.
    ◇ IGF-I mediates growth-promoting actions of the growth hormone (GH); circulating IGF-I is derived mainly from liver and is GH-dependent.

- ○ Can be synthesized in many different tissues, however.
- ○ Binds to type I receptor.
- ◇ IGF-II is important in fetal growth and development.
  - ○ Little GH dependence.
  - ○ Binds to both type I and type II receptors.
- ◇ IGFBPs.
  - ○ Six known nonglycosylated peptides that function as IGFBPs: IGFBP-1 through IGFBP-6.
  - ○ Carry IGF in serum.
    - □ Prolong half-life of IGF.
    - □ Regulate tissue effects.
      - ▲ Bind and sequester IGFs.
      - ▲ Also may have a direct effect.
  - ○ Do not bind insulin.
  - ○ IGFBP-1—principal binding protein in amniotic fluid.
- ◇ IGFBP-3.
  - ○ GH-dependent hepatic synthesis.
  - ○ Main binding protein in the serum.
    - □ Carries 90% of the circulating IGF.
    - □ Circulating levels = total IGF concentration.
  - ○ Decreases in pregnancy (a unique protease is present) and with age.
- ◇ The IGF receptor.
  - ○ Type I receptor preferentially binds IGF-I.
  - ○ Insulin binds to the type I receptor with moderate affinity.
  - ○ IGF-I receptor is similar to insulin receptor.
    - □ Tetramer with 2α, 2β subunits.
    - □ Intracellular component of β subunit is tyrosine kinase.
- ◇ Ovarian actions of IGFs.
  - ○ IGF-I is involved in both estradiol and progesterone synthesis.
  - ○ Stimulates protein synthesis and steroidogenesis in synergy with FSH.
  - ○ Enhances LH-induced progesterone synthesis and stimulates proliferation of granulosa–luteal cells.
  - ○ Stimulates aromatase activity in synergy with FSH.
  - ○ Differences between rodent and primate gene expression.
- ◇ Human studies.
  - ○ IGF-II is expressed in both theca and granulosa cells; highest in the granulosa.
  - ○ Primary IGF in human ovary is IGF-II.

- ○ Theca cells encode receptors for both IGF-I and insulin; these allow for paracrine and autocrine modulation of granulosa and theca, respectively.
- ○ *In vitro* IGF-II increases steroidogenesis; augmented by GH.
- ○ Dominant follicle has increased IGF-II but not IGF-I.
- ○ No menstrual cycle changes in circulating IGF-I, IGF-II, IGFBP-1, or IGFBP-3.
- ◇ Rat studies—IGFBP-3 is made in theca cells.
  - ○ Stimulated by GH.
  - ○ Inhibited by FSH and estradiol (E_2).
    - □ Low concentration of FSH stimulates IGFBPs.
    - □ When FSH is low, increases in IGFBP result in decreased IGF and have a major effect on steroidogenesis.
- ◇ Human tissue.
  - ○ IGFBPs counteract the synergistic action of gonadotropin and growth factors; IGFBP synthesis is inhibited by FSH, IGF-I, and IGF-II.
  - ○ IGFBP-1 is found in the granulosa of growing follicles.
  - ○ IGFBP-3 is seen in the theca and granulosa of the dominant follicle.
  - ○ IGFBP-2, IGFBP-4, and IGFBP-5 are observed in the theca and granulosa of atretic and antral follicles.
  - ○ Predominant binding proteins are as follows:
    - □ IGFBP-2 in the granulosa of growing follicles.
    - □ IGFBP-3 in the theca and granulosa of dominant follicles.
  - ○ IGFBP expression in polycystic ovary (PCO) follicles is similar to that in atretic follicles.
    - □ Increase in IGFBP-2 sequesters IGF, which deprives follicle of an important source of gonadotropin augmentation.
    - □ Decrease in IGFBP-3 in the dominant follicle allows increased IGF levels and activity.
  - ○ Circulating IGFBP-1 decreases in response to insulin.
    - □ Decreases in anovulatory women with PCO.
    - □ IGF-I increased in these patients; probably is secondary to the LH effect on the theca.

- □ Follicular fluid levels in PCO.
  - ▲ Decreased IGFBP-1.
  - ▲ Increased IGFBP-2, IGFBP-4.
- □ IGFBP levels probably not etiologic in PCO.
- ○ IGFBP protease—estrogen-dominant follicles have low levels of IGFBP-4.
  - □ High levels are found in atretic follicles.
  - □ Low levels are the result of a specific protease; decreased IGFBP activity enhances IGF.
- ○ Extraovarian IGF-I.
  - □ May also operate in the pituitary.
  - □ Rat model of pituitary hyperplasia.
- ○ IGF and reproduction.
  - □ Role may be facilitatory, not obligatory; ovulation induction in Laron-type dwarf patients who are deficient in IGF-I can be successful.
  - □ Possibly a dominant role for IGF-II in humans; could explain the Laron dwarf issue.
- Summary of IGF action in ovary.
  - ■ IGF-II stimulates granulosa cell proliferation and aromatase and progesterone synthesis.
  - ■ IGF-II is produced in granulosa cells, theca cells, and luteinizing granulosa cells (in the pig and rat, the primary IGF is IGF-I).
  - ■ Gonadotropins stimulate IGF production, which is enhanced by estradiol and GH in animal experiments.
  - ■ IGF-I receptors are present in theca and granulosa cells; only IGF-II is found in luteinizing granulosa cells; IGF-II can act via both IGF-I and IGF-II receptors.
  - ■ IGF-II is the most abundant IGF in human follicles.
  - ■ FSH inhibits IGFBP synthesis (maximizes growth factor availability).
- Other growth factors potentially playing a role in the menstrual cycle.
  - ■ EGF.
  - ■ TGF.
  - ■ Fibroblast growth factor (FGF).
  - ■ Platelet-derived growth factor.
  - ■ VEGF.
  - ■ Interleukin-1 (IL-1).
  - ■ TNF.
- Prorenin.
  - ■ Inactive precursor to renin.
  - ■ Concentration in follicular fluid 12 times that in plasma.
  - ■ Stimulated by LH and human chorionic gonadotropin (hCG); increases by 10× in early pregnancy.

- Increase in prorenin not responsible for increased plasma levels of renin.
- Role of ovarian prorenin–renin–angiotensin system.
  - ◇ Steroidogenesis.
  - ◇ Regulation of calcium and prostaglandin (PG) metabolism.
  - ◇ Angiogenesis.
- Proopiomelanocortin family.
  - Adrenocorticotropic hormone (ACTH) and β-lipotropin remain constant.
  - β-Endorphin peaks prior to ovulation.
  - Corticotropin-releasing hormone system is present in theca cells; inhibits LH-stimulated androgen production.
- Antimüllerian hormone.
  - Produced by granulosa cells.
  - Possible role in oocyte maturation; inhibition of oocyte meiosis.
- Prevention of meiosis and luteinization.
  - Oocyte maturation inhibitor (OMI).
  - Pregnancy-associated plasma protein A.
  - Endothelin-1.
- Summary of events in the antral follicle.
  - Follicular phase estrogen production is explained by the two-cell, two-gonadotropin mechanism.
  - Selection of dominant follicle is established during days 5 to 7.
  - Estradiol levels increase steadily and provide negative feedback.
  - Midfollicular phase rise in estradiol directs decline in FSH but increase in LH.
  - Estrogen also affects the bioactivity of gonadotropin.
  - LH levels rise steadily during the late follicular phase, stimulating androgen production in the theca.
  - Unique responsiveness to FSH accelerates estrogen production.
  - FSH induces the appearance of LH receptors on granulosa cells.
  - Follicular response to FSH/LH is modulated by a variety of growth factors and autocrine and paracrine peptides.
  - Inhibin B secreted by granulosa in response to FSH directly suppresses FSH secretion.
  - Activin, originating in both the pituitary and granulosa, augments FSH secretion and action.
- ◆ Follicular growth and development in the primate ovary.
  - Evidence that follicular growth and development may be different in primates includes the following:
    - Failure to locate estrogen receptors in any significant ovarian compartment; recently chal-

lenged by discovery of mRNA for estrogen receptor β (ER-β) in monkey granulosa cells.
- No adverse effect on follicular size or number in monkeys treated with aromatase or 3β-HSD inhibitors.
    ◇ Oocyte development is normal.
    ◇ Fertilization is reduced.
- Normal response of women with 17α-hydroxylase deficiency to gonadotropins.
- Response of gonadotropin-deficient women to recombinant FSH.
    ◇ Similarly demonstrated in GnRH antagonist–treated monkeys.
    ◇ Only FSH required for folliculogenesis.
- Autocrine and paracrine peptides have replaced estrogen.
    - Inhibin and activin regulate androgen synthesis in theca cells.
        ◇ Inhibin enhances LH and/or IGF-I.
        ◇ It can overcome the inhibition of activin.
    - Activin augments all FSH activity in immature granulosa cells, especially aromatase activity.
    - In luteinizing granulosa cells, activin has direct mitogenic activity and suppresses steroidogenesis in response to LH; inhibin has no effect on LH-dependent aromatase in mature granulosa cells.
    - Control of inhibin secretion changes.
        ◇ Follicular phase: FSH.
        ◇ Luteal phase: LH.
    - During follicular growth, the following occurs:
        ◇ Activin production decreases.
        ◇ Inhibin production increases.
        ◇ Follistatin levels increase (decrease activin).
- Putting it all together.
    - Early follicular phase—activin produced by granulosa cells in immature follicles enhances FSH action (Fig. 6.3).
        ◇ Increased aromatase activity.
        ◇ FSH-receptor and LH-receptor formation.
        ◇ Decreased theca androgen production.
    - Late follicular phase (Fig. 6.4).
        ◇ Increased inhibin and decreased activin promote theca androgen production in response to LH and IGF-II; estrogen production increases.
        ◇ Activin serves to prevent premature luteinization and progesterone production.
    - Mature and/or dominant follicle (Fig. 6.5).
        ◇ Acquires highest level of aromatase activity.
        ◇ Attains greatest number of LH receptors.
        ◇ Produces highest concentration of estrogen and inhibin (inhibin B).

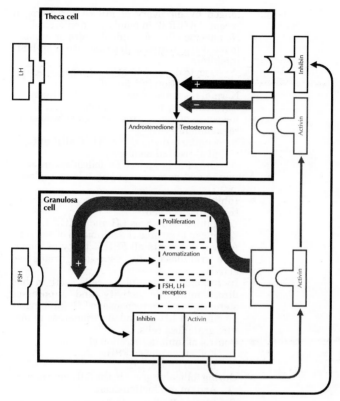

Figure 6.3.   The early follicular phase.

> ◇ Has lowest level of activin.
> ◇ Inhibin: promotes LH stimulation of thecal androgens; comes under LH control.
>   ○ Central FSH suppression.
>   ○ Local LH enhancement.
> ■ Role of IGF.
>   ◇ Important but not essential role.
>   ○ IGF-I deficient patients can produce fertilizable ova.
>   ○ This possibly indicates the role of IGF-II.
>   ◇ May not be GH-dependent.
> ◆ The preovulatory follicle.
>   • Granulosa cells enlarge and acquire lipid inclusions.
>   • The theca becomes vacuolated and richly vascular; the follicle develops a hyperemic appearance.
>   • Oocyte proceeds in meiosis and approaches completion of reduction division.

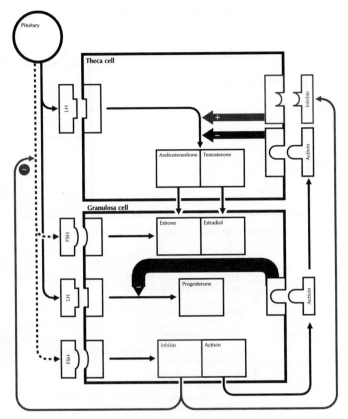

Figure 6.4.   The late follicular phase.

- Increasing amounts of estrogen are produced.
    - Rapid increase, with peak 24 to 36 hours prior to ovulation.
    - Onset of surge with peak estradiol levels.
- LH promotes luteinization.
    - Progesterone is produced as early as day 10.
    - It inhibits further cell growth and enhances steroidogenesis; it is enhanced by IGF.
    - Progesterone receptors appear in the granulosa cells with the dominant follicle in the preovulatory period.
        ◇ Found in response to LH, not estrogen.
        ◇ Inhibit granulosa cell mitosis.
- Progesterone affects positive feedback response to estrogen.
    - Can induce LH surge with subthreshold estrogen levels via direct pituitary action.
    - In high doses, can block LH surge.

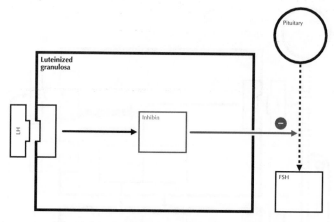

Figure 6.5.   Inhibin activity in the luteal phase.

- Also responsible for FSH surge; ensures full complement of LH receptors.
- 17-Hydroxy progesterone levels also rise in preovulatory phase.
  ◊ These signal LH stimulation of P450scc and P450c17.
  ◊ Some corpus luteum cells lose P450c17 expression.
- Androgens produced in stroma increase in midcycle.
  ◊ Fifteen percent increase in androstenedione; 20% increase in testosterone.
  ◊ Enhanced by rise in inhibin.
  ◊ May enhance atresia of secondary follicles.
  ◊ May stimulate libido.
- Summary of events.
  - Estrogen production reaches levels of the threshold needed to induce the LH surge.
  - LH initiates granulosa cell luteinization and progesterone production.
  - Preovulatory rise in progesterone facilitates positive feedback action of estrogen and induces midcycle FSH.
  - Local and peripheral androgens increase and are derived from the theca of unsuccessful follicles.
II. Ovulation
   ◆ Considerable variation occurs from cycle to cycle and from woman to woman.
   ◆ Ovulation usually occurs 10 to 12 hours after the LH peak.
   - Twenty-four to 36 hours after peak estradiol levels.
   - Thirty-four to 36 hours after onset of LH surge.

- LH concentration must exceed the threshold for 14 to 27 hours in order to assure maturation; the LH surge usually lasts 48 to 50 hours.
- The LH surge usually occurs at 3:00 AM; between midnight to 8:00 AM in two-thirds of women.
- Seasonal variation in timing of ovulation.
  - Evening during autumn and winter.
  - Between 4:00 to 7:00 PM in 90% of women from July through February.
  - Between midnight to 11:00 AM in 50% of women in the spring.
- Action of the LH surge initiates the following:
  - Continuation of meiosis.
  - Luteinization of granulosa cells.
  - Expansion of cumulus.
  - Synthesis of PGs and other eicosanoids necessary for follicular rupture.
  - LH-induced cyclic adenosine monophosphate activity: overcomes action of OMI and luteinization inhibitor (probably endothelin-1).
    - OMI originates in granulosa cells.
    - It requires an intact cumulus.
      - ◇ Cumulus lacks LH receptors.
      - ◇ Cumulus is deficient in progesterone production.
- LH surge induces a continual rise in progesterone.
  - May act to terminate the LH surge.
  - Progesterone increases the distensibility of follicular wall; a rapid increase in volume occurs without a change in pressure.
  - Progesterone and FSH, as well as LH, stimulate activity of proteolytic enzymes; the gonadotropin surge also releases histamine.
- Proteolytic enzyme activity is activated in an orderly sequence as follows:
  1. Granulosa cells and theca cells produce plasminogen activator in response to the FSH and LH surge.
  2. Granulosa cell plasminogen activators induce plasmin production.
  3. Plasmin generates active collagenase.
  4. Collagenase disrupts the follicular wall.
- Plasminogen activator inhibitor systems.
  - Very active in theca and interstitial cells; prevent inappropriate activation.
  - Also present in human granulosa cells and preovulatory follicular fluid; responsive to EGF, IL-1β.
  - With movement and distention of the follicle to the surface of the ovary, the exposed surface is separated from cells rich in plasminogen inhibitor systems; rupture/ovulation occurs at this follicular apex (stigma).
- Role of PGs and eicosanoids.
  - PGE, PGF, and other eicosanoids increase in the preovulatory follicular fluid, peaking at ovulation.

- PG synthesis is stimulated by IL-1β.
- Inhibition of synthesis of these products can block ovulation.
- PGs free proteolytic enzymes within the follicular wall.
- Hydroxyeicosatetraenoic acids may produce angiogenesis and hyperemia.
- PGs may also contract smooth muscle cells.

  The role of PGs is so well demonstrated that infertility patients should be advised to avoid the use of drugs that inhibit PG synthesis.

- ◆ Role of leukocytes—large number of leukocytes enters the follicle prior to ovulation.
  - Mediated by chemotactic mechanisms of the interleukin systems.
  - Probably contribute to the cellular changes associated with ovulation, corpus luteum function, and apoptosis.
- ◆ Estradiol levels.
  - Plunge as LH reaches its peak.
  - May reflect LH down-regulation of its own receptors; theca cells exhibit suppressed steroidogenesis when exposed to high levels of LH.
  - Progesterone may also inhibit estradiol production.
  - Estrogen can directly inhibit P450c17; direct gene action is not receptor-mediated.
- ◆ FSH peak.
  - Partially, and possibly totally, dependent on pre-ovulatory progesterone rise.
  - Plasminogen activator is sensitive to FSH and LH.
  - Stimulates synthesis of hyaluronic acid matrix; allows for cumulus expansion and dispersion.
  - Ensures adequate LH-receptor complement.
- ◆ LH surge.
  - Mechanism attenuating surge is unknown.
  - Precipitous drop in plasma estrogen within hours of LH surge.
  - Etiology of LH decline.
    - ■ Loss of positive stimulation from estrogen.
    - ■ Depletion in pituitary LH content; desensitization of GnRH receptors.
      - ◇ Altered GnRH pulse frequency.
      - ◇ Changes in steroid levels.
  - Short negative feedback loop of LH upon hypothalamus.
  - Gonadotropin surge inhibitor factor in ovary.
    - ■ Produced in granulosa cells under FSH control.
    - ■ Peak in midfollicular phase.
- ◆ Summary of ovulatory events.
  - LH surge stimulates continuation of reduction division in oocytes.
    - ■ Luteinization of granulosa cells.
    - ■ Synthesis of progesterone and PGs in the follicle.
  - Progesterone enhances activity of proteolytic enzymes and PGs.

- Progesterone-influenced FSH rise serves to free oocyte from follicular attachments.
  - Plasminogens → plasmin.
  - Sufficient LH-receptor content.

III. Luteal Phase
  - Prior to rupture, granulosa cells enlarge and assume vacuolated appearance.
  - They continue to enlarge for the first 3 days after ovulation.
  - Capillaries begin to penetrate the granulosa layer after the LH surge.
    - Response to LH-mediated growth factors, such as VEGF.
    - By day 8 to 9 after ovulation peak, vascularization is reached.
    - Unchecked hemorrhage can occur from the corpus luteum.
  - Normal luteal function requires optimal preovulatory follicular development.
    - Determines extent of luteinization.
    - Determines functional capacity of corpus luteum.
  - LDL cholesterol must reach vascularized granulosa cells.
    - LH regulates LDL-receptor binding, internalization, and post–receptor processing.
    - Induction of LH receptors occurs early in luteinization.
  - Corpus luteum lifespan is dependent on continuous tonic LH secretion.
    - Prompt luteolysis is seen after GnRH agonist or GnRH antagonist.
    - Corpus luteum is a heterogeneous tissue.
      - Luteal cells (only 15% to 30% of total cell population).
      - Two distinct cell types as follows:
        ◇ Large cells.
          ○ Possibly derived from granulosa cells.
          ○ Greater steroidogenesis.
          ○ Lack of LH receptors is surprising.
          ○ Produce peptide products: oxytocin, relaxin, and inhibin.
          ○ Greater aromatase activity.
        ◇ Small cells.
          ○ More abundant than large cells.
          ○ Probably derived from theca cells.
          ○ Contain LH and hCG receptors (Fig. 6.6).
  - Progesterone levels.
    - Rise sharply after ovulation.
    - Reach peak 8 days after the LH surge.
    - Locally and centrally suppress new follicular growth.
    - New follicular growth is also inhibited by the action of estrogen and inhibin A.
      - Inhibin A reaches peak at the midluteal phase.
      - Inhibin A peak suppresses FSH to nadir levels.

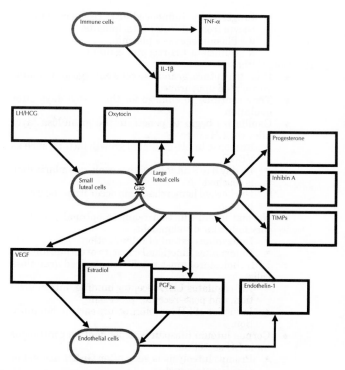

Figure 6.6. Summary of the luteal phase and hormones that are involved.

- ◆ Secretion of progesterone and estradiol is episodic.
  - • Correlates with LH pulses.
  - • Low midluteal progesterone levels sometimes found in normal luteal phases.
- ◆ Luteal phase is consistently close to 14 days.
  - • Range is 11 to 17 days.
  - • Short luteal phase is found in 5% to 6% of women.
  - • Demise of corpus luteum may be due to active luteolytic mechanism.
  - • Corpus luteum rapidly declines in 9 to 11 days after ovulation; the mechanism is unknown.
    - ■ Possible role for estradiol; may also be necessary to allow for synthesis of endometrial progesterone receptors.
    - ■ Possible role of prostaglandin $F_{2\alpha}$ ($PGF_{2\alpha}$), mediated by endothelin-1.
      - ◇ Inhibits steroidogenesis.
      - ◇ Stimulates release of TNF-α.
- ◆ Role of gap junctions—prominent feature of luteal cells.

- Allows for communication and exchange of signals; small cells receive LH signal and transmit it to large cells.
- Regulation is influenced by oxytocin.
- Leuteolysis and LH.
  - LH receptor–binding affinity is unchanged throughout the luteal phase.
  - Decline in steroidogenesis must reflect deactivation of the system.
    - Possible uncoupling of G protein adenylate cyclase system.
    - Alteration in LH pulse frequency or amplitude does not promote luteolysis.
- Luteolysis and proteolytic enzymes—matrix metalloproteinases (MMPs).
  - Under inhibitory control of tissue inhibitors of MMPs (TIMPs).
  - No change in luteal tissue.
    - Luteolysis results in direct increase in MMP expression.
    - hCG prevents increase in MMP expression; may also increase TIMP production.
- Survival of the corpus luteum—prolonged by emergence of hCG.
  - Appears at peak of corpus luteal development.
  - Maintains vital steroidogenic activity of corpus luteum.
    - It is continued until the ninth or tenth week of gestation.
    - Occasionally, placental steroidogenesis is established by the seventh week of gestation.
- Expression of P450scc and P450 3β-HSD is normal at ovulation and declines throughout the luteal phase; lifespan of the corpus luteum is established at the time of ovulation.
- Summary of events in luteal phase.
  - Normal luteal function requires optimal preovulatory follicular development (especially adequate FSH stimulation) and continued tonic LH support.
  - Progesterone acts both centrally and within the ovary to suppress new follicular growth.
  - Regression of the corpus luteum may involve the luteolytic action of its own estrogen production, which is mediated by an alteration in local PG and endothelin-1 concentrations.
  - In early pregnancy, hCG rescues the corpus luteum, maintaining luteal function until placental steroidogenesis is well established.

IV. Luteal Follicular Transition
- Very critical and decisive time—critical factors are GnRH, FSH, LH, E_2, progesterone (P_4), inhibin.
- Selective increase in FSH begins 2 days prior to menses.
  - Decrease in luteal steroids.
  - Change in GnRH pulsatile secretion.
- Inhibin B reaches nadir in midluteal phase.
  - Begins to rise shortly after increase in FSH.

- Peak levels at 4 days after maximal increase in FSH.
♦ Activin levels peak at menses.
  - But highly bound → possible endocrine role?
  - Could contribute to FSH rise; evidence suggests response to GnRH requires activin.
♦ Changes in GnRH pulsatility.
  - Progressive and rapid increase in GnRH pulses.

LH pulsatility	FSH pulsatility
4.5× ↑ in frequency	3.5× ↑ in frequency
2× ↑ in mean level of LH	3.5× ↑ in mean level of FSH

  - Pituitary response to GnRH is also a factor.
    - Estradiol suppresses FSH secretion.
    - Classic negative feedback at the pituitary.
♦ Summary of events.
  - The demise of the corpus luteum results in a nadir in the circulating levels of estradiol, progesterone, and inhibin.
  - The decrease in inhibin A removes a suppressing influence on FSH secretion in the pituitary.
  - The decrease in estradiol and progesterone allows a progressive and rapid increase in the frequency of GnRH pulsatile secretion and a removal of the pituitary from negative feedback suppression.
  - The removal of inhibin A and estradiol and the increasing GnRH pulses combine to allow greater secretion of FSH compared with LH, with an increase in the frequency of the episodic secretion.
  - The increase in FSH is instrumental in rescuing an approximately 60-day-old group of ready follicles from atresia, allowing a dominant follicle to begin its emergence.
V. The Normal Menstrual Cycle
♦ The observations of Vollman and Treloar document cycle parameters.
♦ Menarche is followed by 5 to 7 years of increasingly regular cycles.
♦ Cycles lengthen in patients in their 40s, who have an increased incidence of anovulatory cycles.
♦ Cycle length.
  - Fifteen percent of women: 28 days.
  - Approximately 0.5% of women: < 21 days.
  - Approximately 0.9% of women: > 35 days.
♦ Twenty percent experience irregular cycles.
♦ Diminished inhibin B leads to rapid follicular recruitment.
♦ Accelerated follicular loss when total number of follicles is approximately 25,000 (usually between the ages of 32 to 38 years).
♦ Reduced follicular recruitment is a result of the reduced follicular pool.

Sperm and Egg Transport, Fertilization, and Implantation

I. History
   - Antonj van Leeuwenhoek of Delft, Holland, fascinated by the Galileo microscope, first described sperm (1677).
   - Wilhelm August Oscar Hertwig in Germany demonstrated fertilization in the sea urchin (1875).
II. Sperm Transport
   - Sperm reach epididymis 72 days after initiation of spermatogenesis.
   - Need for capacitation, or the cellular changes that ejaculated sperm must undergo to be able to fertilize, may be an evolutionary consequence in response to the storage of inactive sperm in the caudal epididymis (Figs. 7.1 and 7.2).
   - The head of the sperm contains the acrosome—large vesicle of proteolytic enzymes.
     - Inner acrosomal membrane is closely apposed to the nuclear membrane.
     - Outer acrosomal membrane is next to the surface plasma membrane.
   - Flagellum is a complex microtubular array surrounded at the proximal end by mitochondria.
   - Motility and ability to fertilize are acquired gradually with passage into the epididymis.
   - Caudal epididymis.
     - Stores sperm available for ejaculation.
     - Provides capacity for repetitive fertile ejaculations.
   - Preservation of optimal sperm function requires testosterone and the maintenance of a normal scrotal temperature; epididymis is relegated to role of storage.
   - Semen.
     - Forms a gel following ejaculation.
     - Liquefies 20 to 30 minutes later, secondary to prostatic enzymes.
       - Alkaline pH protects against vaginal acidic pH.
       - Most sperm are immobilized within approximately 2 hours.
   - Sperm enter the cervical mucus within 90 seconds of ejaculation.
     - Questionable role of uterine contractions.
     - Sperm must push through pores in the mucus that are smaller than the sperm head; abnormal sperm are less successful at penetrating the cervical mucus.
     - Sperm are present in the fallopian tube within 5 minutes after insemination.
   - Human sperm have been found in the fallopian tube at 80 hours following insemination; in animals,

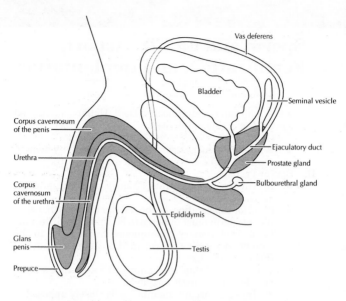

Figure 7.1. The structure of male genitalia involved in reproduction.

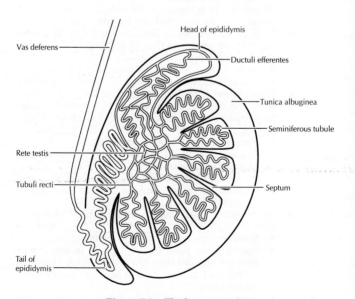

Figure 7.2. The human testis.

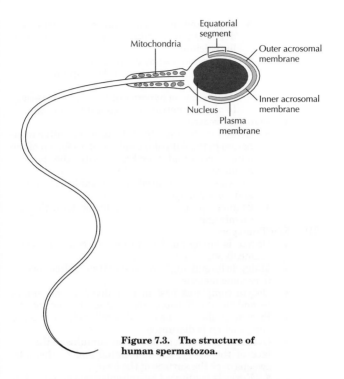

Figure 7.3.   The structure of human spermatozoa.

the fertilizable lifespan = half the motile lifespan (Fig. 7.3).
- ♦ Significant attrition is present: 200 million sperm in ejaculate → 200 sperm reach the proximity of the egg and fallopian tube.
- ♦ Increased motility seen within the fallopian tube—hyperactivated motility.
- ♦ Cervix serves as a sperm reservoir for 72 hours.
- ♦ Capacitation is initiated as sperm pass cervix.
- ♦ Capacitation.
  - • In 1951, rabbit and rat spermatozoa were shown to require several hours in the female genital tract before acquiring the ability to fertilize an egg.
  - • The three features of capacitation are as follows:
    - ■ The ability to undergo the acrosome reaction.
    - ■ The ability to bind to the zona pellucida.
    - ■ The acquisition of hypermotility.
  - • Capacitation may be induced by a zona protein or human follicular fluid.
    - ■ Changes the surface characteristics of sperm.
      - ◇ Removal of seminal plasma factors.
      - ◇ Modification of surface charge.
      - ◇ Restriction of receptor mobility.

- Regulated by redox status of sperm cell; dependent on a critical increase in intracellular calcium.
- Can be induced by defined media.
- *In vitro* capacitation takes approximately 2 hours.
- Acquisition of hypermotility may be necessary to allow penetration of cumulus and zona.

♦ Acrosome reaction.
- Occurs in the vicinity of the oocyte or after incubation in the follicular fluid; involves fusion of the outer acrosomal membrane with the plasma membrane.
- Enzymes are released: hyaluronidase, acrosin, and corona-dispersing enzyme.
- Changes prepare sperm for fusion with the egg membrane.

III. Egg Transport
♦ Oocyte is surrounded by granulosa cells that communicate via gap junctions.
♦ Midcycle luteinizing hormone (LH) surge frees oocyte to resume meiosis.
♦ Oocyte completes first meiotic division and enters second meiotic division; arrests at second metaphase.
♦ Prior to ovulation, the cumulus cells retract and the gap junction is disrupted.
♦ Ovulated eggs adhere with their cumulus to the surface of the ovary; the fimbriated end of the tube sweeps over the surface of the ovary.
- Entry is facilitated by muscular movements that bring fimbriae into contact with the surface of the ovary.
- Eggs can be picked up from the contralateral ovary or cul-de-sac.
- Oocyte pickup is not dependent on negative pressure.
♦ Fallopian tube epithelium.
- Comprised of ciliated and nonciliated cells.
- Nonciliated cells release cytoplasmic contents.
♦ Fimbriae have higher concentration of ciliated cells; cumulus is necessary to ensure egg pickup.
♦ Ampullary cilia beat in synchrony toward uterus; motility of tubal cilia in patients with Kartagener syndrome may be disordered, but not totally absent.
♦ Maturation is induced and cortical granules move to the outer cortex of the oocyte.
♦ Prior to ovulation, the oocyte and cumulus detach from the follicular wall.
♦ Within 2 to 3 minutes of ovulation, the cumulus and oocyte are in the ampulla.
♦ Transvaginal endoscopic observation of ovum and cumulus oophorous pickup in women revealed that this process is relatively slow (more than 15 minutes).
- Fimbriae on the ovulatory side are erect.

- Fimbriae sweep over the surface of the ovary.
- ◆ In most species, tubal transport requires 3 days.
  - In women, the egg spends 80 hours in the tube, 90% of the time in the ampulla.
  - Tubal function is influenced by (a) hormones, (b) adrenergic stimulus, and (c) prostaglandins (PGs).
    - Estrogen has a tube-locking effect that can be overcome by progesterone.
    - Surgical denervation does not affect transport.
    - PGE relaxes tubal musculature; $PGF_{2\alpha}$ stimulates contraction.
- ◆ Tubal incubation.
  - A prerequisite in most species.
  - Toxic endometrial secretions may be present in the first 48 hours.
  - Duration of tubal incubation may not be crucial.
    - Donor-egg data reveal an implantation window that lasts several days.
    - Estes procedure (ovarian implantation to cornua) can result in pregnancy.
- ◆ Embryo development is dependent on the uterus (Fig. 7.4).

IV. Oocyte Maturation
- ◆ In human oocytes, an influx of extracellular calcium occurs in response to estradiol.
- ◆ Followed by a secondary rise in calcium from intracellular stores.
- ◆ Improves oocyte quality, contributes to fertilizability; not an obligate role but an important one.

V. Fertilization
- ◆ Rabbit ovum is fertilizable for 6 to 8 hours.
- ◆ Human ova are estimated to be fertilizable for 12 to 24 hours (Fig. 7.4); immature ova are fertilizable for 36 hours in *in vitro* fertilization.
- ◆ Human sperm can fertilize for approximately 48 to 72 hours.
- ◆ Most pregnancies occur in the 3-day interval prior to ovulation.
- ◆ Sperm–egg contact.
  - Occurs in the ampulla of the tube.
  - May not be random.
    - Evidence exists of sperm–egg communication.
    - Includes chemotactic responsiveness that requires changes that occur in the capacitation process.
  - Cumulus expansion may have the following two roles:
    1. Increases chances of encounter with a sperm.
    2. Facilitates sperm passage to oocyte.
- ◆ The zona pellucida has the following two major functions in the fertilization process:
  1. Contains ligands for sperm.
  2. Zona reaction prevents polyploidy.

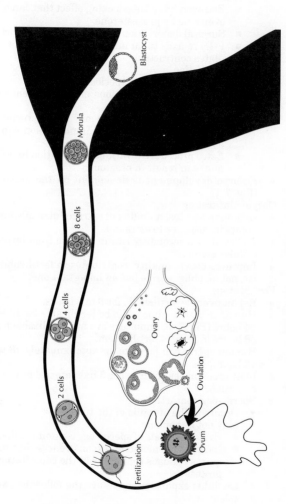

Figure 7.4.   The process of release, fertilization, and transport of an ovum.

- Passage through the zona is mediated by an acrosome reaction via acrosin.
- Sperm motility may be the critical factor; both tail and head motility are necessary.
◆ Acrosome reaction.
  - Exocytotic reaction with the release of vesicle contents.
  - Requires influx of calcium, efflux of hydrogen atoms, increase in pH, and fusion of the membrane.
  - Binding to the zona is required to induce acrosome reaction; probably mediated via the glycoprotein sperm receptor.
◆ Sperm receptors currently identified include the following:
  - Zona pellucida (ZP) 1, 2, 3.
    - ZP3 is the primary ligand for sperm.
    - ZP2 binding occurs after the acrosome reaction.
    - Structural alteration leads to the loss of receptor activity.
    - Inactivation likely is secondary to the cortical granule enzyme release.
  - Disruption of ZP3 renders mice infertile; vaccination against the ZP protein can control reproduction in animals.
◆ Binding to the zona.
  - Initial binding requires sperm recognition of the carbohydrate component of the glycoprotein-receptor molecule.
  - After binding, the acrosome reaction is triggered by the peptide chain component of the receptor glycoprotein.
  - At least one receptor on the sperm head is a tyrosine kinase, which is activated by ZP3 binding initiating the acrosome reaction.
  - The G protein signaling system is activated and opens calcium channels.
◆ Sperm entry into perivitelline space (Fig. 7.5).
  - Entry occurs at an angle.
  - The equatorial region of the sperm makes the initial contact.
  - The egg membrane engulfs the sperm head.
    - Fusion occurs and is mediated by two proteins.
      ◇ PH-20 (hyaluronidase) binds to the zona pellucida, resulting in cumulus dispersion.
      ◇ PH-30 (fertilin) mediates fusion with the oocyte.
    - Integrins are also present.
◆ Membrane fusion is followed by cortical reaction and metabolic activation.
  - Mediated by calcium oscillations that are signaled by oscillin in the equatorial region of the sperm head.
  - Fusion will only occur with sperm that has undergone the acrosome reaction.

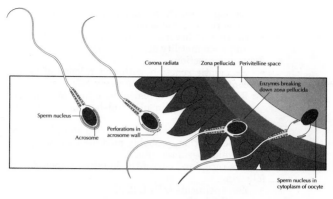

Figure 7.5. Sperm entry into the zona pellucida and fertilization of the oocyte.

- The release of the cortical granules leads to the zona reaction and a block to sperm entry; a transient block is secondary to rapid depolarization.
- ◆ Early pregnancy loss.
    - Thirty percent of embryos are lost following implantation.
    - Forty-six percent of all fertilized eggs will eventually end with early loss.
    - Fifteen percent of clinically recognized pregnancies end in spontaneous loss.
        - ■ Fifty percent to 60% are clinically abnormal.
        - ■ Only 30% of conceptions survive to birth.
- VI. Implantation
    - ◆ At the time of implantation, the endometrium is 10 to 14 mm thick with a large amount of secretions; the window of receptivity in the cycle is from days 16 to 22 (of the natural 28-day cycle) and from days 16 to 19 of cycles with exogenous gonadotropins.
    - ◆ Endometrial receptivity is heralded by the formation of pinopodes; these may absorb the endometrial fluid, forcing the blastocyst to be in contact with the endometrium.
    - ◆ Communication between the mother and early embryo begins very early (early pregnancy factor [EPF]).
        - EPF is secreted initially by ovary.
            - ■ After implantation, derived from the embryo.
            - ■ Has immunosuppressive properties.
        - Blastocysts secrete human chorionic gonadotropin (hCG) 7 to 8 days after fertilization, resulting in enhanced steroid secretions from the corpus luteum.
        - PGE_2 is increased at the implantation site.
    - ◆ Implantation begins 2 to 3 days after embryo entry into the uterus (day 18 to 19 of cycle).

- Five to 7 days after fertilization.
- Usually occurs on the upper posterior wall in the midsagittal plane.
♦ Apposition and adhesion.
- Blastocyst hatches after 1 to 3 days; critical for implantation.
- At least three cytokines are involved in implantation.
  - Colony-stimulating factor–1 (CSF-1). Mice with inactivating mutation are infertile.
  - Leukocyte inhibitory factor (LIF).
    ◊ Same pattern as CSF-1.
    ◊ Mice with LIF mutation are infertile.
  - Interleukin-1 (IL-1).
    ◊ Blocking the IL-1 receptor also prevents implantation.
    ◊ However, mice deficient in the receptor have normal reproduction.
- Adhesive molecules—adhesion due to integrin binding is followed by invasion of the trophoblast via degradation of the extracellular matrix.
  - Peak integrin expression at the time of implantation.
  - Abnormal level of integrin expression may be a cause of infertility.
- Formation of junctional complexes prevents dislodging the embryo by flushing.
♦ Invasion and placentation (Fig. 7.6).
- Three subsequent interactions occur:
  1. Trophoblasts intrude between the uterine epithelial cells.
  2. Epithelial cells are lifted off the basement membrane; trophoblasts can interdigitate underneath.
  3. Fusion of trophoblast with the uterine epithelial cells.
- Process is not destructive.
  - Embryo does contain proteases, but protease activity is confined to the removal of dead cells.
    ◊ Cells move away from the trophoblast → contact inhibition.
    ◊ Trophoblast fills the spaces left.
  - Regulated by many growth factors and cytokines; integrin expression is critical to the early invasion of the trophoblast.
    ◊ Actively migrating cells preferentially bind laminin.
    ◊ Regulation enables directional cell migration.
- Vascular changes—uterine spiral arterioles are invaded by cytotrophoblasts.
  - Maternal endothelium is replaced by cytotrophoblast tissue as far as the first third of the myometrium.

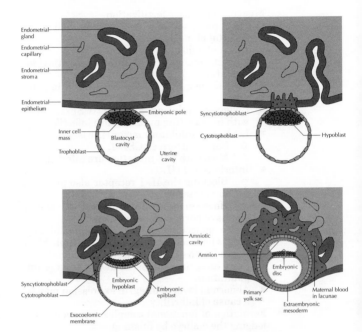

Figure 7.6.   Implantation of an embryo in the uterine wall.

- ■ This replacement may be governed by the selectin family of surface molecules.
- ■ Receptor profile of the trophoblast changes to resemble the endothelial cells.
- ■ Failure of this process is noted in preeclampsia.
- • Matrix metalloproteinases.
    - ■ Involved in menstruation.
    - ■ Also key players in matrix degradation during the trophoblast invasion.
    - ■ Include the following:
        - ◊ Collagenases.
        - ◊ Gelatinases.
        - ◊ Stromelysins.
    - ■ Can be activated by integrin-mediated adhesion.
    - ■ Production is regulated by the following:
        - ◊ Plasminogen activators.
        - ◊ Cytokines.
        - ◊ Tissue inhibitors (TIMPs).
- • Limitation of invasion.
    - ■ Invasion is mediated by serine proteases and metalloproteinases (plasminogen activators); plasmin activator metalloproteinase family.

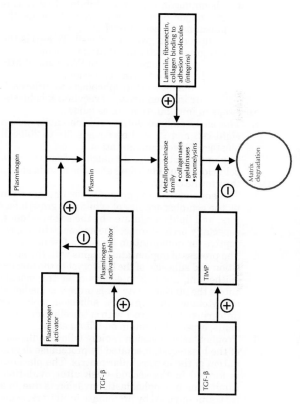

Figure 7.7. Cascade involved in matrix degradation in implantation.

- Binding of plasminogen activator to trophoblast plasminogen activator receptor may control the plasmin proteolysis.
- Cytokine secretion from the endometrial lymphocytes (including natural killer cells) may limit the invasion.
- Invasion is limited by the decidual cell layer.
  ◇ Histamine may initiate the decidual response.
  ◇ Blockage of histamine receptors H_1 and H_2 may decrease the rate of implantation.
- Plasminogen activator inhibitor–1 (PAI-1) is the major decidual cell product; binds the plasminogen activator (Fig. 7.7).
- Transforming growth factor–β (TGF-β) is the key growth factor in limiting invasion.
  ◇ Induces increase in both PAI-1 and TIMP.
  ◇ Inhibits integrin expression.
  ◇ Influences cytotrophoblasts to differentiate into noninvasive syncytiotrophoblasts.

◆ Key steps in implantation are as follows:
  1. The early embryo enters uterine cavity as an eight-cell morula and becomes a 30- to 200-cell blastocyst before implantation.
  2. Implantation begins with hatching from the zona pellucida about 1 to 3 days after the morula enters the uterine cavity.
  3. The endometrium is prepared for implantation by the complex activity of cytokines, growth factors, and lipids modulated by the sex hormones, especially progesterone. The endometrium is receptive for implantation for only a few days.
  4. The process of implantation begins with the apposition and adhesion of the blastocyst to the uterine epithelium, about 2 to 4 days after the morula enters the uterine cavity. This process is mediated by cytokines and involves adhesion molecules (integrins) that interact with extracellular components, especially laminin and fibronectin.
  5. Trophoblastic invasion rapidly follows adhesion of the blastocyst, mediated by proteinase degradation of the extracellular matrix. The placenta is formed in the second week after ovulation. Limitation of trophoblastic invasion is due to a restraint imposed by proteinase inhibitors, especially plasminogen activator inhibitor and tissue inhibitors of metalloproteinases.

8

The Endocrinology of Pregnancy

I. Steroid Hormones in Pregnancy
- ♦ Synthesis does not follow a conventional mechanism; fetal and placental compartments both lack certain enzyme activities.
- ♦ Maternal circulation represents the source of building materials.
- ♦ Cholesterol—enters the trophoblast from the maternal blood by endocytosis as low-density lipoprotein (LDL) cholesterol.
  - • Important role of LDL cell membrane receptors; enhanced by estrogen.
  - • LDL undergoes hydrolysis, forming amino acids and essential fatty acids.
  - • Questionable role of tropic hormones.
  - • Estrogen plays an important role in progesterone (P_4) production.
    - ▪ Increases LDL uptake.
    - ▪ Stimulates cholesterol production in the liver.
    - ▪ Increases P450 activity.
- ♦ Progesterone.
  - • Placenta can use precursors from either mother or fetus to correct its own enzyme deficiency.
    - ▪ Converts little acetate to cholesterol.
    - ▪ Progesterone is formed from maternal circulatory products.
      - ◊ Cholesterol (97%).
      - ◊ Pregnenolone (3%).
    - ▪ Fetal contribution is negligible; after intrauterine fetal demise, progesterone levels remain high.
  - • Progesterone is produced by the corpus luteum until about 10 weeks into pregnancy.
    - ▪ Pregnancy is dependent upon the corpus luteum until 7 weeks.
    - ▪ Progesterone (100 mg/day) is required to support an early pregnancy.
      - ◊ Associated with maternal serum levels of approximately 10 ng/mL.
      - ◊ The predictive value of blood levels is limited because of great individual variation.
  - • Shared function of the corpus luteum and the placenta between 7 and 10 weeks of pregnancy.
  - • Placenta is primary source of progesterone following 10 weeks of pregnancy; progesterone rises to between 100 to 200 ng/mL at term.
    - ▪ Placenta produces 250 mg progesterone per day; most enters the maternal circulation.

- ■ Progesterone production is independent of the fetus.
- Human decidua and fetal membranes also synthesize progesterone; neither cholesterol nor LDL cholesterol is needed.
  - ■ Pregnenolone sulfate possibly the most important precursor.
  - ■ Possible role in parturition.
- Amniotic fluid progesterone.
  - ■ Maximal levels at 10 to 20 weeks, then decreases during the remainder of the pregnancy.
  - ■ Myometrial levels are 3 times greater than in plasma in early pregnancy; they are equal at term.
- 17-Hydroxyprogesterone levels rise early in pregnancy (corpus luteum production).
  - ■ Return to baseline after the tenth week as the placenta has little 17α-hydroxylase activity.
  - ■ Rise again in the 32nd week, representing placental utilization of fetal precursors.
- Progesterone metabolites—two active metabolites of P_4 are as follows:
  - ■ 5α-Pregnene 3,20-dione.
    - ◇ Tenfold increase in pregnancy.
    - ◇ Contributes to the refractory state against angiotensin II; no difference between normal and hypertensive pregnancies.
  - ■ Deoxycorticosterone.
    - ◇ Shows 1,200× increase over nonpregnant state.
    - ◇ Some secondary to elevations in cortisol-binding globulin (which increases by 3 to 4 times in pregnancy).
    - ◇ Most resulting from the increased 21-hydroxylation activity in the kidney.
    - ◇ No known physiologic role (Fig. 8.1).
- Role of progesterone in pregnancy.
  - ■ Maternal immune suppression.
  - ■ Prepare and maintain endometrium to allow implantation; progesterone is required for normal implantation, whereas estradiol is not.
    - ◇ Human chorionic gonadotropin (hCG) must appear by the tenth day after ovulation to rescue the corpus luteum.
    - ◇ Hormone secretion by the corpus luteum continues as a result of hCG.
      - ○ Progesterone: 25 mg daily.
      - ○ Estradiol: 0.5 mg daily; increased placental contribution by 4 to 5 weeks of pregnancy.
  - ■ Progesterone serves as a precursor for fetal adrenal gland glucocorticoids and mineralocorticoids, but cortisol is also derived from LDL cholesterol in fetal circulation.

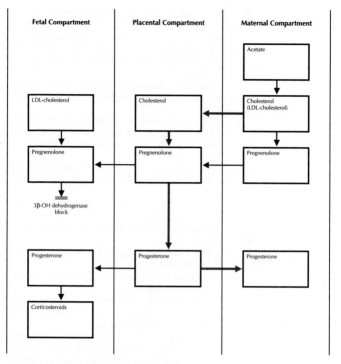

Figure 8.1.   Hormonal interactions between the fetal, placental, and maternal compartments in pregnancy.

> ◊ The fetal zone of the adrenal produces 3β-hydroxy-Δ^5 pregnenolone and dehydroepi-androsterone (DHEA), not Δ^4 steroids like progesterone.
> ◊ The fetus must therefore borrow progesterone.
> ◊ The fetus provides C-19 steroids for estradiol production and draws upon placental progesterone to produce:
>   ○ Cortisol.
>   ○ Corticosterone.
>   ○ Aldosterone.
- Estrogens.
  - Estrogen production is under fetal control.
  - Placenta lacks 17-hydroxylation and 17,20-desmolase activity (as well as 16α-hydroxylase activity); C-21 structures cannot be transformed into C-19 structures.
  - Early pregnancy androgens are derived from the maternal bloodstream.

- By 20 weeks, most are from the fetus—90% of estriol is synthesized in fetal adrenal gland from dehydroepiandrosterone sulfate (DHEAS).
  - ◊ Fetal zone has low (possibly absent) 3β-hydroxysteroid dehydrogenase (HSD) activity.
  - ◊ Increased activity is noted in cell culture.
- The fetus rapidly conjugates steroids with sulfate.
  - ◊ This is possibly a protective mechanism.
  - ◊ Placenta must cleave sulfate conjugates; sulfatase activity is therefore critical for steroid production.
- DHEAS is provided by the fetal adrenal gland.
  - ◊ The placenta lacks 16α-hydroxylation activity.
  - ◊ Estriol must be derived from fetal precursors: 16α-hydroxy DHEAS; after birth, neonatal 16α-hydroxylase activity disappears.
  - ◊ The fetal adrenal gland produces 200 mg/day of DHEAS.
    - ○ This is 10 times greater than maternal production.
    - ○ Maternal contribution is limited as is demonstrated by pregnancies with anencephalic fetuses.
      - □ No fetal adrenal activity is present.
      - □ Very low estradiol and estriol levels are found in these pregnancies (Fig. 8.2).
- Estrogens in pregnancy.
  - Estrone (increases by 100 times over nonpregnant state).
    - ◊ Rises by approximately 6 to 10 weeks of pregnancy.
    - ◊ Two to 30 ng/mL at term.
    - ◊ Wide range of values can be seen.
  - Estradiol (100 times increase over nonpregnant state).
    - ◊ Rise begins at 6 to 8 weeks of pregnancy.
    - ◊ Varies between 6 and 40 ng/mL.
      - ○ At 36 weeks, an accelerated increase in levels is seen.
      - ○ At term, an equal amount is formed from maternal and fetal DHEAS production; its importance in fetal monitoring is negligible.
  - Estriol (increased by 1,000 times over nonpregnant state).
    - ◊ First detected at 9 weeks of pregnancy concurrent with fetal adrenal 16-hydroxy DHEAS production.
    - ◊ Plateaus at 31 to 35 weeks.
    - ◊ Increases again at 35 to 36 weeks.

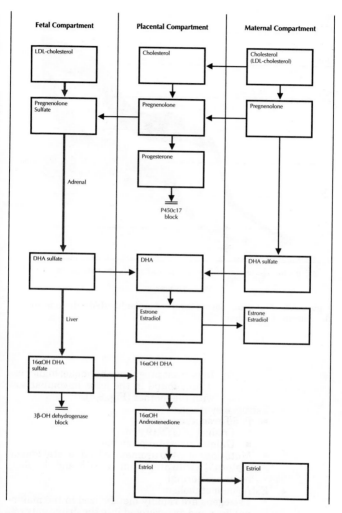

Figure 8.2.   Estrogen production in the fetal, placental, and maternal compartments in pregnancy. Abbreviation: DHA, dehydroepiandrosterone.

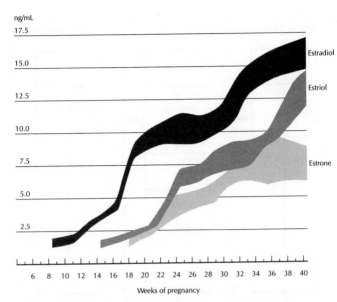

Figure 8.3.   Maternal plasma levels of unconjugated estrogens over the course of gestation.

◇   Important pregnancy hormone; higher estriol is found in the fetus in comparison with the mother (Fig. 8.3).
- ♦ Estrogen synthesis.
  - P450 aromatase enzyme.
    - Product of CYP19 gene.
    - Unique placental promoter.
  - Mutations of P450 aromatase lead to fetal and/or maternal virilization, but growth and development are normal.
- ♦ Estrogen metabolism.
  - Estrogens are rapidly metabolized in the maternal liver and are excreted into the urine; only 8% to 10% of maternal estriol is unconjugated.
  - Usually glucosiduronates are conjugated at 16; also 3-glucosiduronate and 3-sulfate-16-glucosiduronate.
- ♦ The fetal adrenal cortex.
  - Differentiated by 8 to 9 weeks of pregnancy into the thick fetal zone and thin outer definitive zone (cortisol source).
  - Gland increases to the size of the fetal kidney by the end of the first trimester; the secondary growth spurt occurs at 34 to 35 weeks.
  - Involutes following delivery; is replaced by the expansion of the adult adrenal cortex.

- Fetal DHEA and DHEAS rise steadily as 3β-HSD activity and gene expression are suppressed.
- Early in pregnancy, the adrenal can grow and function without adrenocorticotropic hormone (ACTH) stimulation, possibly in response to hCG.
- After 15 to 20 weeks, fetal ACTH is required.
- During the last 12 to 14 weeks of pregnancy, a large increase in the size of the gland is seen, while fetal ACTH levels are decreased.
  - Perhaps a growth-initiating mechanism.
  - Possibly resulting from fetal production versus the ACTH effect.
- ACTH actions.
  - Essential for morphologic development.
  - Activates steroidogenesis via adenylate cyclase.
  - Increases the concentration of LDL receptors.
    - ◇ Usual source of cholesterol.
    - ◇ Some synthesis of cholesterol is possible in association with low levels of LDL.
- Maintenance of ACTH stimulation from the fetal pituitary.
  - It is protected by placental estrogen.
  - Estradiol stimulates placental 11β-HSD activity and prevents maternal cortisol from reaching the fetus.
  - In late gestation, fetal ACTH increases, the fetal adrenal gland undergoes greater maturation, and fetal cortisol increases (from endogenous cholesterol).
- Autocrine and paracrine regulation.
  - The fetal adrenal produces inhibin.
    - ◇ α Subunit is preferentially increased by ACTH.
    - ◇ β Subunit is not expressed.
  - Activin enhances ACTH, stimulates steroidogenesis, and inhibits mitogenesis.
    - ◇ Shifts fetal adrenal cells from DHEAS to cortisol production.
    - ◇ Possible mechanism of fetal adrenal remodeling after birth; specific action for inhibin in the fetal adrenal cells has not been described.
- Insulin-like growth factors (IGFs).
  - IGFs are important in mediating the tropic effects of ACTH.
    - ◇ IGF-II production very significant in the fetal adrenal.
    - ◇ Mediation of ACTH-induced growth.
  - Adult adrenal secretes mainly IGF-I.
    - ◇ IGF-II transcription is stimulated by ACTH.
    - ◇ IGF-II increases P450c17.
- Estrogen environment.
  - Estrogens at a high concentration inhibit 3β-HSD.

- DHEAS secretion is enhanced by ACTH and IGF-II.
- Estradiol concentrations of between 10 to 100 ng/mL inhibit cortisol secretion; the mechanism is independent of estrogen reception.
- Baboon experiments.
  - Treatment of neonatal baboons with estrogen and progesterone did not halt the regression of the fetal zone and DHEAS production.
  - Treatment of a pregnant baboon with estradiol reduced DHEAS production; the possible suggestion is that exogenous steroids can affect the fetal adrenal microenvironment.
  - This estrogen explanation is challenged by *in vitro* human fetal adrenal studies.
    - ◇ Estradiol and IGF-II direct steroidogenesis to DHEAS in a mechanism that is NOT due to inhibition of 3β-HSD.
    - ◇ Also, no estradiol receptors in the fetal zone of monkeys.
- Measurement of estrogen in pregnancy.
  - The amount of estrogen in maternal blood and urine is indicative of placental function and fetal health.
  - About 90% of maternal estriol is derived from fetal precursors.
  - Increased adrenal androgen production is secondary to increased fetal ACTH.
  - Chronic fetal stress differs from acute stress; decreased androgen production occurs in chronic stress.
- Measurement of estriol (maternal).
  - Twenty-four–hour urine collection was the standard assay of fetal well-being for many years.
  - Replaced by radioimmunoassay of unconjugated estriol in plasma.
    - Short half-life (5 to 10 minutes).
    - Less variation than urinary or total blood estriol.
  - Estriol measurement has been superseded by various biophysical fetal-monitoring techniques.
- Amniotic fluid estriol.
  - Correlates with the fetal estrogen pattern.
  - Not present as 16-glucosiduronate or 3-sulfate-16-glycosiduronate.
  - Very little unconjugated estriol is present; free estriol is rapidly transferred across the placenta.
  - Glucosiduronates predominate in the fetal urine and amniotic fluid.
  - No clinical usefulness has been identified.
- Estetrol.
  - 15α-Hydroxyestriol is formed from a fetal precursor; dependent upon 15α-hydroxylation activity in the fetal liver.
  - No clinical use of measurements.

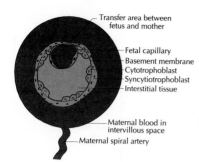

Transfer area between
fetus and mother

Fetal capillary
Basement membrane
Cytotrophoblast
Syncytiotrophoblast
Interstitial tissue

Maternal blood in
intervillous space
Maternal spiral artery

**Figure 8.4. Transfer of
substances between the
fetus and the mother in
the placenta.**

- ♦ Placental sulfatase deficiency.
  - • X-linked metabolic disease occurring in from 1 of 2,000 to 1 of 3,000 newborn males.
  - • Cannot hydrolyze DHEAS or 16α-hydroxy DHEAS; placenta cannot form normal amounts of estrogen.
  - • May present clinically as cervical dystocia that is resistant to oxytocin in a postdate fetus.
  - • Genetic locus maps to the distal short arm of the X chromosome.
  - • Characteristic findings.
    - ■ Low estriol and estetrol in mother.
    - ■ Greatly increased amniotic fluid concentration of DHEAS; normal levels of DHEA, androstenedione.
  - • Diagnosis.
    - ■ Suggested by hormone assays.
    - ■ Definitive diagnosis by demonstration of decreased sulfate activity *in vitro* with assessment of placental tissue.
  - • Clinical manifestations.
    - ■ Ichthyosis occurs between birth and the age of 6 months.
    - ■ Associated with corneal opacities, pyloric stenosis, and cryptorchidism.
    - ■ Perinatal outcome is usually good, so the need for antenatal diagnosis is difficult to justify.
II. Protein Hormones of Pregnancy
  - ♦ Cytotrophoblast.
    - • Separate mononuclear cells in early pregnancy.
    - • Represents the basic placental stem cell.
  - ♦ Syncytiotrophoblast.
    - • Continuum of multinucleate layer on surface.
    - • Functional cell of the placenta (Fig. 8.4).
      - ■ Makes activated inhibin, activin, and neurohormones.
      - ■ Direct contact with maternal blood in the intervillous space (Fig. 8.5).
  - ♦ Hypothalamic-like releasing hormones found in the placenta.
    - • Gonadotropin-releasing hormone (GnRH).

Fetal Compartment	Placental Compartment	Maternal Compartment
Alpha-fetoprotein	Hypothalamic-like hormones 　GnRH 　CRH 　TRH 　Somatostatin 　GHRH	Decidual proteins 　Prolactin 　Relaxin 　IGFBP-1 　Interleukin-1 　Colony stimulating factor-1 　Progesterone-associated 　endometrial protein
	Pituitary-like hormones 　HCG 　HPL 　HGH 　HCT 　ACTH 　Oxytocin	Corpus luteum proteins 　Relaxin 　Prorenin
	Growth factors 　IGF-I 　IGF-II 　Epidermal growth factor 　Platelet-derived growth factor 　Fibroblast growth factor 　Transforming growth factor-α 　Transforming growth factor-β 　Inhibin 　Activin 　Follistatin	
	Cytokines 　Interleukins 　Interferons 　Tissue necrosis factor-α 　Colony stimulating factor-1	
	Other 　Opiates 　Prorenin 　Pregnancy-specific 　β_1-glycoprotein 　Pregnancy-associated 　plasma protein A	

Figure 8.5. Proteins associated with pregnancy, according to compartment.

- Localized in the cytotrophoblast and syncytiotrophoblast.
- Regulation of the placental steroid, prostaglandin (PG) release, and hCG.
- Levels are highest in early pregnancy according to some, but constant levels have been found by others.
- Placental binding site has lower affinity than other receptors (e.g., pituitary, ovaries, testis); high concentrations are not needed given the proximity—high serum concentration is related to proximity.
- Receptor is produced in a pattern that parallels hCG secretion; further evidence of the role of placental GnRH and its receptor in hCG secretion.
- GnRH release.

◇ Increased by estrogen, activin A, insulin, and PG.
◇ Decreased by progesterone, opiates, inhibin, and follistatin.
- Corticotropin-releasing hormone (CRH).
  - Produced by trophoblast, fetal membranes, and decidua.
  - Production decreased by progesterone and increased by glucocorticoids; consistent with increased levels of ACTH, cortisol is found in late pregnancy.
  - Regulated by vasopressin, norepinephrine, angiotensin II, PGs, neuropeptide Y, and oxytocin.
  - Stimulated by activin; inhibited by inhibin and nitric oxide.
  - Increase in CRH during pregnancy.
    ◇ Binding protein is produced in the placenta, membranes, and decidua; maternal levels decrease until term.
    ◇ Maternal CRH increases in stressed pregnancies; represents a possible increase in placental CRH in response to fetal pituitary ACTH and adrenal cortisol.
◆ Human chorionic gonadotropin (Fig. 8.6).
- Glycoprotein: a peptide framework with carbohydrate side chains.
  - Alterations in carbohydrate component alter biologic properties.
    ◇ hCG half-life is 24 hours versus 2 hours for luteinizing hormone (LH).
    ◇ Greatest sialic acid content is found in hCG.
  - Structure is similar to follicle-stimulating hormone (FSH), LH, and thyroid-stimulating hormone (TSH) with α, β components.
- α Subunit gene on chromosome 6, which is identical in all glycoproteins (92 amino acids).
- β Subunit gene on chromosome 19; source of biologic and immunologic variation (145 amino acids with unique 24-amino-acid tailpiece).
- β Subunit of hCG.
  - One hundred forty-five amino acids residues, including unique C-terminal 24-amino-acid tail; allows highly specific antibodies; detected by immunoassays.
    ◇ In carboxyl terminal tailpiece four glycosylation sites exist, which explains the increased half-life.
    ◇ Only the placenta produces glycosylated hCG; hCG is synthesized in all human tissues.
  - hCG β subunit promoter does not have steroid hormone response elements.
- Genetic aspects.
  - Single human α subunit gene at 6p21.1-23.
    ◇ Single promoter site is subject to multiple signals.

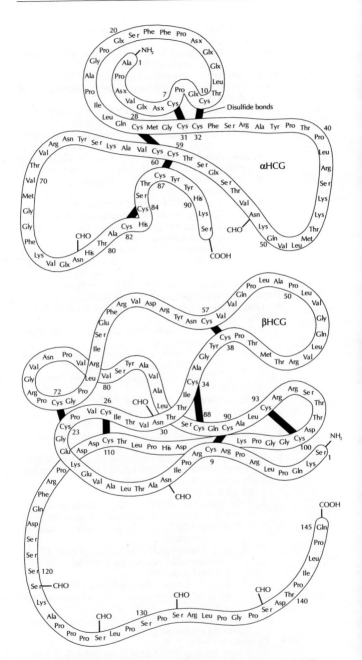

Figure 8.6.   Structure of human chorionic gonadotropin (hCG).

◇ Regulation of α subunit gene expression depends on cell type.
  ○ Gonadotrophs → GnRH signaling via diacylglycerol, inositol 1,4,5-trisphosphate (IP_3), and calcium, which increase protein kinase C activity and regulate the promoter; growth factor and steroids appear to regulate expression.
  ○ Placenta—primary signal via adenosine monophosphate–protein kinase A pathway.
◇ β Subunits are restricted in all types.
■ Six genes for the β-hCG component (only one gene for β-LH); only two genes are actively transcribed; β subunit genes of LH, hCG, and TSH are located in a cluster on 19q13.3.
• Only primates and horses have β-hCG genes; in horses, β–chorionic gonadotropin = β-LH gene.
  ■ β-hCG is 96% homologous with β-LH.
  ■ Single mutation creates a read-through mutation.
• Regulation of hCG production.
  ■ Placental function is more complex, and a simple presentation is not possible.
    ◇ GnRH synthesized in placental cells stimulates hCG production.
    ◇ Inhibin restores and activin enhances GnRH–hCG system.
  ■ Locally produced hormones, growth factors, and peptides work together to regulate placental function; the role of hCG is to maintain the corpus luteum function and to support pregnancy.
  ■ hCG gene expression is present in both the cytotrophoblast and syncytiotrophoblast (mainly in syncytiotrophoblast).
    ◇ Maternal levels.
      ○ Approximately 100 IU/L at missed menses.
      ○ Reaches 100,000 IU/L maximum at 10 weeks; questionable down-regulation by corpus luteum receptors.
      ○ Decreases to 10,000 to 20,000 IU/L at 18 to 20 weeks, at which level it remains until term.
    ◇ With advancing gestation, increased levels of "nicked" hCG are found.
      ○ Also decreased glycosylation.
      ○ In addition, increase in secondary isoforms.
    ◇ Clearance is via the renal system.
    ◇ Levels are higher in female fetuses; the mechanism and purpose are unknown.
  ■ Clinical uses of measurement of β-hCG.
    ◇ Gestational trophoblastic neoplasia (GTN) is distinguished by β-hCG production, and whole hCG production may not occur.

- ○ Rate of hydatidiform mole is between 1 in 600 to 1 in 1,000 to 2,000.
- ○ β-hCG should fall to a nondetectable level by the 16th week after evacuation of the mole.
- ◇ Ectopic pregnancy (see Chapter 32).
  - ○ Normal rise in hCG usually indicates a normal pregnancy.
  - ○ When titer >1,000 to 1,500 IU/L, the gestational sac should be visible on an endovaginal sonogram.
- ■ hCG in nonpregnant state.
  - ◇ Secreted in men and women in pulsatile fashion similar to LH.
  - ◇ Pituitary gland origin; only rarely reaches detectable levels.
  - ◇ Free α subunit is also produced in healthy individuals.
- ♦ Human placental lactogen (HPL).
  - • Also called human chorionic somatomammotropin.
  - • Secreted by syncytiotrophoblast; 191–amino-acid single chain held together by two disulfide bonds.
  - • Similar to human growth hormone (HGH), but only 3% of HGH has somatotropin activity.
    - ■ HPL–HGH gene family consists of five genes on chromosome 17q22-q24.
      - ◇ Two are for HGH; three, for HPL.
      - ◇ Only two HPL genes are active in the placenta; the third gene generates a protein of limited activity.
    - ■ Lactogenic contribution is uncertain in the human pregnancy.
      - ◇ Short half-life (approximately 15 minutes).
      - ◇ Levels correlate with fetal and placental weight.
      - ◇ Increases during pregnancy, plateaus during the last 4 weeks (5 to 7 mg/mL); very high levels are found in a multiple pregnancy (up to 40 mg/mL).
  - • Physiologic function.
    - ■ Neither growth hormone–releasing hormone (GHRH) nor somatostatin influences placental HPL secretion.
    - ■ In the mother, HPL stimulates IGF-I production and insulin secretion and induces insulin resistance and carbohydrate intolerance.
    - ■ HPL increases with hypoglycemia and decreases with hyperglycemia.
  - • Metabolic role.
    - ■ HPL mobilizes lipids as free fatty acids.
    - ■ Pregnancy represents a state of accelerated starvation.

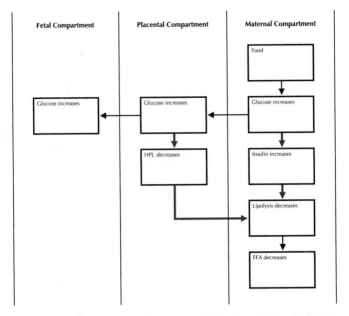

Figure 8.7. Human placental lactogen (HPL) levels in the fed state.

    ◇ Constant flow of glucose from mother to fetus.

    ◇ Human HPL (and estrogen and progesterone) interfere with maternal insulin activity.

■ In the fasting state, HPL stimulates lipolysis so the mother can have metabolic fuel while conserving amino acids and glucose for the fetus.

    ◇ Maternal ketones rise.

    ◇ The fetus can also use ketones for energy source.

■ HPL results in a free fatty acid increase.

■ This directly decreases insulin-directed entry of glucose into the cells; it involves IGF at the cellular level (Figs. 8.7 and 8.8).

■ It provides fuel for the fetus between maternal meals.

■ Fetal undernutrition results in an elevated fetal IGF-I and in a possible risk of diabetes as an adult.

■ HPL may be fetal HGH as normal growth is seen in anencephalic fetuses.

■ Clinical uses of HPL: although blood levels are related to placental function, it has no clear-cut role in clinical management.

♦ Human chorionic thyrotropin (HCT).

    • Similar in size and action to TSH.

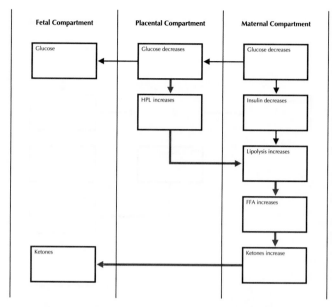

Figure 8.8.   Human placental lactogen (HPL) levels in the fasting state.

- Placental content very small; unlikely to have physiologic importance.
- Does not share common α subunit.
- hCG also has thyrotropic activity.
  - Activity is 1/4,000th of that of TSH.
  - A correlation exists between elevated thyroid function and hyperemesis gravidarum; hCG with reduced sialic acid content is increased in patients with hyperemesis.
- Human chorionic adrenocorticotropin.
  - Maternal free cortisol rises throughout pregnancy due to ACTH and CRH production.
  - Placental ACTH is higher than is expected.
    - Pregnant women also have an increased resistance to dexamethasone suppression.
    - It is probably stimulated by locally produced CRH in the cytotrophoblast.
  - Placental proopiomelanocortin (POMC) gene expression is present throughout pregnancy, possibly to raise maternal adrenal activity, thus providing increased substrate for placental steroidogenesis.
  - Maternal ACTH response to CRH is blunted during pregnancy.
  - CRH levels in maternal plasma are elevated.

- Oxytocin is a powerful stimulator of CRH and ACTH placental production; fall in CRH-binding protein levels near term allows for increased cortisol availability during parturition.
- Pathologic states during pregnancy also increase maternal and fetal CRH, which can stimulate PG synthesis in the placenta and fetal membranes.
- Growth hormone, growth hormone–releasing hormone, and somatostatin.
  - GHRH and somatostatin are found in the placenta.
  - Somatostatin is found in the decidua; it is decreased with increasing gestation.
  - One of the two growth hormone (GH) genes on chromosome 17 is expressed only in the syncytiotrophoblast.
  - Placental GH gradually replaces maternal GH; by term, maternal GH is undetectable.
  - Changes in maternal IGF and insulin-like growth factor–binding proteins (IGFBPs) reflect placental GH regulation.
  - Maternal IGF-I levels increase during pregnancy.
  - Placental GH is not regulated by placental GHRH but by maternal glucose levels.
- α-Fetoprotein (AFP).
  - Relatively unique glycoprotein.
    - Five hundred ninety amino acids.
    - Four percent carbohydrate.
  - Derived from fetal liver and yolk sac.
  - Function unknown; may serve as steroid hormone protein carrier.
  - Levels peak in fetal blood by end of first trimester; levels gradually decrease until 32 weeks when the decrease becomes rapid.
  - Highly concentrated in the fetal nervous system; elevated maternal blood levels associated with the following:
    - Neural tube defects.
    - Intestinal obstruction.
    - Omphalocele, gastroschisis.
    - Congenital nephrosis.
    - Multiple pregnancy.
    - Adverse pregnancy outcome.
    - Miscarriage.
    - Stillbirth.
    - Pregnancy-induced hypertension.
    - Preterm birth.
  - Multiple marker screening.
    - Low maternal AFP is associated with trisomy 21; extensive overlap occurs.
    - Several other placental products are associated with trisomy 21.
      - ◇ hCG, HPL, and free β-hCG.
      - ◇ Lower levels of estriol in trisomy 21.
    - Use of triple marker screening: AFP, hCG (or β-hCG), and unconjugated estriol.

◇ Detects 85% of neural tube defects.
◇ Detects 80% of Down syndrome; only 50% of chromosomal abnormalities are detected.
- Use of AFP and free β-hCG may be more accurate and less expensive.
- Gestational dating is critical for risk assessment.

◆ Relaxin.
  • Peptide hormone produced by the corpus luteum in pregnancy.
  • Two short peptide chains (24 and 29 amino acids) linked by disulfide bridges.
  • May also be produced in the placenta, decidua, and chorion.
  • Role in early pregnancy unknown.
  • May be helpful as a cervical ripening agent.

◆ Prolactin.
  • Synthesized by endometrium after decidualization.
  • Control of synthesis uncertain; may require the combined effects of progestin and estrogen plus other placental and decidual factors.
  • Not produced by the trophoblast or fetal membranes during pregnancy.
    - Decidua prolactin is the source of amniotic fluid prolactin.
    - Transcribed by the gene with an additional exon.
  • Prolactin levels rise during pregnancy.
    - Peak between 200 to 400 ng/mL at 8 weeks.
    - Probably the result of estrogen suppression of prolactin-inhibiting factor (dopamine).
  • Amniotic fluid levels parallel maternal concentrations until the tenth week.
    - They rise markedly until the 20th week; decrease until delivery.
    - Levels remain unaffected by dopamine agonist therapy.
  • Prolactin receptor is expressed in fetal and maternal tissues; decreasing order of intensity as follows:
    - Chorionic cytotrophoblast.
    - Decidua.
    - Amnion.
    - Syncytiotrophoblast.
  • Decidual and amniotic fluid prolactin levels are lower in hypertensive pregnancies and in patients with polyhydramnios; receptors are decreased in the chorion of patients with polyhydramnios.
  • Amniotic fluid prolactin regulates fetal water and electrolyte balance.

◆ Cytokines and growth factors.
  • Placenta synthesizes many proteins.
  • Communication occurs between the maternal decidual and fetal tissue cytokines.

- ■ IL-1β is produced by the decidua.
- ■ Colony stimulating factor–1 is produced by the decidua and the placenta.
- ■ IL-6 is also produced by the placenta; stimulates hCG release.
- ■ IL-1 and tumor necrosis factor–α synergistically release IL-6.
- IGF and IGFBP system.
  - ■ Both IGF-I and IGF-II are involved in prenatal and postnatal growth; they do not cross into fetal circulation.
  - ■ The fetus can influence maternal IGF-I levels via HPL secretion; no major changes in IGF-II levels seen during pregnancy.
  - ■ IGFBPs modulate IGF availability; IGFBP-1 is equivalent to placental protein 12.
    - ◊ Decidual products regulated by progesterone.
    - ◊ The dominant binding protein in pregnancy.
  - ■ IGF and IGFBP systems modulate the fetal growth state; the newborn's weight correlates positively with maternal IGF-I levels and inversely with IGFBP-1 levels.
- ◆ Inhibin, activin, and follistatin.
  - Placental production of inhibin leads to high maternal inhibin levels.
  - Inhibin A is the principal bioactive inhibin during pregnancy (inhibin B levels are very low); peaks at 8 weeks, then decreases, but rises in the third trimester to levels 100 times greater than during the normal cycle.
  - Maternal gonadotropins are profoundly suppressed.
  - Activin A also increases in maternal circulation.
  - Placental actions: regulate GnRH, hCG, and steroids.
  - Follistatin binds activin and antagonizes the stimulatory effects of activin.
- ◆ Endogenous opiates.
  - Originate from fetal and maternal pituitary glands.
  - Intermediate lobe of the pituitary may be the major source of endorphins.
  - The syncytiotrophoblast can also respond to CRH with all the products of POMC metabolism.
  - Their function during pregnancy remains unclear.
- ◆ Renin–angiotensin system.
  - Levels of prorenin increase tenfold in early pregnancy; from an ovarian source in response to hCG stimulus.
  - No change in blood renin levels is observed.
  - Possible role in ovarian system includes steroidogenesis, regulation of calcium metabolism, or angiogenesis.
  - Potential role of prorenin is seen in early pregnancy.

- Maternal renin activity increases fourfold by midgestation.
- ♦ Atrial natriuretic peptide.
  - Derived from atrial tissue and the placenta.
  - Potent natriuretic, diuretic, and smooth muscle relaxant.
  - Circulates as a hormone in the fetus.
- ♦ Other proteins.
  - Early pregnancy factor is detected 1 to 2 days after coitus in the conception cycle.
    - Produced by the ovary in response to the embryo.
    - Has immunosuppressive properties.
  - Pregnancy-specific γ1-glycoprotein.
    - Physiologic function unknown.
    - Coded for on chromosome 19.

III. Prostaglandins
- ♦ Prostaglandin biosynthesis.
  - The family with the greatest biologic activity is derived from arachidonic acid (AA).
    - AA is obtained from direct dietary sources (meats) or from precursors (linoleic acid) in vegetables.
    - The majority of AA is covalently found in esterified form in phospholipids.
  - The rate-limiting step in synthesis is the release of free AA.
    - Phospholipase A_2 is an important initiator of synthesis; AA is abundant in position 2 of phospholipids.
    - Phospholipase C can also provide AA.
  - Eicosanoids—all 20-carbon derivatives.
  - Prostanoids—only those containing a structural ring.
  - The two pathways after the release of AA are the following:
    - Lipoxygenase pathway.
    - Cyclooxygenase (COX) pathway (PG endoperoxide H synthase pathway).
  - Lipoxygenase pathway—three enzymes that lead to active compounds are as follows:
    - 5-Lipoxygenase.
      - ◇ Leads to leukotrienes.
      - ◇ Potent increases in microvascular permeability.
    - 12-Lipoxygenase—leads to 12-hydroxyeicosatetraenoic acid (leukostatic agent).
    - 15-Lipoxygenase—lipoxins produced (Fig. 8.9).
  - COX pathway.
    - Leads to PGs—PGG_2 and PGH_2, which are the "mothers" of all other PGs.
    - Numerical subscript refers to the number of double bonds.
      - ◇ Linoleic acid leads to the PG_1 series.
      - ◇ Pentanoic acid leads to the PG_3 series.

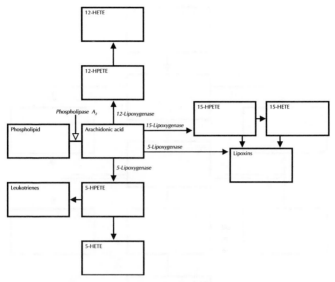

Figure 8.9. Arachidonic acid metabolism.

- ■ PGs of importance in reproduction are PGE_2 and $PGF_{2\alpha}$ (and possibly PGD_2).
- ■ COX enzyme (PG synthase) exists in two forms: COX-1 and COX-2.
  - ◇ Prostacyclin is produced by COX-1.
  - ◇ Inflammatory stimuli induce COX-2 (Fig. 8.10).
- ♦ Thromboxane and prostacyclin.
  - • Thromboxanes (half-life 30 seconds) are not true PGs; lack pentane ring.
  - • PGI_2 (half-life 2 to 3 minutes) is a legitimate PG.
  - • These two can be viewed as opponents.
    - ■ Thromboxane A_2 (TXA_2) is the most potent vasoconstrictor known.
    - ■ PGI_2 is potent vasodilator.

TXA_2 production	PGI_2 production
Platelets	Heart
Lungs in response to	Stomach
pathologic stimuli	Normal lungs
Spleen	Vessels

  - • Platelets.
    - ■ Primary function is preservation of the vascular system.
    - ■ Stick to foreign surfaces or tissue (adhesion).
    - ■ Stick to each other (aggregation).
    - ■ Vascular endothelium produces PGI_2 to prevent the sticking of platelets, which is the defensive role for PGI_2 (Fig. 8.11).

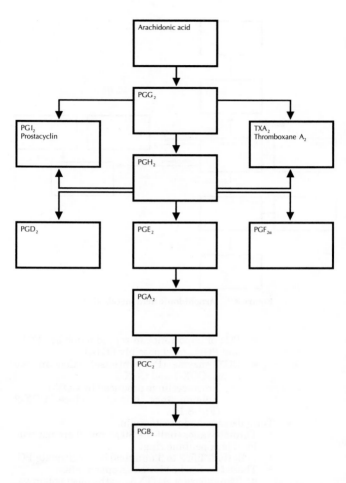

Figure 8.10. Derivation of various prostaglandins from their precursor, arachidonic acid.

- ■ PGI_2 may play an important role in pregnancy.
- ■ Pathologic conditions may result in vascular disease through the effects on PGI_2 action.
  - ◇ LDL inhibits PGI_2 action.
  - ◇ Smokers who use oral contraceptives demonstrate decreased levels of PGI_2.
  - ◇ Pregnant diabetics release more TXA_2.
  - ◇ Onion and garlic inhibit platelet aggregation and TXA_2 synthesis.
- • Dietary effects.
  - ■ High content of pentanoic acid in Eskimo and Japanese diets (fish are 8% to 12% pentanoic acid).

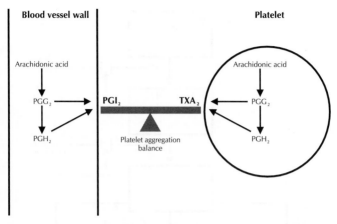

**Figure 8.11.   The balance between the roles of prostacyclin (PGI₂)
and thromboxane A₂ (TXA₂) in platelet function.**

- ■ Pentanoic acid is the precursor of PGs with
  three double bands.
- ■ PGI₃ is active, but TXA₃ is not.
- ◆ Metabolism.
  - • Initiated by 15-hydroxyprostaglandin dehydroge-
    nase.
  - • Occurs mainly in lungs, kidneys, and liver;
    nearly all active PGs are metabolized in the lungs
    during one passage.
  - • Rapid half-lives: require the measurement of
    inactive end-products to evaluate the efficiency of
    drugs.
- ◆ Prostaglandin inhibition.
  - • Corticosteroids.
    - ■ Induce synthesis of lipocortins or annexins
      that block the action of phospholipase.
    - ■ Reduce the availability of AA for both path-
      ways.
  - • Aspirin—selectively inhibits COX in an irre-
    versible fashion.
  - • Nonsteroidal antiinflammatory drugs (NSAIDs).
    - ■ Form a reversible bond with the active site of
      the enzyme.
    - ■ Acetaminophen inhibits COX in the central
      nervous system.
      - ◇ No antiinflammatory properties.
      - ◇ Good analgesic and antipyretic properties.
    - ■ Analgesic, antipyretic, and antiinflammatory
      action is mediated by inhibition of COX-1 and
      COX-2; aspirin, indomethacin, and ibuprofen
      are more potent inhibitors of COX-1.
    - ■ Reduction in gastric mucosa COX-1 and, thus,
      in PGE₂ formation leads to ulcers.

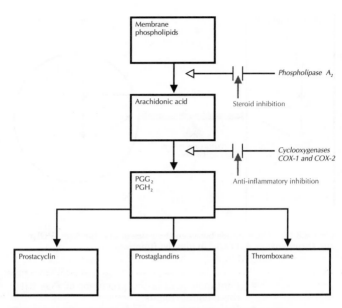

Fig. 8.12. The antiinflammatory and steroid inhibition of prostaglandins.

■ Platelets are exclusively COX-1.
  ◇ Aspirin inhibits activity for the lifetime of platelets (8 to 10 days).
  ◇ Higher aspirin doses will decrease PGI_2 synthesis as well as TXA_2 synthesis (Fig. 8.12).

IV. Endocrinology of Parturition
  ♦ Hormonal changes in the uteroplacental environment lead to the eventual development of uterine contractions.
  ♦ Ovine parturition.
    • Fetal pituitary ACTH increases, leading to fetal cortisol elevation; maternal stimulation of the fetal adrenal is not a factor.
    • Cortisol secretion initiates a chain of events.
    • P450c17 activity increases (possibly as a result of PGE_2); progesterone declines.
    • Increased progesterone metabolism and progesterone withdrawal lead to increased myometrial activity.
    • Dihydroxyprogesterone serves as a precursor for estrogen synthesis.
    • Final event is rise in $PGF_{2\alpha}$ as a result of rise in estrogen.
  ♦ Human parturition.
    • Steroid events are not identical to those in the ewe.

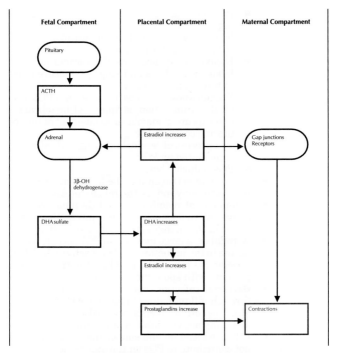

Figure 8.13.   Hormonal changes leading to contractions in human parturition in fetal, placental, and maternal compartments.

- ■ More extended time scale.
- ■ Proportionally similar.
- • Cortisol in the amniotic fluid rises dramatically beginning at 34 to 36 weeks; cord blood levels decrease after the induction of labor or elective cesarean.
- • Maternal cortisol is metabolized to cortisone by the placenta; the fetal lung and liver can convert cortisone to cortisol.
- • Estrogen production plays an important role in human parturition.
- • The role of progesterone is less clear; the removal of local progesterone could lead to uterine contractions (Fig. 8.13).
- ◆ Prostaglandins.
  - • Evidence for a role for PG in parturition includes the following:
    - ■ PG levels in maternal blood and amniotic fluid increase in association with labor.
    - ■ AA levels in the amniotic fluid also rise in labor, and arachidonate injected into the amniotic sac initiates parturition.

- Patients taking high doses of aspirin have a highly significant increase in the average length of gestation, the incidence of postmaturity, and the duration of labor.
- Indomethacin prevents the normal onset of labor in monkeys and stops premature labor in human pregnancies.
- Stimuli known to cause the release of PGs (cervical manipulation, stripping of membranes, and rupture of membranes) augment or induce uterine contractions.
- The process of cervical ripening and softening is mediated by PGs.
- PGs induce labor.

- The role of estrogen may be key; a marked rise near term may induce the release of AA.
- Human fetal membranes and decidua are very active; steroidogenic and PG interactions may result in the changes needed for parturition.
- With labor, a large increase in PGE_2 occurs; could be due to the induction of COX-2 activity by CRH.
- Specific PG inhibitors are absent in tissues from patients with spontaneous labor.
- Bacterial infection may initiate preterm labor through inflammatory induction of COX-2.
- Multiple other agents may also play a role, including activin, inhibin, and cytokines.
- PGs produced on one side of the membranes do not contribute to PGs on the other side.
  - Uterine contractions must be primarily influenced by decidual or myometrial PGs.
  - Chorion usually forms a barrier, blocking the passage of bioactive PG (Fig. 8.14).
- The role of placental CRH is as follows:
  1. CRH is produced in trophoblast, the fetal membranes, and decidua.
  2. During pregnancy, CRH levels in the amniotic fluid and the maternal circulation progressively increase. Although amniotic fluid levels do not further increase with labor, the highest maternal levels are found at labor and delivery.
  3. Levels of the CRH-binding protein (also produced in the trophoblast, membranes, and decidua) are decreased in the amniotic fluid and the maternal circulation prior to labor. This decrease in CRH-binding protein would allow an increase in CRH activity.
  4. CRH stimulates PG release in the fetal membranes, decidua, and myometrium.
  5. Increased CRH and decreased CRH-binding protein have been measured in women with preterm labor and in women with threatened preterm labor who subsequently deliver within 24 hours.

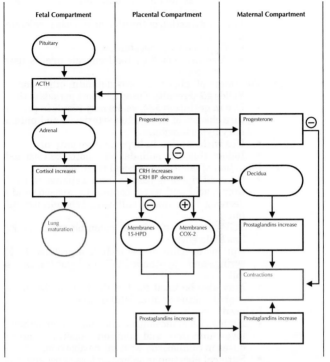

Figure 8.14. Hormonal changes leading to lung maturation and contractions in human parturition in fetal, placental, and maternal compartments.

6. Cortisol, in the presence of progesterone, stimulates (probably by blocking progesterone inhibition) trophoblastic CRH synthesis.

♦ Oxytocin and myometrial responses.

• Oxytocin levels rise significantly, especially during the second stage of labor.

• Monkey studies fail to show a role for fetal oxytocin in parturition.

• Cervical dilation seems to be dependent upon the oxytocin stimulation of PG production, probably in the decidua.

• Oxytocin-receptor concentration increases steadily during pregnancy; the mechanism for increase is likely due to the change in the PG and hormonal milieu.

• The formation of gap junctions in the myometrium is important.

■ A pore (consisting of six special proteins called connexins) forms within the gap junction.

- Provides means of communication between myometrial cells.
- Final contraction of the uterine muscle is calcium-dependent.
  - Opposed by progesterone.
  - Also decreased by β-adrenergic agents used for tocolysis.
- ◆ Treatment of labor with prostaglandin inhibition.
  - Yields good results if used for short periods of time.
  - Use in gestation >34 weeks may result in premature closure of the ductus arteriosus and pulmonary hypertension.
  - Use with caution in hypertensive patients.
  - Indomethacin or sulindac have both been studied.
- ◆ Induction of labor and cervical ripening.
  - Cervical ripening results from a change in hyaluronic acid and water content (increased) and a decrease in dermatan sulfate and chondroitin sulfate.
  - PGF_2 is very effective at ripening, while $PGF_{2\alpha}$ has little effect.
  - Options for clinical use include a prefilled PGE_2 syringe and a synthetic PGE_2 analogue (misoprostol).
  - May also be used for termination of the anencephalic fetus or after fetal demise.
- ◆ Induced abortion.
  - Higher risk of incomplete abortion or hemorrhage, fever, infection, and additional operative procedures in comparison with saline abortion.
  - Surgical abortion is safer and less expensive.
  - Use of PG and RU486 has been proven both effective and safe.
- ◆ Prostaglandins and postpartum hemorrhage.
  - The use of a $PGF_{2\alpha}$ analogue has proven very effective in cases of uterine atony.
  - Administer 0.25 to 0.5 mg up to 4× either intramuscularly or intramyometrially.
  - Avoid use in asthmatics and in patients with severe hypertension.
  - Prostin 15M is (15-S)—15-methyl $PGF_{2\alpha}$.
- V. Prostaglandins and the Fetal Circulation
  - ◆ The ductus arteriosus is very important—59% of cardiac output flows through this connection.
  - ◆ Control of ductal patency and closure is PG-mediated.
  - ◆ Ductal patency can be maintained after birth by the use of PGE_2.
    - Indomethacin can close a patent ductus in 40% of premature infants.
    - This is most effective in infants <30 weeks of gestation and <10 days old.
  - ◆ A fetus exposed to indomethacin can develop a syndrome with premature ductal closure, cardiomegaly, and persistent pulmonary hypertension; this is rare

in pregnancies with exposure at <27 weeks of gestation or with <2 weeks of exposure.
- ◆ PGs also reduce fetal breathing movements; this could explain the decrease of fetal breathing movements in labor.

VI. Fetal Lung Maturation
- ◆ Pulmonary alveoli are lined with surfactant.
  - • Decreases surface tension and facilitates lung expansion.
  - • Present in lesser amounts in preterm infants.
- ◆ Lecithin is the most active and abundant lipid in surfactant; phosphatidylglycerol is the second most active and abundant.
- ◆ Sudden surge in lecithin at about 35 weeks.
- ◆ Ratio of lecithin to sphingomyelin predicts fetal lung maturity; a ratio of >2 indicates primary lung maturity.
- ◆ Final maturation of the lung is marked by phosphatidylglycerol; measurement is not affected by meconium, blood, or vaginal secretions.
- ◆ Accelerated maturation is caused by the following:
  - • Hypertension.
  - • Advanced diabetes.
  - • Hemoglobinopathies.
  - • Heroin addiction.
  - • Poor nutrition.
- ◆ Delayed maturation occurs with the following:
  - • Diabetes.
  - • Rh disease.
- ◆ Fetal cortisol is a requisite for surfactant biosynthesis; results in synergistic action between numerous factors for possible lung maturity.
- ◆ Corticosteroid therapy reduces neonatal mortality, respiratory distress syndrome, and intraventricular hemorrhage.
  - • Administer at 24 to 32 weeks of gestation.
  - • Optimum effect is found after 48 hours and is lost after 7 days.
  - • It is an effective additive to postnatal surfactant administration.

VII. Postpartum Period
- ◆ About 10% to 15% of women become clinically depressed.
- ◆ A 5% to 10% incidence of postpartum thyroiditis is observed.

9

Normal and Abnormal Sexual Development

I. Normal Sexual Differentiation
- ♦ Gender identity.
  - • Genetic sex.
  - • Gonadal sex.
  - • Internal genitalia and external genitalia.
  - • Secondary sexual characteristics.
  - • Societal role (Fig. 9.1).
- ♦ Prenatal events.
  - • Genetic sex → gonadal differentiation → hormonal environment.
  - • Central nervous system (CNS) and external and internal genitalia.
- ♦ Gonadal differentiation.
  - • Gonads begin development as protuberances overlying mesonephric ducts at 5 weeks.
  - • Germ cells migrate at 4 to 6 weeks of gestation; germ cells do not induce gonadal development.
  - • At 6 weeks of gestation, gonad is bipotential.
  - • Composed of the following:
    - ■ Germ cells.
    - ■ Special epithelial cells.
      - ◊ Potential granulosa cells.
      - ◊ Potential Sertoli cells.
    - ■ Mesenchyme.
      - ◊ Potential theca cells.
      - ◊ Potential Leydig cells.
    - ■ Mesonephric duct system.
      - ◊ Wolffian.
      - ◊ Müllerian.
  - • The distal end of the short arm of the Y chromosome contains the sex-determining region and pairs with the distal short arm of the X, the pseudoautosomal region (Xp22.3).
    - ■ Homologous pairing of X and Y at this region.
    - ■ Genes doubly present → no X inactivation.
    - ■ Deletion → contiguous gene syndrome.
      - ◊ Short stature.
      - ◊ Mental retardation.
      - ◊ X-linked ichthyosis.
      - ◊ Kallmann syndrome.
    - ■ Testis-determining factor (TDF) gene is immediately adjacent on the distal short arm of Y.
    - ■ The loss of TDF results in gonadal dysgenesis.
    - ■ Transfer of this gene to the X chromosome results in an XX male.
    - ■ The two previous contenders for TDF were H-Y histocompatibility antigen and the zinc finger protein (ZFY).

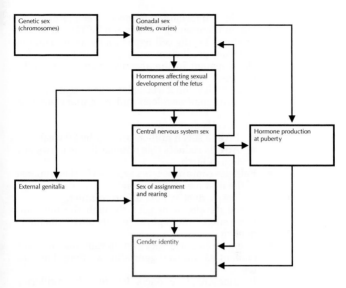

Figure 9.1. Factors that influence the development of gender identity.

- ♦ SRY—potential candidate for TDF.
  - • Single gene copy in the smallest Y chromosome region is capable of sex reversal.
  - • Expressed at appropriate times in sexual differentiation.
  - • Present in XX males and absent in XY females.
  - • Can sex-reverse mice.
  - • Protein product of this gene: 204 amino acids.
    - ■ Contains 80–amino-acid domain that binds DNA.
    - ■ High mobility group (HMG) box of SRY binds P450 aromatase and antimüllerian hormone (AMH; also known an müllerian-inhibiting substance [MIS]) promoters.
  - • Other genes are also necessary for correct sexual differentiation; autosomal genes govern the migration of germ cells and the correct expression of steroidogenic enzymes. Presumably controlled by SRY.
  - • SF-1 and DAX-1: orphan nuclear receptors.
    - ■ SF-1 is involved in the expression of steroidogenic enzymes and AMH.
    - ■ DAX-1 mutations result in adrenal hypoplasia.
- ♦ Testicular differentiation begins at 6 to 7 weeks.
  - • Sertoli cells aggregate to form spermatozoic cords; *seminiferous* tubules form following the formation of cord.

- Leydig cell formation follows 1 week later.
- Human chorionic gonadotropin (hCG) stimulation produces Leydig-cell hypertrophy; peak fetal testosterone production is present in 15 to 18 weeks.

◆ XX development in the absence of the active influence of the Y chromosome.
  - Ovaries develop 2 weeks later than testes.
  - Cortical zone develops and medullary zone regresses.
  - Germ cells proliferate.
    - Five to seven million present by 20 weeks.
    - Atresia reduces this number to one to two million at birth.
  - Follicles contain oocytes arrested in the prophase of the first meiotic division.

◆ Reproductive duct system differentiation.
  - Renal development goes through the following three stages: pronephric, mesonephric, and metanephric.
  - The mesonephric duct system remains for development as internal genitalia (wolffian duct system).
  - Paramesonephric ducts become the müllerian ducts.
  - Both systems temporarily coexist at 8 weeks.

◆ Alfred Jost performed classic studies demonstrating the role of testicular products (AMH and testosterone) in the sexual differentiation in rabbits.
  - Antimüllerian hormone.
    - It is a member of the transforming growth factor–β family of glycoprotein differentiation factors.
    - Inhibin and activin are also members of this family.
    - The gene is found on the short arm of chromosome 19; the receptor, on chromosome 12.
    - It is synthesized by Sertoli cells (activated by SRY).
      ◊ Induces ipsilateral regression of müllerian ducts by 8 weeks.
      ◊ Occurs before emergence of testosterone and stimulation of wolffian ducts.
    - Gene mutation results in the lack of regression of the uterus and tubes.
    - Extra müllerian functions.
      ◊ Inhibitory effect on oocyte meiosis.
      ◊ Facilitates testicular descent up to passage through inguinal canal; passage through inguinal canal mediated by androgens.
      ◊ Surfactant production inhibited in pregnancy.
      ◊ Cleavage product—inhibits growth of various tumors.
    - AMH is not present in adult females until the second decade of life.

- It can be a useful marker for intersex disorders.
- Testosterone inhibits AMH after puberty.
  ◊ Patients with androgen inactivity syndrome have high levels of AMH.
  ◊ Sertoli cells lack the testosterone receptor during the fetal and newborn period.

♦ Testosterone.
- Secreted by Leydig cells soon after formation (8 weeks).
- Peak secretion at 15 to 18 weeks.
- Stimulates development of wolffian system into the following:
  - Epididymis.
  - Vas deferens.
  - Seminal vesicles.
- Testosterone levels correlate with the following:
  - Leydig cell development.
  - Gonadal weight.
  - 3β-Hydroxysteroid dehydrogenase (HSD) activity.
  - hCG concentration—after 20 weeks, luteinizing hormone (LH) produced by the fetal pituitary is more important than hCG for Leydig-cell stimulation.
- Wolffian ducts do not form dihydrotestosterone (DHT).
  - Direct high local paracrine effect of testosterone is essential for ipsilateral differentiation.
  - Development cannot be stimulated in females by the adrenal or by exogenous androgens.
  - Estrogen may play a role in the degeneration of the wolffian system (Fig. 9.2).

♦ External genitalia differentiation.
- Neutral primordia are able to differentiate into either male or female genitalia.
  - Differentiation depends upon the gonadal steroid signals.
  - Masculinization manifests at 10 weeks; it is completed by 14 weeks.
  - Masculine development is dependent on the DHT formed from testosterone by 5α-reductase.
- Exposure to androgens at the critical time (9 to 14 weeks) results in variable masculinization of female fetus.
- Sex steroids may influence CNS differentiation; inappropriate fetal hormonal programming may contribute to the range of human psychosexual behavior.

II. Abnormal Sexual Differentiation
  ♦ True hermaphrodite has both testicular and ovarian tissue.
  ♦ Male pseudohermaphrodite has testes but an external female phenotype.

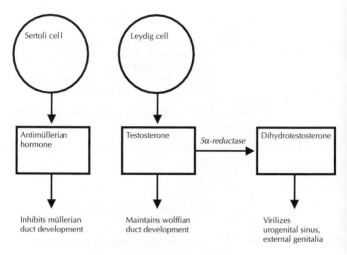

Figure 9.2.   Male sexual development.

- ♦ Female pseudohermaphrodite has ovaries but an external male phenotype (Table 9.1).
- ♦ Congenital adrenal hypoplasia (adrenogenital syndrome).
  - • Masculinized external genitals in females; diagnosed by demonstrating excessive androgen production by the adrenal cortex.
  - • Normal female internal genitals with absence of wolffian duct tissue (high local androgens are not present).
  - • External genitalia can be substantially altered.
  - • Fusion of labia (anterior → posterior) can occur.
  - • Clitoral hypertrophy.
  - • Absence of palpable testes: possibly the only clinical marker suggesting female pseudohermaphroditism.
  - • Timing depends upon the level of masculinization.
    - ■ Early exposure (7 to 12 weeks) may fully masculinize.
    - ■ Later exposure (18 to 20 weeks) results in limited ambiguity.
    - ■ Clitoral size is dependent on quantities, not timing, of androgen access.
    - ■ If untreated, the potential for progressive virilization exists.
      - ◊ At age 2 to 4 years → pubic hair → axillary hair, then body hair and beard.
      - ◊ Advanced bone age can occur by age 2; early epiphyseal closure results in short stature as an adult.

Table 9.1.   Disorders associated with abnormal sexual differentiation

Disorders of Fetal Endocrinology
Masculinized females (female pseudohermaphroditism)
   Congenital adrenal hyperplasia
      21-Hydroxylase (P450c21) deficiency
      11β-Hydroxylase (P450c11β) deficiency
      3β-Hydroxysteroid dehydrogenase deficiency
   Elevated androgens in the maternal circulation
      Drug intake
      Maternal disease
   Aromatase (P450arom) deficiency
Incompletely masculinized males (male pseudohermaphroditism)
   Androgen insensitivity syndromes
   5α-Reductase deficiency
   Testosterone biosynthesis defects
      3β-Hydroxysteroid dehydrogenase deficiency
      17α-Hydroxylase (P450c17) deficiency
      17β-Hydroxysteroid dehydrogenase deficiency
   Gonadotropin-resistant testes
   Antimüllerian hormone deficiency
Disorders of Gonadal Development
Male pseudohermaphroditism
   Primary gonadal defect—Swyer syndrome
   Anorchia
True hermaphroditism
Gonadal dysgenesis
   Turner syndrome
   Mosaicism
   Normal karyotype—Noonan syndrome

P450, cytochrome P450.

◇ Metabolic disorders include salt wasting, hypertension, or, rarely, hypoglycemia.
    ○ Two-thirds of patients with virilization usually present within a few days of birth with addisonian-like crisis characterized by hyponatremia, hyperkalemia, and acidosis.
    ○ Five percent present with hypertension.
◇ Virilizing congenital adrenal hyperplasia (CAH) results from the inability to synthesize glucocorticoids.
    ○ Elevated levels of adrenocorticotropic hormone (ACTH) occurs secondary to low levels of cortisol.
    ○ Hyperplastic adrenal cortex attempts to compensate for the lack of feedback and produces excessive androgens and corticoid precursors.
◇ The most common enzymatic defects include the following:

- ○ 21-Hydroxylase deficiency (P450c21).
- ○ 11β-Hydroxylase deficiency (P450c11).
- ○ 3β-HSD deficiency.
- ○ Rarely P450c17.

- ♦ Enzyme defect in the adrenal only (P450c21).
  - • Ninety-five percent of cases.
  - • Most frequent cause of sexual ambiguity.
  - • Most frequent endocrine cause of neonatal death.
  - • Three forms are observed as follows:
    - ■ Salt wasting—linked to female pseudohermaphroditism.
    - ■ Simple virilizing—linked to female pseudohermaphroditism.
    - ■ Nonclassic—previously known as late-onset, attenuated, or acquired.

- ♦ Genetics.
  - • Monogenetic autosomal recessive.
  - • HLA antigen typing can determine carrier status, allowing genetic diagnosis.
  - • The two genes involved are CYP21A and CYP21B.
    - ■ Both present on chromosome 6.
    - ■ Localized between HLA-B and HLA-DR.
    - ■ Genes in tandem duplication with the fourth component of the compliment.
    - ■ **Only** CYP21B is an active gene; CYP21A (also called CYP21P) is a pseudogene and is inactive.
  - • A variety of mutations affect CYP21B.
    - ■ Eighty-five percent gene conversion.
    - ■ Most patients compound heterozygotes; severity depends on the activity of the least affected allele.
    - ■ Heterozygotes exhibiting the mildest enzyme deficiency are clinically asymptomatic (Fig. 9.3).

- ♦ Enzyme defect in the adrenal only: 11β-hydroxylase deficiency.
  - • This enzyme represents the final step in cortisol synthesis → failure of conversion of 11-deoxycortisol to cortisol.
  - • Deficiency results in virilization, hypertension, hypokalemic alkalosis, and fluid overload ($\uparrow$ deoxycorticosterone [DOC], $\downarrow$ renin, and $\downarrow$ aldosterone).
    - ■ 11-DOC conversion is blocked, so no aldosterone is produced ($\uparrow$ dehydroepiandrosterone [DHEA], dehydroepiandrosterone sulfate [DHEAS], androstenedione [A_4]).
    - ■ Aldosterone levels are affected in a variable manner.
  - • Between 5% and 8% of cases of CAH are due to 11β-hydroxylase deficiency.
  - • It is diagnosed by high levels of DOC and compound S (deoxycortisol).

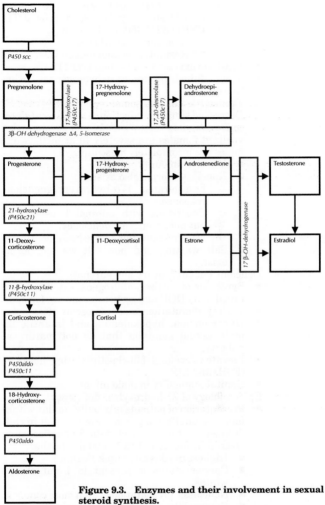

Figure 9.3.   Enzymes and their involvement in sexual steroid synthesis.

- Two-thirds of untreated patients become hypertensive.
- A mild form is also recognized; the patient is mildly virilized, but no (or rare) cases of hypertension are seen.
- 11β-Hydroxylase gene is present on chromosome 8.
  - Remote from the HLA antigen locus.
  - Transmitted as autosomal recessive.
  - Two isozymes are encoded by the following two genes:

        ◇   CYP11B1 (P450c11)—classically referred to as 11β-hydroxylase; regulated by ACTH.

        ◇   CYP11B2 (P450c18, P450 also).

            o   Aldosterone synthesis.

            o   Regulated by angiotensin II.

- 11β-Hydroxylase results from CYP11B1.

♦ Deficient 3β-hydroxysteroid dehydrogenase (ovary and adrenal).

- Transmitted as autosomal recessive.
- Decreased steroid production in all classes (*glucocorticoids*, *mineralocorticoids*, and sex steroids); virilized females are severely ill at birth, while males are incompletely masculinized.
  - Massive amounts of DHEA.
  - Nonclassic forms also exist.
    - ◇ Exaggerated 17α-hydroxypregnenolone response.
    - ◇ Consistent with adrenal hyperactivity but not an enzyme deficiency.
    - ◇ No gene mutations have been identified.
  - Salt wasting and non–salt wasting forms exist.

♦ Deficient P450c17 (ovary and adrenal).

- Synthesis of cortisol, androgens, estrogens curtailed; only DOC and corticosterone are formed.
- Variety of mutations on chromosome 10.
- Hypertension, hypokalemia, and infantile female sexual genitalia that do not mature at puberty.
- Elevated levels of follicle-stimulating hormone (FSH) and LH.
- Genital ambiguity in male infants.

♦ Epidemiology of 21-hydroxylase deficiency.

- Presentation of patients is usually similar within families; unaffected parents would result in children with ratio of 1 affected–to–3 nonaffected.
- Overall incidence is 1 in 14,000 live births.
  - Highest in Alaskan Yupik Eskimos.
  - Carrier status is present in 1 out of 100 whites.
  - Nonclassic presentation is even more common.
  - Extrapolations from ACTH testing suggest the following frequency:

	Nonclassic Disease	Heterozygous Carrier
Eastern European Jews	$\frac{1}{30}$	$\frac{1}{3}$
Hispanic	$\frac{1}{40}$	$\frac{1}{4}$
Slavs	$\frac{1}{50}$	$\frac{1}{5}$
Italians	$\frac{1}{333}$	$\frac{1}{9}$
Others	$\frac{1}{1,000}$	$\frac{1}{14}$

- Prenatal diagnosis—amniotic fluid steroids.

- Diagnosis is made based on elevated levels of 17-hydroxyprogesterone, 21-deoxycortisol, and androstenedione in amniotic fluid; 17-hydroxyprogesterone may be the only abnormal steroid in the salt wasting form, while androstenedione is increased in all forms.
- 11β-Hydroxylase deficiency is diagnosed based on elevated levels of 11-deoxycortisol in amniotic fluid and of tetrahydro-11-deoxycortisol in maternal urine.
- Molecular genetic diagnosis.
- Chorion villus sampling for 21-hydroxylase deficiency allows termination or *in utero* therapy.
  - ◊ Begin at 4 to 5 weeks of gestation; multiple daily doses (1.5 mg QD) of dexamethasone.
  - ◊ Maternal side effects can be extreme; include severe striae, hyperglycemia, hypertension, and gastrointestinal symptoms.
  - ◊ Attempt to reduce dose in the second half of pregnancy.
  - ◊ Monitor with estriol production → titrate to keep maternal serum estriol in the normal range.
- Only one-eighth of fetuses require treatment; treatment should be governed by appropriate research-type institutional protocols.
- Diagnosis of congenital adrenal hyperplasia.
  - Immunoassay for 17-hydroxyprogesterone (50 to 400 times the normal level) and plasma renin activity assesses the degree of mineralocorticoid deficiency.
  - In normal infants, 17-hydroxyprogesterone decreases to 100 to 200 mg/dL after 24 hours.
    - ◊ In affected infants, the level is 3,000 to 4,000 ng/dL.
    - ◊ The Texas screening program detected classic CAH in 1 in 16,000 births (ratio of salt wasting to simple virilization of 2.7 to 1).
  - Diagnosis of adults for 21-hydroxylase deficiency.
    - ◊ Measure 17-hydroxyprogesterone in the morning.
      - ○ Avoids the diurnal ACTH increase.
      - ○ Baseline level should be <200 ng/dL.
        - □ Levels >800 ng/dL are diagnostic.
        - □ ACTH stimulation test useful for evaluating patients with 17-hydroxyprogesterone level of 200 to 800 ng/dL.
    - ◊ DHEAS levels are usually in the normal range.
    - ◊ Increased renin serum levels can be seen in the salt wasting form.

◇ ACTH stimulation test.
  ○ Measure at 0 minutes and at 60 minutes after ACTH infusion.
  ○ Examine levels of pregnenolone, 17-hydroxypregnenolone, 17-hydroxyprogesterone, DHEAS, 11-deoxycortisol, cortisol, and testosterone.
- Diagnosis of 3β-HSD deficiency in adults.
  ◇ 17-Hydroxyprogesterone levels will be normal.
  ◇ DHEA and DHEAS will be increased; plasma renin will be increased in the salt wasting form.
- Adult diagnosis of 11β-hydroxylase deficiency.
  ◇ 17-Hydroxyprogesterone levels will be elevated; elevated 11-deoxycortisol levels are diagnostic.
  ◇ Plasma renin will be decreased when compared with increased plasma renin in 21-hydroxy and 3β-hydroxysteroid deficiencies.

III. Treatment
  ♦ Overview.
    • Cornerstone of treatment is to supply the deficient hormone: cortisol.
      - Treatment with cortisol will decrease ACTH and will therefore decrease the production of androgens.
      - Treatment with mineralocorticoid will help to normalize plasma renin and will also decrease ACTH and androgen production.
      - Commonly used drugs and dosages are as follows:
        ◇ Hydrocortisone, 10 mg/day (12 to 18 mg/m^2 or 3 to 5 mg/m^2 of prednisone).
        ◇ 9-Fluorohydrocortisone, 100 µg/day.
      - Monitor 17-hydroxyprogesterone level to maintain it in the 500 to 4,000 ng/dL range; also monitor androstenedione, testosterone, and plasma renin.
    • Surgical treatment is used to reconstruct normal female external genitalia as needed.
    • Prenatal exposure to androgens may explain the increased rates of homosexual behavior.
    • During labor and delivery, patients may be counseled regarding elective cesarean section to avoid excessive perineal scarring.
    • Continue maintenance dose of steroids during pregnancy.
      - Use stress doses in labor.
      - Observe newborn for adrenal insufficiency due to steroid crossover.
  ♦ Treatment problems.

- Overtreatment can result in iatrogenic Cushing disease with short stature, hirsutism, and infertility.
- The mineralocorticoid should keep plasma renin in the low-normal range; it should eliminate hypovolemia as the stimulus for ACTH secretion via angiotensin II pathway.
- A gonadotropin-releasing hormone (GnRH) agonist may be a useful adjuvant to treatment in cases where increased androgens have led to preventive pubertal maturation.
- Newer strategies may involve the use of flutamide and testolactone in addition to steroids.
♦ Incomplete masculinization (male pseudohermaphrodite).
  - Genetically, the fetus is male (XY).
  - External genitalia are not normal male genitalia.
  - The four etiologies are the following:
    - Defective receptor (androgen insensitivity syndrome).
    - Abnormal androgen synthesis.
    - Gonadotropin-resistant testes.
    - Absent or defective müllerian-inhibiting substance.
♦ Syndromes—factors influencing androgen target cell responsiveness.
  - Intracellular androgen concentration.
  - Binding affinity of steroid to nuclear receptor.
  - Binding capacity of receptor.
  - Nuclear content of receptor.
  - Cellular concentration of 5α-reductase, aromatase, 17β-HSD.
  - Adequacy of nuclear (chromatin) acceptor site.
  - Adequacy of regulatory molecules (adapter proteins) controlling chromatin "read" of the androgen message.
  - RNA processing and translation.
  - Quality of protein gene product.
♦ Complete androgen insensitivity syndrome (testicular feminization).
  - Congenital insensitivity to androgens.
  - Transmitted via maternal X-linked recessive gene.
  - Phenotypically female but uterus and tubes are absent; scant pubic hair.
  - Karyotype is 46,XY.
  - No müllerian structures present; normal AMH production.
  - Testes are present to the level of the inguinal ring; descent is mediated by AMH.
  - Testosterone production normal or slightly increased.
  - Androgen insensitivity syndrome represents 10% of all cases of primary amenorrhea (third most

common cause after gonadal dysgenesis and congenital absence of the vagina).
- Hormone profile.
  - High LH.
  - Normal to slightly elevated male testosterone.
  - High estradiol (for men).
  - Normal to ↑ FSH.
  - Gonadal tumors in 5% of patients, rarely prior to age 25; perform gonadectomy at the age of 16 to 18 years to allow feminization to occur with puberty.
- Genetic implications.
  - X-linked recessive disorder.
    ◊ Apparent sisters of affected individuals have a one-third chance of being karyotypically XY.
    ◊ Female offspring of a normal sister have a one-sixth chance.
  - One-third of patients have no family history of the syndrome.
♦ Incomplete androgen insensitivity.
  - One-tenth as common as the complete form; a spectrum of clinical disorders.
  - Wide range of presentations, from complete failure of virilization to near-normal masculinization.
    - Reifenstein syndrome is the moniker applied to all intermediate forms.
    - Incidence may approach 40% in men with azoospermia or oligospermia.
  - Receptor-gene mutation.
    - Localized to q11–12 of X chromosome.
    - Two hundred unique mutations have been identified.
    - Two classes of defects.
      ◊ Abnormalities of androgen binding.
      ◊ Abnormalities of receptor binding.
    - Poor correlation between receptor levels and androgen binding with clinical syndrome; only a few patients respond to androgen therapy.
  - Sex assignment—can have normal phallus with hypospadias but inadequate response to pubertal androgens will result in gynecomastia.
    - Karyotype XY.
    - Cannot respond to exogenous androgens.
    - High levels of estradiol (Table 9.2).
♦ 5α-Reductase deficiency.
  - Familial incomplete male pseudohermaphroditism.
  - Autosomal recessive.
  - Severe perineal hypospadias.
  - Underdevelopment of the vagina.
    - Previously known as pseudovagina–pseudoscrotum–hypospadias (PPH).
    - Masculinization will occur at puberty (the breasts remain male).

Table 9.2. The androgen insensitivity syndromes

	5α-reductase	Complete	Incomplete	Reifenstein	Infertile
Inheritance	Autosomal recessive	X-linked recessive	X-linked recessive	X-linked recessive	X-linked recessive
Spermatogenesis	Decreased	Absent	Absent	Absent	Decreased
Müllerian	Absent	Absent	Absent	Absent	Absent
Wolffian	Male	Absent	Male	Male	Male
External	Female	Female	Female clitoromegaly	Male hypospadias	Male
Breasts	Male	Female	Female	Gynecomastia	Gynecomastia

- Normal testicular function and no lack of response to endogenous or exogenous androgen.
- Diagnosis.
  - External genitalia at birth are similar to incomplete androgen insensitivity syndrome.
    - ◇ No müllerian ducts.
    - ◇ Normal steroid levels.
  - Elevated testosterone to DHT ratio; evaluate with hCG stimulation test.
  - Karyotype is XY.
  - Can rear as female after gonadectomy.
  - Early correction of cryptorchidism and hypospadias can allow a male life.
- Three types of enzyme deficiency are seen as follows:
  - Abnormal low concentration.
  - Reduced enzyme stability.
  - Normal concentration but defective testosterone affinity and/or essential cofactors leading to reduced enzyme deficiency.
- Genetic defect.
  - The following two 5α-reductase genes have been isolated:
    - ◇ 5α-Reductase-1 on chromosome 5.
    - ◇ 5α-Reductase-2 on chromosome 2.
      - ○ Affected gene in 5α-reductase deficiency.
      - ○ Relatively easy switch to new gender identity suggests gene is active in brain.
  - Treatment.
    - ◇ Intersex results in tricky assignment of sex of rearing.
    - ◇ DHT is necessary only for external genitalia; testosterone is present for wolffian structure and brain development.
- ♦ Abnormal androgen synthesis.
  - Accounts for 4% of male pseudohermaphroditism.
  - Caused by the following:
    - Defects in testosterone biosynthesis.
    - Gonadotropin-resistant testes (LH-receptor mutations).
    - Congenital lipoid adrenal hyperplasia.
    - Defective synthesis, secretion, or response to müllerian-inhibiting substance.
  - Defect in hormone biosynthesis.
    - 3β-HSD, P450c17, 17β-HSD—inherited as autosomal recessive with decreased testosterone levels.
    - Increased blood levels of androstenedione and estrogens.
    - All blocks except 17β-HSD are very bad → involve adrenal failure.

- 17β-HSD.
  - Male internal genitalia.
  - No müllerian structures.
  - Testes are in the inguinal canal.
  - May virilize with puberty.
  - Conversion of androstenedione by unaffected isoenzymes; early gonadectomy is required to avoid virilization at puberty and testicular neoplasia.
- Gonadotropin-resistant testes.
  - Receptor deficiency or postreceptor defect to LH and/or hCG.
  - Female but has ambiguous genitalia.
  - Male cryptorchid testes with degenerated Leydig cells (Leydig-cell hypoplasia).
  - No müllerian ducts.
  - Vas deferens and epididymis present.
  - Elevated gonadotropins.
- Congenital lipoid adrenal hyperplasia.
  - Rate-limiting step in steroidogenesis is transfer of cholesterol from outer mitochondrial membrane to inner membrane; mediated by protein activation stimulated by tropic hormones.
    - ◇ Long-term steroidogenesis requires gene transcription.
    - ◇ Short-term, acute responses also occur.
  - Several proteins have been proposed as regulators.
    - ◇ Sterol carrier protein 2.
    - ◇ Steroidogenesis-activator polypeptide.
    - ◇ Peripheral benzodiazepine receptor.
    - ◇ Steroidogenic acute regulator (StAR) protein.
  - Evidence that StAR is involved includes the following:
    - ◇ StAR mRNA and protein are induced in response to cyclic adenosine monophosphate.
    - ◇ StAR increases steroid production.
    - ◇ StAR is imported and localized to mitochondria.
    - ◇ StAR mutations result in congenital lipoid adrenal hypoplasia and failure in adrenal and gonadal steroidogenesis.
  - StAR mutation.
    - ◇ Gene is found on chromosome 8p11.2.
    - ◇ Mutation results in premature truncation of message, preventing proteolytic cleavage.
    - ◇ StAR is absent in the placenta and the brain.
- Abnormal antimüllerian hormone (uterine hernia syndrome).

- Appear to be normal males but have well-differentiated müllerian duct structures in the inguinal hernia sac.
- Recessive X-linked or autosomal; either a failure of AMH secretion or of müllerian ducts to respond.
- Fertility is usually preserved.
- Abnormal gonadogenesis.
- Bilateral dysgenesis of the testes (Swyer syndrome).
  - XY karyotype.
    - ◇ Normal XX external (infantile).
    - ◇ Normal XX internal.
  - Gonads are replaced by fibrous bands.
  - Removal of the gonads is recommended to avoid virilization or neoplasm.
  - Must have complete testicular loss between 6 and 12 weeks; if loss occurs later, then genitalia are ambiguous with present müllerian and wolffian components.
  - One cause is mutation of the SRY gene.
- Anorchia.
  - Infantile male external genitalia.
  - Absent müllerian ducts.
  - Male internal genitalia (wolffian ducts).
  - No testes present: "disappearing-testes syndrome."
  - Sex of rearing secondary to external genitalia development.
- ◆ True hermaphrodites.
  - Individuals with both ovarian and testicular tissue present.
    - Both can be present in one gonad → ovotestis.
    - **Or**, can have one side ovarian and one side testicular.
    - Internal structure corresponds to the adjacent gonad.
  - Three-fourths develop gynecomastia; half menstruate.
  - Approximately 60% XX with a few XY; the rest are mosaics with at least one cell line of XX.
- ◆ Gonadal dysgenesis.
  - Turner syndrome = absence and/or abnormality of one of the X chromosomes in all cell lines, resulting in rudimentary streak gonads.
    - About 60%—a total loss of the X chromosome.
    - Remaining 40%—a structural anomaly or are mosaic with an abnormal X.
    - Phenotypically female.
    - Short stature (56 to 58 inches).
    - Streak gonads, sexual infantilism present.
    - Webbed neck, cubitus valgus, and high arched palate.
    - Shield-like chest, widely spaced nipples, and low hairline on the neck.

- Renal abnormalities may be present, including horseshoe kidney and unilateral pelvic kidney.
- Hashimoto thyroiditis common (hypothyroid in 10% of young patients; 50%, later in life).
  ◇ Especially vitiligo.
  ◇ Seen in 46,XXqi cases.
  ◇ Disease and alopecia also common.
- One-third of patients—cardiovascular abnormality.
  ◇ Bicuspid aortic valve.
  ◇ Aortic aneurysm.
  ◇ Coarctation of the aorta.
  ◇ Mitral valve prolapse.
- Normal intelligence present.
- Pregnancy wastage—99% of fetuses with Turner syndrome abort, 1% survive (1 in 2,000 to 1 in 5,000 live births).

- Yearly evaluation and initial evaluation.
  - Thyroid function, intravenous pyelogram, renal sonogram, echocardiogram, audiology evaluation, and lipid and glucose profile (annual).
  - Spontaneous puberty found in 10% to 20%; spontaneous menstruation in 2.5%. Likely from an undetected mosaic cell line.
  - In rare pregnancies, a 30% risk of congenital anomalies, including trisomy 21, spina bifida, congenital heart disease.
  - Phenotype secondary to the region of the X chromosome that is lost (Fig. 9.4).
  - 45,XO karyotype may possibly represent 46,XY with a mitotic error resulting in 45,XO; suggest close evaluation with yearly pelvic examinations.
    ◇ Development of breasts or sexual hair may represent gonadoblastoma or dysgerminoma.
    ◇ Three percent to 4% of 45,X patients have Y-derived DNA from a polymerase chain reaction (PCR).
    ◇ Seek chromosomal material in patients with virilization or with identification of chromosomal fragment of uncertain origin.

- Pure gonadal dysgenesis.
  - No Turner syndrome stigmata.
  - May result from autosomal-gene mutation.
- Perrault syndrome.
  - XX gonadal dysgenesis.
  - Associated with neurosensory deafness.
- XY gonadal dysgenesis (Swyer syndrome).
  - Most are without stigma of Turner.
  - Puberty is delayed.
    ◇ Elevated gonadotropins.
    ◇ Normal female androgens.
    ◇ Low level of estrogens.

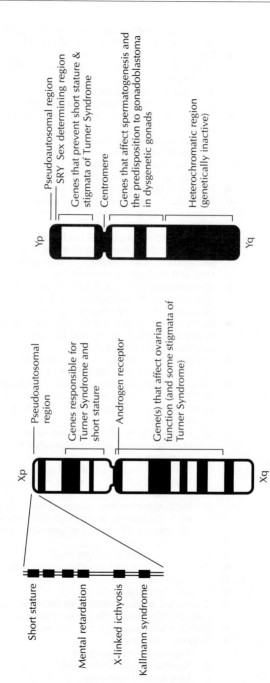

Figure 9.4.   The X and Y chromosomes and affected regions in abnormal sexual development.

- ◊ Female external gestation.
- ◊ Uterus and fallopian tubes.
- Gonads should be removed as early in life as possible.
- Gonadal tumors occur in 20% to 30%.
- Risk of tumor in mosaicism is from 15% to 20%.
- Bilateral gonadoblastoma is most common; dysgerminoma and embryonal carcinoma are also seen.
- Etiology of defect.
  - Deletion of the short arm of the Y involving SRY.
  - **Or** mutation in SRY that inhibits functions.
  - **Or** XXqi mutation of SRY.
    - ◊ *Or* impaired function of the X chromosome gene necessary for SRY function.
    - ◊ Some protection from stigma of Turner syndrome in these patients.
  - Partial gonadal dysgenesis in some degree of testicular development.
  - Sex-reversed male.
  - SRY mutations in 46,XY gonadal dysgenesis.
    - ◊ Not very common.
    - ◊ Other mutations.
      - ○ Duplication of the short arm of X.
      - ○ LH-receptor-gene mutation.
        - □ Male pseudohermaphrodites.
        - □ 46,XX sisters present with the female phenotype and primary amenorrhea.
    - ◊ Usually have SRY; if SRY is negative, an additional genetic defect *yields* 46,XX maleness.
- Mixed gonadal dysgenesis (45,X; 46,XY most common).
  - Mosaicism with Y associated with abnormalities of sexual differentiation.
  - Mixed picture.
    - ◊ Ranges from ambiguous genitalia to fertile males to normal females with streak gonads.
    - ◊ Normal on one side, streak on the other.
  - Incidence of gonadal tumors is 25%.
  - Most have short stature; one-third have Turner stigmata.
  - Can use PCR to find any evidence of the Y chromosome.
- Hormonal treatment.
  - Treatment with estradiol is indicated for:
    - ◊ Formation of female secondary sexual characteristics.
    - ◊ Bone density.
    - ◊ Promotion of attainment of full adult height.

- Current recommendations.
  - ◇ Begin at age 12 to 14 with 0.3 mg conjugated equine estrogens or 0.5 mg estradiol.
  - ◇ After 6 months to 1 year, increase dose to 0.625 mg or 1 mg and add progestin 14 days/month.
  - ◇ Some clinicians increase further to 1.25 mg and 2.0 mg to enhance bone and breast effects.
  - ◇ Defer treatment until bone age of 11 or 12 years with Turner syndrome to avoid early epiphysial closure.
- Stimulation of growth.
  - ◇ Short stature occurs in virtually all 45,XO patients and in nearly all with Turner stigmata and other karyotypes.
  - ◇ Probably this is caused by insufficiency of growth hormone production.
  - ◇ Deficiency of sex steroids.
  - ◇ End-organ resistance to insulin-like growth factor–I (IGF-I).
  - ◇ The use of recombinant growth hormone (50 µg/kg/day, with lesser doses of anabolic steroid) yields best results.
  - ◇ Adolescents with Turner syndrome do not lose bone mineral density; one does not need to start too early and risk early epiphyseal closure.
- Risks of pregnancy.
  - Thirty percent incidence of congenital anomalies in offspring.
  - Use of donor ova has been successful, but fatal aortic events can occur.
- Noonan syndrome.
  - Conduct an early screening of all growth-retarded girls.
  - This includes boys and girls with normal chromosomes but a phenotypic appearance of Turner syndrome.
  - Cardiac lesion is different.
    - ◇ Pulmonary stenosis most frequent.
    - ◇ Probably transmitted as autosomal dominant with variable expression.
- ◆ Diagnosis of ambiguous genitalia.
  - Social and medical emergency.
  - The presumed diagnosis must be congenital adrenal hyperplasia, given the life-threatening nature of this disease.
  - Questions to address include the following:
    1. Are the gonads palpable?
       - Most important part of the physical examination.
       - Gonads in inguinal regions or scrotal folds almost certainly testes.

2. What is the phallus length in diameter?
    - Less than 2.5 cm is 2.5 standard deviation below the mean.
    - The normal clitoris <1 cm.
    - The normal phallus is 2.8 to 4.2 cm.
3. Where is the urethral meatus?
4. Are the labioscrotal folds fused?
    - Distance from the anus to the edge of vagina/base of clitoris; the ratio should be <0.5.
    - Ratio of >0.5 indicates some element of fusion.
5. Is there a vagina, vaginal pouch, or urogenital sinus present?

- Other physical signs should be examined, including hyperpigmentation, secondary to increased melanocyte-stimulating hormone production (ACTH production).
- Tests to perform.
    - Ultrasound (US) to detect a uterus, ovaries, or undescended testes.
    - Retrograde injection of contrast dye.
    - Magnetic resonance imaging (MRI)—can supplant both the US and contrast dye study.
    - Karyotype.
    - Electrolytes.
    - Androgens (androstenedione, testosterone, DHEA, DHEAS, 17-hydroxyprogesterone, 11-DOC, 11-deoxycortisol).
    - In selected circumstances, ACTH testing and hCG stimulation testing.
- Differential diagnosis.
    - Check gonads, *uterus*, and karyotype to place in one of four categories.
    - Abnormal electrolytes must be an enzyme defect.
        ◊ Decreased aldosterone will result in hyperkalemia and hyponatremia.
        ◊ Increased DOC will result in hypokalemia and hypertension.
- Female pseudohermaphroditism.
    - 21-Hydroxylase deficiency; diagnosed with elevated 17-hydroxyprogesterone.
    - 11β-Hydroxylase deficiency; diagnosed with elevated 11-deoxycortisol, 11-DOC levels.
    - 3β-HSD deficiency; associated with elevations in DHEA or 17-hydroxypregnenolone.
- Male pseudohermaphroditism may result from enzyme biosynthetic errors.
    - P450scc—no cortisol or androgens.
    - P450c17—elevated progesterone.
    - 3β-HSD—elevated DHEA, 17-hydroxypregnenolone.
    - 17β-HSD.

◇ No adrenal insufficiency in patient with electrolyte disturbance.
◇ hCG stimulation → increased androstenedione and DHEA.
■ Leydig cell hypoplasia.
◇ No response to hCG.
◇ No adrenal defects.
• Other enzymes that may be involved.
■ 5α-Reductase diagnosed via culture fibroblast of genital stimulation.
■ Increased testosterone: DHT with hCG stimulation.
• Androgen-insensitive patient.
■ Normal ACTH, hCG stimulation tests.
■ Abnormal androgen-binding-gene or androgen-receptor-gene mutation in cultured cells (Fig. 9.5).
♦ Laparotomy may be only means to reach definitive diagnosis.
• XX infant with ambiguous genitalia, normal androgens, and no history of maternal drug exposure: questionable hermaphrodite versus mixed gonadal dysgenesis.
• XY infant with ambiguous genitalia.
■ No palpable gonads.
■ Normal androgens.
■ Possibilities.
◇ Incompletely masculinized male (variant of androgen insensitivity syndrome).
◇ True hermaphrodite.
◇ Mixed gonadal dysgenesis.
◇ 5α-Reductase deficiency.
■ Sex of rearing—female; gonadectomy needed to avoid pubertal virilization and propensity for neoplasia.
♦ Assignment of sex of rearing.
• This important decision should be based upon the following:
■ Future fertility.
■ Appearance of genitals after puberty.
■ Penile adequacy.
• All masculinized females should be raised as females.
■ Future fertility is unaffected.
■ Males with reproductive capability include the following:
◇ Isolated hypospadias.
◇ Male with repaired isolated cryptorchidism.
◇ Uterine hernia syndrome.
• All others are sterile.
■ Sex of rearing depends on penis size and factors as described above.
■ Reassignment can probably be made safely up to 18 months of age.

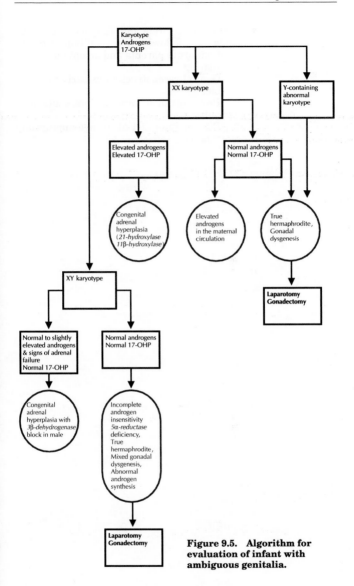

Figure 9.5. Algorithm for evaluation of infant with ambiguous genitalia.

- Future gender role and assigned sex can be made if the following four conditions are met:
  - ◇ Comfort of parents and acceptance of sex rearing.
  - ◇ Genital reconstruction as early as possible.
  - ◇ Properly timed hormonal interventions at puberty.
  - ◇ Patient informed at an age-appropriate time.

Abnormal Puberty and Growth Problems

I. Introduction
   - Early teenage pregnancies have become a new and emerging health problem.
   - Abnormalities of puberty include premature puberty, attenuated puberty, and delayed puberty.
II. Physiology of Puberty
   - Period of infancy and childhood.
     - Midgestation luteinizing hormone (LH) and follicle-stimulating hormone (FSH) levels in the fetus are high; these levels fall secondary to the increased levels of circulating steroids in pregnancy.
     - At birth, negative feedback is released.
       - Prompt increases in FSH and LH are seen (to levels higher than in an adult).
       - Inhibin B levels also increase.
       - Transient estradiol increases as a result of gonadotropin stimulation.
     - Full negative feedback is rapidly attained.
       - Levels of FSH and LH fall rapidly until age 6 to 8 years.
       - The endogenous gonadostat is very sensitive to the negative feedback of very low levels of estradiol.
     - Gonadotropins are also suppressed in hypogonadal children (gonadal dysgenesis).
       - Therefore, suppression cannot be solely a function of estradiol.
       - A central nonsteroidal suppression of endogenous gonadotropin-releasing hormone (GnRH) secretion must also exist.
   - Prepubertal period.
     - FSH and LH remain low but do show some pulsatile activity.
     - The following three changes in low endocrine hematostatic function emerge as puberty approaches:
       1. Adrenarche (pubarche).
       2. Decreased repression of gonadostat.
       3. Gonadal amplification of peptide–peptide and peptide–steroid interactions leading to gonadarche.
   - Adrenarche (pubarche).
     - Growth of pubic/axillary hair is secondary to increased adrenal androgens.
     - Premature adrenarche is sometimes seen in isolation.
     - Premature thelarche is very rare.

- It can occur in late childhood (6 to 7 years old) → adolescence (13 to 15 years old).
  - Increased adrenal cortical function, increased 17α-hydroxylase, increased 17,20-lyase activity, and all of the following are related to the increased size of the reticularis zone:
    ◊ Increased dehydroepiandrosterone (DHEA).
    ◊ Increased dehydroepiandrosterone sulfate (DHEAS).
    ◊ Increased androstenedione.
  - Adrenarche usually occurs 2 years before the growth spurt.
    ◊ Possibly, this is due to an initiating event in the pubertal transformation.
    ◊ Most evidence, as follows, supports dissociation between pubarche and gonadarche:
      ○ Premature adrenarche is not associated with premature gonadarche.
      ○ In hypergonadotropic hypogonadotropism (gonadal dysgenesis) or hypogonadotropic states (Kallmann syndrome), adrenarche still occurs.
      ○ In true precocious puberty before the age of 6 years, gonadarche occurs first.
  - Adrenarche is not under the direct control of adrenocorticotropic hormone (ACTH) or gonadotropins.
  - Candidates for the agent initiating adrenarche that have failed on close inspection include the following:
    ◊ All proopiomelanocortin peptides—ACTH, β-endorphin, β-lipoprotein.
    ◊ Melatonin.
- The kinetics of adrenal enzyme activity may play a role.
  - 3β-Hydroxysteroid dehydrogenase activity.
  - 17,20-Lyase activity following serine phosphorylation of P450c17.

III. Decreasing Repression of the Gonadostat—Progressive Responsiveness of the Anterior Pituitary to GnRH
  ◆ Mechanisms of gonadotropic restraint.
    • Highly sensitive negative feedback of estradiol.
    • Central negative influence on GnRH secretion.
  ◆ Similar pattern observed in children who are agonadal.
  ◆ Reversal of central intrinsic suppression may explain pathogenesis of the central nervous system (CNS) etiologies of precocious puberty.
  ◆ Pineal gland melatonin reduction may reverse central suppression; no evidence that normal timing in humans depends on it.
  ◆ Research continues for this agent.

IV. Alteration/Amplification of GnRH–Gonadotropin and GnRH–Sex Steroid Interactions

- ◆ FSH/LH serum levels increase during progress through puberty.
  - • FSH response to GnRH initially is pronounced in prepubertal girls.
  - • It decreases steadily throughout the onset of puberty.
  - • LH response is low prepubertally but increases strikingly during puberty.
- ◆ GnRH pulses increase in amplitude and frequency.
- ◆ GnRH induces its own receptor in gonadotropes.
- ◆ Midpuberty.
  - • Estrogen: enhances LH response to GnRH.
  - • Negative feedback on FSH in combination with inhibin.
- ◆ Increased biologic availability of LH; changes in the glycosylation pattern result in the increased bio-availability.
- ◆ The onset of augmented GnRH pulses occurs during sleep cycles.
  - • Early puberty → nocturnal augmentation in FSH and LH pulses both in amplitude and especially in frequency.
  - • Late puberty → diurnal differences increase with the onset of puberty.
- ◆ Sleep-related LH pulses.
  - • Also seen in idiopathic precocious puberty.
  - • Found in anorexia patients during intermediate stages of exacerbation and recovery.
  - • Agonadal when gonadotropin levels are returning from midchildhood reductions.
V. Puberty
  - ◆ Usually occurs between the ages of 10 and 16 years.
    - • The pattern is as follows:
      - ■ Increased pulsatile pattern of LH during sleep.
      - ■ Smaller pulses of lower amplitude during the day.
      - ■ Episodic peaks of estradiol.
      - ■ Menarche appears.
      - ■ Maturation of response to pulsatile secretion results in ovulatory cycles.
    - • Timing of puberty—major determination is genetic.
    - • Other factors.
      - ■ Geographic location.
      - ■ Exposure to light.
      - ■ General health and nutrition.
        - ◇ Possibly a critical body weight of 47.8 kg (Frisch hypothesis).
        - ◇ A greater percentage of body fat (16% to 23.5%) may serve as the initiating signal.
          - ○ Moderately obese girls have earlier menarche.
          - ○ Anorectics have delayed menarche.
        - ◇ Puberty is delayed in patients with morbid obesity; other factors are also involved.

- Other exceptions:
  - Blind girls enter puberty with a total body fat of 19%.
  - Girls with central precocious puberty may undergo menarche.
  - Girls with no sign of puberty may have a measured total body fat of 27%.
- ◆ Leptin and puberty.
  - Leptin is a peptide secreted by adipose tissues; it acts on CNS neurons, regulating eating behavior and energy balance.
  - Evidence of supporting role for leptin in reproductive physiology includes the following:
    - Leptin accelerates onset of puberty in rodents.
    - Leptin levels increase at puberty in boys.
    - Low leptin levels are present in athletes, anorexics, and patients with pubertal delay.
    - Mice with leptin gene knock-out undergo normal sexual development but remain prepubertal without ovulating; fertility is restored with leptin.
    - Higher levels of leptin correspond to earlier menarche.
    - Girls with idiopathic precocious puberty have higher leptin levels.
  - Leptin levels in girls decrease with increasing Tanner stage.
    - They have increased sensitivity to leptin.
    - The decrease may allow greater food intake.
- ◆ Stages of pubertal development.
  - The pubertal sequence requires 4.5 years (range, 1.5 to 6 years) (Table 10.1).
  - The first sign of puberty is usually the growth spurt, followed by breast budding.
  - In 20% of children, adrenarche is the first sign; adrenarche usually appears after the breast bud, with axillary hair 2 years later.

Table 10.1. Pubertal development in American girls

	Black Americans	White Americans
Breast budding and/or pubic hair at age 7	27.2%	6.7%
at age 8	48.3%	14.7%
Menarche at age 11	27.9%	13.4%
at age 12	62.1%	35.2%
Mean age for thelarche	8.87 yr	9.96 yr
Mean age for adrenarche	8.78 yr	10.51 yr
Mean age for menarche	12.16 yr	12.88 yr

- ♦ Growth.
  - Growth.
    - The growth spurt occurs earlier in girls than in boys (age 11 to 12 years).
    - The growth rate doubles in year 1 (6- to 11-cm height increase).
    - Growth peaks 2 years after breast budding, 1 year prior to menarche.
    - Growth spurts are associated with increased levels of growth hormone and a secondary increase in insulin-like growth factor–I (IGF-I).
    - Adrenal androgens are not involved, as the normal pattern in Addisonian patients demonstrates.
    - The short stature of African pigmies is due to growth failure in puberty.
    - Increased sex steroid concentration results in elevations of growth hormone, which, in turn, increases IGF-I.
    - Laron-type dwarfs have a genetic absence of the growth hormone receptor.
      - Cannot stimulate IGF-I.
      - Can undergo pubertal growth spurt with sex steroids, but final height is decreased because of decreased growth hormone response.
    - Estrogens can cause epiphyseal fusion, limiting final height; true for boys and girls.
- ♦ Growth hormone.
  - Most abundant hormone produced by the pituitary.
  - Not a single form—one predominant form of the hormone and one smaller hormone.
  - Growth hormones coded by five genes.
    - Chromosome 17q22-q24.
    - One gene for the predominant form; three genes are expressed in the placenta.
  - Regulation of pituitary gene by growth hormone–releasing hormone (GHRH), thyroid function, and glucocorticoids.
  - Pulsatile secretion of the growth hormone.
    - Increased pulses are seen during sleep.
    - Age of onset of increased pulse frequency corresponds to age of most rapid growth.
    - Growth response does not correlate with baseline changes, only with pulsatile changes.
  - Pulsatile pattern stimulated by GHRH and inhibited by somatropin release–inhibiting hormone.
  - Influenced by sex steroids.
  - At puberty, growth hormone secretion critically dependent on sex steroids.
    - Very sensitive to estrogens in both sexes.
      - ◇ The response is prior to any signs of sexual development.
      - ◇ Secretion of 100 ng/kg will increase the amplitude of growth hormone pulses.

- Too low to induce secondary sexual changes.
  - ◊ Low doses stimulate growth hormone–induced IGF-I secretion.
  - ◊ Males with estrogen receptor mutation or aromatase deficiencies grow slowly with reduced bone densities.
- Actions of the growth hormone.
  - Stimulates IGF-I in cartilage.
  - Stimulates IGF-I production in liver.
  - Insulin-like growth factor–binding protein–1 (IGFBP-1) is decreased by insulin, which allows increased IGF-I during puberty.
- Bone density.
  - Pubertal increase is greater in black girls.
  - This increase explains reduced osteoporosis in black women.
  - Calcium supplementation in adolescence helps.
  - Almost all bone mass is accumulated by late adolescence (age 18).
- ◆ Menarche.
  - In affluent cultures, the age dropped until 1960s.
  - It occurs after peak growth velocity.
  - The normal range is from 9 to 17.7 years of age; the median age is 12.8 years.
  - The final endocrine hallmark is the development of positive estrogen feedback on the pituitary and hypothalamus.
  - Midcycle LH surge occurs.
  - Anovulatory cycles often occur for 12 to 18 months; 20% to 50% of adolescents are anovulatory 4 years after menarche (Fig. 10.1).

VI. Summary of Pubertal Events
  1. FSH and LH rise moderately before the age of 10 years, followed by a rise in estradiol.
     - This results in increased levels of estradiol.
     - LH pulse frequency increases are first seen in sleep but then are extended throughout the day.
     - The final adult pattern is 1.5- to 2-hour intervals between pulses.
  2. Increased levels of estradiol (gonadarche) result in the maturation of secondary sexual characteristics.
     - Also increased skeletal growth occurring at low levels of estradiol.
     - Increased estradiol results in increased growth hormone and increased IGF-I.
  3. Adrenal androgens cause adrenarche (pelvic and axillary hair).
     - No major role in growth.
     - An independent event.
  4. Midpuberty levels of estradiol are sufficient to induce vaginal bleeding.
  5. Postmenarchal periods are irregular for 12 to 18 months—LH surge responses are late pubertal events.

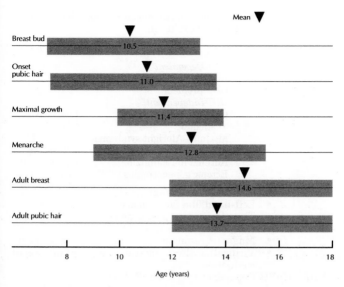

Figure 10.1.   Average age of appearance of pubertal events.

VII.   Precocious Puberty
- ♦ Pubertal changes in child < 8 years old = precocious puberty (2.5 standard deviation).
  - • However, recent data show that normal girls often begin pubertal development before the age of 8 years.
  - • Often the growth spurt is the first sign, followed by breast development and pubic hair.
  - • Menarche can occasionally be the first sign of precocious puberty.
  - • Adrenarche, thelarche, and growth can occur simultaneously.
- ♦ Two classifications follow. However, *these classifications are of little practical use.*
  - • GnRH-dependent → activation of hypothalamic–pituitary–gonadal axis—also called complete, isosexual, central, or true precocious puberty.
  - • GnRH-independent → extrapituitary human chorionic gonadotropin (hCG) or sex steroid exposure—also known as incomplete, isosexual or heterosexual, and peripheral or precocious pseudopuberty.
  - • Precocity is 5 times more common in girls.
    - ■ Approximately 75% of girls have idiopathic precocious puberty (girls >4 years of age rarely demonstrate any etiology).
    - ■ In younger girls, a CNS lesion is usually present.

■ However, the diagnosis of idiopathic precocity is one of exclusion.

	Girls	Boys
GnRH-Dependent		
Idiopathic	74%	41%
CNS problem	7%	26%
GnRH-Independent		
Ovarian cyst	11%	N/A
Testicular	N/A	10%
McCune–Albright syndrome	5%	1%
Adrenal feminizing	1%	0%
Adrenal masculinizing	11.1%	22.1%
Ectopic gonadotropins	0.5%	0.5%

- ◆ Evaluation is as follows:
  - Left-hand film for bone age.
  - Thyroid function assessment.
  - Gonadotropin/sex steroid levels.
  - Magnetic resonance imaging (MRI) of the brain.
  - Virilization always indicates need for full adrenal evaluation.
- VIII. GnRH-Dependent Precocious Puberty
  - ◆ Premature maturation of the hypothalamic–pituitary–ovarian axis.
  - ◆ Increased growth is associated with IGF-I levels.
  - ◆ Constitutional precocious puberty.
    - Usually runs in families.
    - Usually occurs close to the normal age of 8 years.
  - ◆ Idiopathic precocious puberty.
    - Does not usually run within families.
    - Occurs earlier in childhood.
    - Sequence of pubertal events possibly disordered.
    - *Overall, the most serious problem with precocious puberty is lack of attainment of a normal adult height*—approximately 50% are <5 feet tall.
  - ◆ Central nervous system etiologies of precocious puberty.
    - Abnormal skull development (rickets).
    - Brain tumors (especially hamartomas); also craniopharyngiomas, astrocytomas, and gliomas.
    - Pineal tumors in male precocious puberty.
    - Encephalitis, meningitis, hydrocephalus, and von Recklinghausen disease.
    - Skull injury.
    - Evaluation for growth hormone deficiency necessary because of recognized association.
  - ◆ Theories.
    - Possibly transforming growth factor–α induction of GnRH release occurs in areas of trauma.
    - Hamartomas can produce GnRH pulses.
  - ◆ Ectopic hCG production.
    - Chorioepithelioma and dysgerminoma of the ovary.
    - Liver hepatoblastoma.

- ♦ Thyroid function: long-standing hypothyroidism.
  - • May result in true sexual precocity.
  - • High levels of thyrotropin (TSH) can stimulate FSH receptor.
  - • Short stature (not bone-age accelerated).
  - • Galactorrhea.
  - • Sella turcica enlargement is frequent.

IX. GnRH-Independent Precocious Puberty
- ♦ Approximately 11% of girls have ovarian tumors.
  - • Five percent of granulosa cell tumors and 1% of thecal cell tumors occur before puberty.
  - • Bleeding is anovulatory in nature.
  - • About 80% of patients will have a palpable pelvic mass.
  - • Estrogen, androgens, and hCG secretion occur; feminizing adrenal tumor with increased dehydroepiandrosterone sulfate (DHEAS) is very rare.
  - • Drug ingestion.
    - ■ Especially in cases with dark pigmentation of nipples and breast areolae.
    - ■ Oral contraceptives, steroids, and hair or facial cream.
- ♦ McCune–Albright syndrome.
  - • Five percent of female precocity.
    - ■ Multiple disseminated cystic bone lesions that can easily fracture.
    - ■ Café-au-lait spots.
    - ■ Manifestation—varied and subtle.
    - ■ Can be associated with ovarian cysts, growth hormone adenomas, prolactin-secreting adenomas, hyperthyroidism, adrenal hypercortisolism, and osteomalacia.
    - ■ Premature menarche—first sign.
  - • Sexual precocity.
    - ■ Autonomous ovarian estrogen production is seen.
    - ■ FSH and LH levels are low.
    - ■ Technetium 99 bone scan may be necessary to demonstrate bone lesions.
    - ■ Patients respond poorly to GnRH stimulation.
    - ■ An absence of nocturnal GnRH secretion exists.
  - • A cellular regulatory defect has been classified.
    - ■ It involves G protein and cyclic adenosine monophosphate kinase function.
      - ◇ α Subunit is abnormal.
        - ○ Attenuates guanosine triphosphatase activity.
        - ○ Autonomous activity of adenylate cyclase activation.
      - ◇ "Inherited $G_s\alpha$ deficiency"—nonendocrine manifestation can be seen.
    - ■ Eventual fertility is impaired.
    - ■ Height is normal.
    - ■ Patients will not suppress with a GnRH agonist.

- Familial male precocious puberty: activating mutations of LH receptor.
- Ovarian follicular or luteal cysts.
  - Absence of gonadotropin pulsations.
  - Variable responses to GnRH.
  - Lack of suppression by GnRH.

Nearly every cause of peripheral precocious puberty can eventually activate the hypothalamic pituitary ovarian axis (Table 10.2).

X. Special Cases
  - Premature thelarche.
    - Usually occurs in the first few years of life.
    - Usually self-limiting; requires no therapy.
    - Normal puberty and normal reproduction.
    - Can be unilateral.
  - Premature menarche.
    - Very rare.
    - Check for infection, foreign bodies, and abuse, as well as trauma and a local neoplasm.
    - Normal growth, development, fertility are ultimately unaffected.
  - Premature adrenarche.
    - Consequence of early modest increase in adrenal androgens, dehydroepiandrosterone (DHEA), DHEAS.
    - Excludes adrenal enzyme defect, but such defects are rare; laboratory testing includes the following:
      - Early morning 17-hydroxyprogesterone test will suffice.
      - ACTH stimulation test is not necessary in most cases, except in cases of advanced bone age and circulating androgens > than early stages of puberty.
    - Treatment indicated only for unequivocal cases of 21-hydroxylase deficiency (Table 10.3; Figs. 10.2 and 10.3).
  - Diagnosis of precocious puberty.
    - Rule out life-threatening disease (neoplasm).
    - Define the velocity.
  - Diagnostic steps: physical examination and history.
    1. Growth, Tanner staging, height and weight percentiles.
    2. External genitalia changes.
    3. Abdominal, pelvic, and neurologic examination.
    4. Signs of androgenization.
    5. Other findings: McCune–Albright syndrome and hypothyroidism.
  - Laboratory diagnosis.
    1. Bone age.
    2. Computed tomography (CT) and/or MRI of the head; ultrasonography of the abdomen and pelvis.
    3. FSH, LH, and hCG.
    4. Thyroid function tests (TSH and free thyroxine [T_4]).
    5. Steroids (estradiol [E_2], progesterone [P_4], 17-hydroxyprogesterone, DHEAS, testosterone).

Table 10.2. Laboratory findings in disorders producing precocious puberty

	Gonadal Size	Basal FSH/LH	Estradiol or Testosterone	DHEAS	GnRH Response
Idiopathic	Increased	Increased	Increased	Increased	Pubertal
Cerebral	Increased	Increased	Increased	Increased	Pubertal
Gonadal	Unilaterally increased	Decreased	Increased	Increased	Flat
Albright	Increased	Decreased	Increased	Increased	Flat
Adrenal	Small	Decreased	Increased	Increased	Flat

Abbreviations: DHEAS, dehydroepiandrosterone sulfate; FSH, follicle-stimulating hormone; GnRH, gonadotropin-releasing hormone; LH, luteinizing hormone.

Table 10.3. Tanner staging

	Breast	Pubic Hair
Stage 1 (prepubertal)	Elevation of papilla only	No pubic hair
Stage 2	Elevation of breast and papilla as small mound, areola diameter enlarged. Median age: 9.8 yr	Sparse, long, pigmented hair chiefly along labia majora. Median age: 10.5 yr
Stage 3	Further enlargement without separation of breast and areola. Median age: 11.2 yr	Dark, coarse, curled hair sparsely spread over mons. Median age: 11.4 yr
Stage 4	Secondary mound of areola and papilla above the breast. Median age: 12.1 yr	Adult-type hair, abundant but limited to the mons. Median age: 12.0 yr
Stage 5	Recession of areola to contour of breast. Median age: 14.6 yr	Adult-type spread in quantity and distribution. Median age: 13.7 yr

6. GnRH stimulation testing.
- GnRH test.
  - Give GnRH, 100 µg, subcutaneously.
  - Check serum LH 40 minutes later; it should be <8 IU/L.
- Differential diagnosis.
  - Idiopathic sexual precocity is a diagnosis of exclusion.
  - Consider ectopic hCG production if gonadotropins are decreased and estradiol is elevated.
  - Look for an ovarian tumor or cyst if no virilization is present.
  - Check for adrenal or ovarian tumor if virilization is present.
  - Breast development usually correlates with bone age of 11 years.
  - Menarche usually correlates with bone age of 13 years.
  - If all signs are present in a short child with delayed bone growth → primary hypothyroidism is most likely.
    - Galactorrhea may be present.
    - Increased serum prolactin is observed.
    - FSH and LH levels are usually in the pubertal range; these will decline following thyroid treatment.
- Treatment objectives.
  1. Diagnose and treat intracranial disease.
  2. Arrest maturation until normal pubertal age.

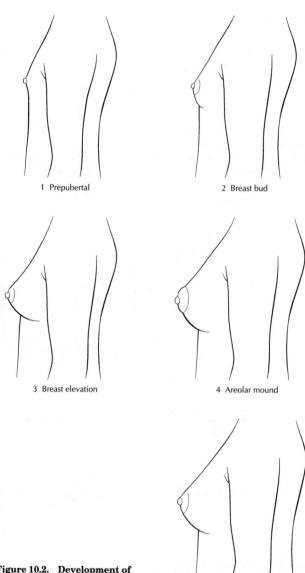

Figure 10.2.   Development of breasts in the female by Tanner stage.

1 Prepubertal

2 Breast bud

3 Breast elevation

4 Areolar mound

5 Adult contour

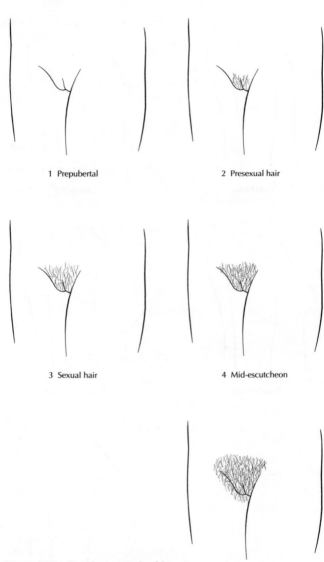

1 Prepubertal

2 Presexual hair

3 Sexual hair

4 Mid-escutcheon

Figure 10.3.   Development of pubic hair in the female by Tanner stage.

5 Female escutcheon

3. Attenuate and diminish established precocious characteristics.
4. Maximize adult height.
5. Avoid abuse, reduce emotional and social problems, and provide counseling regarding contraception.

♦ Treatment with GnRH agonist.
  • Substitute native GnRH at position 6 with replacement C-terminal glycine amide.
  • Regression of symptoms occurs in the first year.
    ■ Regression of pubertal characteristics, amenorrhea, and ↓ growth velocity.
    ■ Delay epiphyseal fusion; treatment more effective if begun before bone age >12 years.
  • Maintain estradiol at <10 pg/mL; this can also be confirmed by gonadotropin levels in response to GnRH.
  • Children require higher doses than adults for suppression.
  • Adrenarche will continue.
  • Treatment is continued until the epiphyses are fused or the appropriate pubertal and chronologic ages are matched.
  • The GnRH agonist can also shrink hamartomas.
  • GnRH is not effective in the following:
    ■ McCune–Albright syndrome.
    ■ Congenital adrenal hyperplasia.
    ■ GnRH-independent precocious puberty.
    However, if these three activate true precocious puberty, then there is benefit to the use of GnRH agonist.

♦ McCune–Albright syndrome treatment options.
  • Testolactone (aromatase inhibitor).
  • Medroxyprogesterone acetate (Depo-Provera) to suppress LH.

♦ Treatment of ovarian tumor.
  • Excision.
  • GnRH testing resolves question of GnRH responsiveness.

♦ Treatment of hypothyroidism and congenital adrenal hypoplasia are discussed elsewhere.

♦ Psychosocial issues.
  • Libido is age-related.
  • Careful evaluation of unrealistic expectations is needed with regard to parents' dealings with a child.

♦ Prognosis.
  • Depends on the underlying cause.
    ■ Prognosis in primary hypothyroidism is excellent.
    ■ Patients with congenital adrenal hyperplasia usually have short stature as adults.
    ■ Ovarian tumor outcomes are good with benign tumors but poor in aggressive malignant neoplasms.

◇ Granulosa cell tumors are malignant in 20% of cases.
◇ Sertoli–Leydig cells are malignant in 25% of cases.

- CNS causes.
    - Completely resectable CNS tumors have good prognosis.
    - However, this is the exception, not the rule.

XI. Delayed Puberty
- ♦ Nearly all females enter puberty by age 13; if puberty is delayed until age 17, a problem likely exists.
- ♦ The history and physical examination are useful.
    - Physiologic delay tends to be familial.
    - Persistent decidual teeth indicate probable hypothyroidism.
    - Absent pubic hair suggests hypopituitarism if the uterus is present.
    - Absent pubic hair with a vaginal pouch suggests androgen insensitivity syndrome.
    - Isolated growth hormone deficiency is associated with somewhat delayed sexual maturity.
    - Gonadal dysgenesis is associated with sexual infantilism, ↑ gonadotropin levels, and normal to slightly reduced bone age.
- ♦ Laboratory assessment.
    - Hand film for bone age.
    - Skull imaging if hypogonadotropic.
    - Gonadotropin and prolactin levels.
    - Thyroid function testing.
    - Adrenal and gonadal steroids.
    - Karyotype if gonadotropins are elevated.
    - Measurements of IGF-I, IGFBP-3, IGFBP-2; can distinguish between delayed puberty and growth hormone deficiency.
- ♦ Gonadotropin findings (Table 10.4).
- ♦ Hypergonadotropic hypogonadism.
    - Gonadal dysgenesis.
        - 45,XO.
        - 46,XX.
            ◇ Pure gonadal dysgenesis.
            ◇ 17α-Hydroxylase deficiency; hypertension, elevated progesterone, and sexual infantilism.
    - Sickle cell also results in hypertension.
- ♦ Hypogonadotropic hypogonadism.
    - LH <6 IU/L is associated with depressed FSH.
    - Hypothalamic amenorrhea.
    - Poor nutrition.
    - Kallmann syndrome.
    - Hyperprolactinemia.
    - Pituitary tumor.
    - Physiologic delay (only in 10%); short with appropriate bone maturation delay.
    - MRI of brain—craniopharyngioma.
        - Most common neoplasm associated with delayed puberty.

**Table 10.4.   Relative frequency of delayed
pubertal abnormalities**

Hypergonadotropic Hypogonadism		**43.0%**
Ovarian failure, abnormal karyotype		26.0%
Ovarian failure, normal karyotype		17.0%
46,XX	15.0%	
46,XY	2.0%	
Hypogonadotropic Hypogonadism		**31.0%**
Reversible		18.0%
Physiologic delay	10.0%	
Weight loss/anorexia	3.0%	
Primary hypothyroidism	1.0%	
Congenital adrenal hyperplasia	1.0%	
Cushing syndrome	0.5%	
Prolactinomas	1.5%	
Irreversible		13.0%
GnRH deficiency	7.0%	
Hypopituitarism	2.0%	
Congenital CNS defects	0.5%	
Other pituitary adenomas	0.5%	
Craniopharyngioma	1.0%	
Malignant pituitary tumor	0.5%	
Eugonadism		**26.0%**
Müllerian agenesis		14.0%
Vaginal septum		3.0%
Imperforate hymen		0.5%
Androgen insensitivity syndrome		1.0%
Inappropriate positive feedback		7.0%

Abbreviations: CNS, central nervous system; GnRH, gonadotropin-releasing hormone.

- ■ Tumor of Rathke pouch.
    - ◊ Originates from pituitary stalk with suprasellar extension.
    - ◊ Peak incidence between the ages of 6 to 14 years.
    - ◊ Abnormal sella and calcification in 70%.
    - ◊ Treated with radiation or surgery.
- ♦ Eugonadotropic hypogonadism.
    - • Müllerian abnormality—müllerian agenesis in one-seventh of cases of primary amenorrhea.
    - • Anovulation and polycystic ovaries.
    - • Androgen-producing adrenal disease.
    - • Virilization—congenital adrenal hyperplasia or intersex problem possible.
- ♦ Treatment.
    - • Correct the etiology.
        - ■ Thyroid disease.
        - ■ Growth hormone dysfunction.
        - ■ Treatment of nutritional problems (ileitis).
        - ■ Gonadectomy of XY individuals.

- Hormone treatment.
  - Initiate and sustain maturation of secondary sexual characteristics; reduce psychological stress.
  - Promote full height.
  - Increase bone density.
- Usual doses of conjugated estrogens (Premarin) are 0.3 mg for 6 months, increasing to 0.625 mg; add medroxyprogesterone acetate (Provera), 10 mg × 12 days/month; patients with physiologic delay will continue on their own once bone age reaches 13 years.
- Use of pulsatile GnRH is possible but not practical.

XII. Growth Problems in Normal Adolescent
  - Evaluate by left-hand film.
  - Bayley–Pinneau tables; x-ray, age, and present height allow for prediction of final adult stature.
  - Short stature.
    - Bone age only 1 year behind chronologic age suggests a constitutional pattern.
    - Thyroid disease.
    - Exogenous corticosteroids.
  - Treatment of short stature.
    - Usually give reassurance only.
    - Steroids can limit growth, which is an emerging issue of anabolic steroid use.
  - Tall stature.
    - This can be an issue for girls.
    - Perform a hand–wrist x-ray.
    - Consider treatment if predicted height is >6 feet, but treatment must be initiated before age 12 and even as early as age 8 to 9.
    - Use 50 µg of estradiol-containing oral contraceptives.
    - The overall goal is to close epiphyseal plates; check x-rays every 6 months.
    - Consider 1.25 mg conjugated estrogen if the patient is unable to tolerate high-dose oral contraceptives.

Amenorrhea

I. Definition of Amenorrhea
    ♦ No period by the age of 14 years in the absence of growth or development of secondary sexual characteristics.
    ♦ No period by the age of 16 years regardless of the presence of normal growth and development with the appearance of secondary sexual characteristics.
    ♦ In a previously menstruating woman, the absence of periods for a length of time equivalent to three of the previous cycle intervals or 6 months.
    ♦ Strict adherence may be inappropriate depending on the clinical situation (e.g., a girl with obvious stigmata of Turner syndrome).
II. Basic Principles in Menstrual Function
    ♦ Intact outflow tract is necessary.
    ♦ Outflow requires endometrial shedding.
    ♦ Endometrium depends upon ovarian steroids.
    ♦ Ovarian function is dependent upon the anterior pituitary.
    ♦ Pituitary function is dependent upon gonadotropin-releasing hormone (GnRH).
    ♦ Diagnostic compartments are helpful.
      • Compartment I—disorders of outflow tract or uterine target organ.
      • Compartment II—disorders of the ovary.
      • Compartment III—disorders of the anterior pituitary.
      • Compartment IV—disorders of the hypothalamus.
III. Evaluation of Amenorrhea
    ♦ Galactorrhea (nonpuerperal breast secretions) can be present and is associated with amenorrhea.
    ♦ Step 1.
      1. Measure thyroid-stimulating hormone (TSH).
      2. Measure prolactin.
      3. Progestational challenge.
      4. (Addition of coned-down view of the sella turcica.)
         • Hypothyroidism.
           ■ Longer duration usually results in increased incidence of galactorrhea and elevations of prolactin.
           ■ This is associated with declining hypothalamic dopamine and unopposed thyrotropin-releasing hormone effect on the pituitary.
           ■ Prolactin levels are always less than 100 ng/mL in cases of primary hypothyroidism.
           ■ Distortion of the sella can be seen in hypothyroidism.

◇ Results from pituitary hypertrophy and hyperplasia.
◇ Can also be seen in patients with elevated gonadotropins and premature ovarian failure.
- Can present as primary amenorrhea or secondary amenorrhea.
- Progestational challenge.
  - Useful to assess level of endogenous estrogen and assure patency of outflow tract.
  - Three choices for initiating the progestational challenge are as follows:
    1. 200 mg intramuscular progesterone.
    2. 300 mg oral micronized progesterone.
    3. 10 mg oral medroxyprogesterone acetate × 5 days.
  - Bleeding should occur within 2 to 7 days.
  - If bleeding occurs, then the diagnosis is anovulation.
  - Bleeding should be considered anything greater than a few spots of blood.
  - Failure of withdrawal bleeding can occur in two special cases:
    ◇ Elevated androgens with polycystic ovary syndrome → results in decidualized endometrium.
    ◇ Elevated progesterone levels present in patients with congenital adrenal hyperplasia.
  - The anovulatory patient must be managed appropriately.
    ◇ Protect her from endometrial hyperplasia; give 10 mg/day medroxyprogesterone acetate × 10 days/month.
    ◇ A low-dose oral contraceptive is also helpful.
  - If the patient has failure of withdrawal bleeding after previous withdrawal, then continue the evaluation and look for additional sources. Consider ovulation in response to the progestin challenge as a possible etiology.
  - *In the absence of galactorrhea and with a normal prolactin level and withdrawal bleeding, further evaluation to rule out a pituitary tumor is unnecessary.*
- ♦ Step 2.
  - Conduct if no progestin withdrawal flow.
  - Either outflow tract problem or no preliminary estrogen proliferation of the endometrium.
  - Step 2 clarifies the situation.
  - Method.
    - Administer oral estrogen for 21 days.
      ◇ 1.25 mg conjugated estrogens.
      ◇ 2 mg estradiol.

- ■ Add 10 mg medroxyprogesterone acetate ×
      5 days.
    - ■ Repeat sequence if no bleeding occurs.
  - • If patient has normal external and internal geni-
    talia and no history of infection or trauma to the
    outflow tract, then Step 2 may be excluded.
  - ◆ Step 3.
    - • Determine whether problem lies with gonado-
      tropins or with follicular activity.
    - • Wait 2 weeks after Step 2 to allow gonadotropins
      to return to baseline (Table 11.1).
- IV. High Gonadotropins
  - ◆ Clinical implications are very important.
    - • Repeat several months apart.
    - • Relationship with absent ovarian follicles is very,
      but not totally, reliable.
    - • Rare situations occur where high gonadotropins
      can be found in patients whose ovaries contain
      follicles. This can be caused by the following:
      - ■ Production of gonadotropins by tumors (very
        rare).
      - ■ Single gonadotropin deficiency—high follicle-
        stimulating hormone (FSH) or normal or low
        luteinizing hormone (LH).
        - ◊ Elevated α subunit can be found.
        - ◊ Presence of pituitary mass—gonadotrope
          adenoma.
      - ■ Gonadotropin-secreting adenoma.
        - ◊ Not associated with amenorrhea.
        - ◊ Evaluate by checking α subunit levels.
      - ■ Perimenopausal changes.

Table 11.1.   Assessment of serum gonadotropins

Clinical State	Serum FSH	Serum LH
Normal adult female	5–20 IU/L, with the ovulatory midcycle peak about 2 times the base level	5–20 IU/L, with the ovulatory mid-cycle peak about 3 times the base level
Hypogonadotropic state: prepuber-tal, hypothalamic, or pituitary dys-function	Less than 5 IU/L	Less than 5 IU/L
Hypergonadotropic state: post-menopausal, cas-trated, or ovarian failure	Greater than 20 IU/L	Greater than 40 IU/L

Abbreviations: FSH, follicle-stimulating hormone; LH, luteinizing hormone.

◇ Declining inhibin production → elevated FSH levels.
◇ Not an absolute indicator of infertility.
- Resistant or insensitive ovary.
  ◇ Absent or defective gonadotropin receptors.
  ◇ Possibly a subtle form of autoimmune failure.
  ◇ Laparotomy not recommended.
- Premature ovarian failure due to autoimmune disease.
  ◇ Normal-appearing primordial follicles; developing follicles surrounded by nests of lymphocytes and plasma cells.
  ◇ Mechanism unknown.
  ◇ Complete thyroid testing indicated.
  ◇ Rare polyglandular syndrome occasionally present.
  ◇ Adrenal insufficiency seen at times.
    ○ Antibodies against P450scc.
    ○ Premature ovarian failure; predates adrenal failure.
    ○ Continued adrenal surveillance suggested.
  ◇ Other rare conditions associated with premature ovarian failure:
    ○ Myasthenia gravis.
    ○ Idiopathic thrombocytopenic purpura.
    ○ Rheumatoid arthritis.
    ○ Vitiligo.
    ○ Autoimmune hemolytic anemia.
  ◇ Ovulation induction difficult; some success with use of a GnRH agonist, steroids, and high-dose gonadotropins.
- Galactosemia.
  ◇ Rare autosomal-recessive disorder.
  ◇ Deficiency in galactose-1-phosphate uridyl transferase.
  ◇ Excessive galactose—possible direct toxic effect on germ cell migration.
- Enzyme deficiencies.
  ◇ 17α-Hydroxylase deficiency.
    ○ Absent secondary sexual characteristics.
    ○ Hypertension and hypokalemia.
    ○ Elevated progesterone levels.
  ◇ Aromatase deficiency.
♦ The need for chromosomal evaluation.
  • All patients under age 30 with elevated gonadotropins should have one.
  • The presence of mosaicism with Y chromosome requires excision of gonadal areas—a risk for malignant germ cell transformation.
    - Gonadoblastoma.
    - Dysgerminoma.

- ■ Yolk sac tumor.
- ■ Choriocarcinoma.
- • Thirty percent of patients with a Y chromosome will not virilize.
- • Even if the patient has a normal karyotype, perform a yearly pelvic examination.
- • In patients over 30 years old, the diagnosis is premature menopause.
- • Tumors appear prior to age 30 and usually prior to age 20.
- • Also karyotype women with premature ovarian failure who are <63 inches tall as this may indicate Turner syndrome or Turner mosaic.
- ♦ Premature ovarian failure: a clinical dilemma.
  - • Normal ovarian function may resume in 10% to 20% of patients.
  - • Recovery is probably spontaneous.
    - ■ Questionable association with estrogen therapy.
    - ■ No impact determined in one study.
  - • Detection of ovarian antibodies is of little clinical value.
  - • Perform a few selected blood tests for autoimmune disease.
    - ■ Calcium.
    - ■ Phosphorus.
    - ■ Fasting glucose.
    - ■ A.M. cortisol.
    - ■ Free thyroxine (T_4).
    - ■ TSH.
    - ■ Thyroid antibodies.
    - ■ Complete blood cell count and sedimentation rate.
    - ■ Total protein.
    - ■ Rheumatoid factor.
    - ■ Antinuclear antibody.
  - • Adrenocorticotropic hormone (ACTH) response testing is not necessary.
  - • Hypothyroidism is commonly associated with premature failure.
  - • Consider induction of ovulation if the following are true:
    - ■ FSH:LH ratio <1.
    - ■ Estradiol >50 pg/mL.
- V. Normal Gonadotropins
  - ♦ How can a patient have negative withdrawal but normal levels of FSH and LH? The answer lies in the heterogenicity of glycoprotein molecules.
    - • Increased amounts of sialic acid are present.
    - • Hormones are rendered biologically inactive.
  - ♦ Take-home lesson.
    - • FSH and LH levels in the normal range in a patient with negative withdrawal bleeding are consistent with pituitary and central nervous system (CNS) failure.

- • Evaluation should follow the guidelines for low gonadotropins.

VI. Low Gonadotropins
- ♦ Need to distinguish between pituitary and CNS hypothalamic etiology.
- ♦ Imaging of the sella turcica.
  - • Employ thin computed tomography (CT) or magnetic resonance imaging (MRI); use contrast on both.
  - • MRI is preferred.
  - • A conservative approach is used for small pituitary tumors.
    - ▪ Majority of these never change.
    - ▪ Tumors <10 mm may require no treatment.
  - • If prolactin is >100 ng/mL (or the coned-down view is abnormal), then consider an MRI.
  - • A double floor on the coned-down view is a normal variant.
  - • A history of visual problems and/or headache should prompt a CT or MRI.
  - • Prolactin levels >100 ng/mL require a more aggressive approach; large mass with prolactin <100 ng/mL is not likely to be prolactin-secreting, but it may cause stalk compression and therefore can decrease dopamine delivery, leading to hyperprolactinemia.
- ♦ Microadenoma.
  - • Prolactin <100 ng/mL.
  - • Normal coned-down view.
  - • Give a dopamine agonist for pregnancy; otherwise, conduct an annual prolactin and coned-down view for surveillance.
- ♦ Seven reasons why the diagnosis of microadenoma is not necessary are as follows:
  1. Microadenomas are very common.
  2. They rarely grow in pregnancy.
  3. They rarely progress to macroadenoma.
  4. The rate of recurrence after surgery is significant.
  5. The natural course is unaffected by dopamine treatment.
  6. No contraindication exists for hormone replacement therapy or oral contraceptive use.
  7. Overall, this avoids the problem of the incidentaloma.
- ♦ The pituitary incidentaloma.
  - • Pituitary microadenomas are found in 9% to 27% of autopsies.
  - • Silent microadenomas do not grow.
  - • Reassess at 1, 2, and 5 years for microadenoma; at 0.5, 1, 2, and 5 years for macroadenoma.
  - • Growth requires treatment.
  - • Minimal hormone screening includes prolactin; TSH; insulin-like growth factor–I (IGF-I); and 24-hour urinary cortisol or overnight dexamethasone-suppression test.

♦ Evaluation of the abnormal sella turcica and/or high prolactin.
  • Endocrine testing beyond prolactin and a coned-down view of the sella turcica is not helpful.
  • Further evaluation is needed for prolactin >100 ng/mL and/or an abnormal sella turcica.

VII. Hypogonadotropic Hypogonadism
  ♦ Diagnosis of exclusion.
  ♦ Provocative testing not helpful.

VIII. Specific Disorders within Compartments
  ♦ Frequency in secondary amenorrhea (Table 11.2).
  ♦ Compartment I: disorders of the outflow tract of the uterus.
    • Asherman syndrome.
      ■ Secondary amenorrhea following the destruction of the endometrium.
      ■ Typical pattern is multiple synechiae on a hysterogram; hysteroscopic diagnosis is more accurate.
      ■ Despite cervical stenosis in some cases, hematometra does not inevitably occur; possibly a response to increased intrauterine pressure.
      ■ Etiology.
        ◊ Often postpartum curettage.
        ◊ Other uterine surgery may contribute, including cesarean section, myomectomy, and metroplasty.
      ■ Rare problems.
        ◊ Tuberculous endometritis.
        ◊ Uterine schistosomiasis.
        ◊ Intrauterine device–related infections and pelvic inflammatory disease.
      ■ Treatment.
        ◊ Hysteroscopy is preferred to "blind" dilation and curettage.
        ◊ A pediatric Foley catheter is placed inside the uterine cavity after resection.

Table 11.2. Frequencies of etiology of amenorrhea by compartment

Compartment I	
Asherman syndrome	7.0%
Compartment II	
Abnormal chromosomes	0.5%
Normal chromosomes	10.0%
Compartment III	
Prolactin tumors	7.5%
Compartment IV	
Anovulation	28.0%
Weight loss/anorexia	10.0%
Hypothalamic suppression	10.0%
Hypothyroidism	1.0%

- ○ Fill with 3 mL fluid.
- ○ Maintain in place for 10 days.
- ○ Cover with broad-spectrum antibiotics.
- ○ Encourage endometrial regrowth with high-dose estrogen × 2 months.
  - □ Conjugated equine estrogens, 2.5 mg daily.
  - □ Medroxyprogesterone acetate, 10 mg daily, during the third week of treatment for each month.
- ◇ Persistent attempts at surgical correction are worthwhile.
- ◇ Treatment has approximately a 70% to 80% eventual success rate with regard to pregnancy; a pregnancy may be complicated by preterm labor, placenta accreta, placenta previa, and/or postpartum hemorrhage.
- Müllerian anomalies.
  - Need to rule out segmental disruption of the müllerian tube in primary amenorrhea.
    - ◇ Direct observation.
      - ○ Imperforate hymen.
      - ○ Obliteration of the vaginal orifice.
      - ○ Lapses in the continuity of the vaginal canal.
    - ◇ These obstructive abnormalities may result in hematocolpos, hematometra, and hematoperitoneum.
  - MRI may be very helpful.
- Müllerian agenesis.
  - Mayer–Rokitansky–Küster–Hauser syndrome.
    - ◇ Primary amenorrhea with no apparent vagina; a relatively common cause of primary amenorrhea (1 in 4,000 female live births).
    - ◇ A wide range of upper reproductive tract abnormalities (upper vagina, tube, uterus).
      - ○ Can resemble some forms of male pseudohermaphroditism.
      - ○ Worthwhile to demonstrate a normal female karyotype.
  - Normal ovarian function.
  - Normal growth and development.
  - Etiology.
    - ◇ Exact causes are unknown.
    - ◇ Likely causes are a mutation in the gene for antimüllerian hormone (AMH) or AMH receptor.
      - ○ No activating mutation has yet been identified.
      - ○ Inactivating mutations lead to the abnormal persistence of müllerian structures.

- Occurrence is usually sporadic, but occasionally it is found within a family; mutations in the galactose-1-phosphate uridyl transferase gene have been identified.
  ◇ Differs from classic galactosemia.
  ◇ Premature ovarian failure possibly more common in these patients.
- Further evaluation.
  ◇ One-third of patients have urinary tract abnormalities.
    ○ Ectopic kidney.
    ○ Renal agenesis.
    ○ Horseshoe kidney.
    ○ Abnormal collecting ducts.
  ◇ Approximately 12% have skeletal abnormalities.
    ○ Most involve the spine.
    ○ Absent digits or syndactyly can also occur.
  ◇ MRI is better than ultrasound and is less expensive and less invasive than laparoscopy.
- Treatment—vaginal dilation (Frank method) is preferred over surgical construction of an artificial vagina.
  ◇ Begin in a posterior direction; after 2 weeks, change to the normal axis of the vagina.
  ◇ Perform for 20 minutes daily to the point of moderate discomfort.
  ◇ Gradually increase dilator size.
  ◇ This method has good success over several months of persistent dilation.
- Surgical options.
  ◇ Vecchietti operation applies a traction device either transabdominally or by laparoscopy; a functional vagina is created in 7 to 9 days.
  ◇ Surgical treatment is usually reserved for women who meet the following criteria:
    1. Failure of the Frank method.
    2. Refusal to perform Frank method.
    3. A well-formed uterus is present and patient desires to attempt fertility preservation.
      ○ However, if cervix is atretic, hysterectomy is recommended.
      ○ Most experts warn against attempts to preserve fertility in cases of complete vaginal agenesis.
- Transverse vaginal septum—failure of cannulization of the distal one-third of vagina.
  ◇ Patients usually present with symptoms of menstrual obstruction and/or urinary frequency.

- ◇ No introital distention with Valsalva maneuver.
- ◇ May be accompanied by anomalies of the upper reproductive tract.
- Distal obstruction.
  - ◇ Considered an emergency.
  - ◇ A delay in treatment can lead to inflammatory changes and endometriosis.
  - ◇ Diagnostic needling can lead to the conversion of hematocolpos into pyocolpos.
- Reproductive potential.
  - ◇ Reassurance and support are needed.
  - ◇ Genetic offspring can be produced; in 34 live births (through use of a gestational surrogate), no evidence of inheritance in a dominant fashion was seen.
- Androgen insensitivity (testicular feminization).
  - Overview.
    - ◇ Complete androgen insensitivity syndrome (AIS) is the likely diagnosis in a patient with an absent uterus and a blind vaginal canal.
    - ◇ Third most common cause of primary amenorrhea after gonadal dysgenesis and müllerian agenesis.
    - ◇ May be considered a form of male pseudohermaphroditism.
      - ○ Male karyotype.
      - ○ Pseudohermaphrodite = genitalia opposite of the gonads (Table 11.3).
    - ◇ Genetic and/or gonadal male with failure of virilization.
    - ◇ Transmission by X-linked recessive.
    - ◇ Consider this diagnosis in the following cases:
      1. Female child with inguinal hernias (testes partially distended).
      2. Patient with primary amenorrhea and absent uterus.
      3. Patient with absent body hair.
    - ◇ Growth and development are normal.
      - ○ Overall height usually greater than average.
      - ○ Eunuchoid tendency.
      - ○ Large breasts—somewhat abnormal with small nipples and a pale areolae area.
    - ◇ Approximately 50% of patients present with an inguinal hernia.
    - ◇ The blind vagina is less deep than normal.
    - ◇ Rudimentary fallopian tubes only occasionally have an epithelial lining.
    - ◇ Horseshoe kidneys have been reported.
  - Testes.

Table 11.3. Differences between Müllerian agenesis and testicular feminization

	Müllerian Agenesis	Testicular Feminization
Karyotype	46,XX	46,XY
Heredity	Not known	Maternal X-linked recessive; 25% risk of affected child, 25% risk of carrier
Sexual hair	Normal female	Absent to sparse
Testosterone level	Normal female	Normal to slightly elevated male
Other anomalies	Frequent	Rare
Gonadal neoplasia	Normal incidence	5% incidence of malignant tumors

   ◊ May be intraabdominal or in the hernia sac.
   ◊ Similar to cryptorchid testes but may be nodular.
   ◊ After puberty, immature tubular development.
      ○ Germ cells and Sertoli cells are immature.
      ○ No spermatogenesis.
   ◊ High incidence of neoplasm.
      ○ Twenty-two percent incidence of malignancy (more recent studies suggest 5% to 10%).
      ○ Fifty-two percent incidence of neoplasia (more recent studies suggest 5% to 10%).
   ◊ In AIS, remove the gonads at age 16 after full sexual development has been attained. *AIS represents the only exception to the rule that gonads with the Y chromosome require immediate removal.*
 ■ Hormone levels.
   ◊ Plasma testosterone levels are in the normal-to-high male range.
   ◊ Plasma clearance and metabolism are normal.
   ◊ AMH is present, so müllerian development is inhibited; the uterus, tubes, and upper vagina are absent.
 ■ Incomplete androgen insensitivity.
   ◊ One-tenth as common as the complete form.

◇ Individuals present with some androgen effect; axillary and pubic hair development with breast growth.
◇ Immediate gonadectomy needed to prevent further virilization.
◇ Patients with a deficit in 17β-hydroxysteroid dehydrogenase activity present in a similar fashion.
- Gender identity.
  ◇ Fully female gender identity in AIS.
  ◇ Best course of action—truthful education with appropriate psychological counseling.
  ◇ Resource A^{L}I^{A}S (www.medhelp.org/www/ais/).
♦ Compartment II: disorders of the ovary.
  • Overview.
    - Problem in gonadal development can present with either primary or secondary amenorrhea.
    - Approximately 30% to 40% of primary amenorrhea cases have streak gonads due to a developmental abnormality.
    - Karyotypes in primary amenorrhea:
      ◇ 45,X—50%.
      ◇ Mosaic—25%.
      ◇ 46,X—25%.
    - Karyotypes in secondary amenorrhea:
      ◇ 46,XX.
      ◇ Mosaics (45,X/46,XX).
      ◇ X deletion.
      ◇ 47,XXX.
      ◇ 45,X.
    - Both X chromosomes must be present and active to avoid accelerated follicular loss.
    - Ovarian failure in a 46,XX patient may reflect specific gene alterations, probably on the X chromosome.
    - It can be linked to neurosensory deafness (Perrault syndrome); consider an auditory evaluation in all 46,XX gonadal dysgenesis cases.
    - Pure gonadal dysgenesis refers to presence of bilateral streak gonads regardless of karyotype.
    - Mixed gonadal dysgenesis applies in cases with testicular tissue on one side and a streak gonad on the other.
  • Turner syndrome.
    - Diagnosis often possible on superficial evaluation.
      ◇ Short stature.
      ◇ Webbed neck.
      ◇ Shield chest.
      ◇ Increased carrying angle at the elbow.
      ◇ Hypergonadotropic hypoestrogenic amenorrhea.

- No gonadal sex hormone production; present with primary amenorrhea.
- Check karyotype to rule out mosaics; 40% have mosaics or structural abnormalities of the X or Y chromosome.
- Evaluate for autoimmune, cardiovascular, and/or renal anomalies.
- Mosaicism.
    - Presence of a Y chromosome must be ruled out.
    - Approximately 30% of patients with a Y chromosome will not develop virilization.
    - If standard cytogenetic analysis is uncertain, then pursue X-specific and Y-specific DNA probes; these are also needed in cases of virilization even if Y is not apparent in the karyotype.
    - Impact of mosaicism is also significant in the absence of a Y-containing cell line.
        - ◊ Some reproductive function is possible.
        - ◊ These patients are short (<63 inches).
        - ◊ Menopause is early.
    - All patients with absent ovarian function and quantitative alterations in the sex chromosomes are characterized as having gonadal dysgenesis.
- Swyer syndrome.
    - Female phenotype with palpable müllerian system, normal female testosterone, and lack of sexual development.
    - XY karyotype.
    - Gonads must be removed in these cases.
- Gonadal agenesis (empty pelvis syndrome).
    - No complicated clinical problems.
    - Other causes of absent development open to conjecture.
    - Hypergonadotropic hypogonadism.
    - Development is typically female.
    - Remove gonadal streaks in cases of XY karyotype.
- Resistant ovary syndrome.
    - Normal growth and development.
    - Amenorrhea.
    - Presence of rare follicles.
    - Elevated gonadotropins.
    - No evidence of autoimmune disease.
    - Laparotomy needed for diagnosis; rarely done because of lack of utility.
- Premature ovarian failure.
    - Surprisingly common phenomenon.
        - ◊ One percent of women enter menopause at <40 years of age.
        - ◊ Ten percent to 28% prevalence in patients with primary amenorrhea.
    - Etiology is usually unknown.

◇ Probably genetic basis; sex chromosome abnormalities may be identified, including 45,XO; 45,XXY; and mosaicism.
◇ Increased atresia of oocytes seen.
◇ Other etiologies: postinfection, postradiation, and postchemotherapy.
■ Spectrum of presentations, depending on timing.
■ Resumption of usual ovarian function: may occur in 10% to 20% of patients.
■ Further evaluation.
  ◇ Survey for autoimmune disease.
  ◇ Assess ovarian–pituitary activity.
■ Treatment.
  ◇ Hormone replacement therapy—oral contraceptives are preferred because of the possibility of spontaneous recovery.
  ◇ Oocyte donation for pregnancy—siblings may be poor candidates for egg donation in these cases.
■ Explanations for ovarian failure.
  ◇ Molecular explanations for ovarian failure.
    ○ Finnish population with recessive inheritance pattern.
    ○ Point mutation in FSH receptor has been found.
      □ Accounted for 29% of patients with premature ovarian failure in Finland.
      □ No such mutation has been found in the U.S. population or in the Brazilian population of women with premature ovarian failure.
    ○ Most likely a heterogenous condition with multiple causes.
    ○ Isolated cases of LH-receptor mutation and also XY translocations; also premutations of the site that transmits the fragile X syndrome.
  ◇ The effect of radiation and chemotherapy.
    ○ Radiation effect is dose-dependent.
    ○ Steroid levels fall and gonadotropins rise within 2 weeks of ovarian irradiation.
    ○ Ovaries of younger women are more resistant.
      □ Function can resume after years of amenorrhea.
      □ Damage may also present as premature ovarian failure.
    ○ If patients conceive, the risk to pregnancy is no greater than normal.
    ○ Transposition of the ovaries out of the radiation field can prevent damage.

- ○ Microwave ovens do not damage ovaries (Table 11.4).
- ○ Chemotherapy.
  - □ Alkylating agents are very toxic.
    - ▲ Combination chemotherapy is similar to alkylating agents.
    - ▲ Two-thirds of premenopausal breast cancer patients who are treated with cyclophosphamide, methotrexate, and 5-fluorouracil lose ovarian function.
  - □ Some suggestion that GnRH agonist protects follicles.
  - □ Oocyte cryopreservation may represent the best bet to preserve future fertility.
- ♦ Compartment III: disorders of the anterior pituitary.
  - • Overview.
    - ■ Pituitary tumors.
      - ◇ Malignant tumors are almost never encountered.
      - ◇ However, growth of a benign tumor can present problems because of limited space; upward growth compresses the optic chiasm.
      - ◇ Extrapituitary tumors can also affect vision.
        - ○ Craniopharyngiomas (associated with calcification on x-ray).
        - ○ Meningiomas.
        - ○ Gliomas.
        - ○ Chordomas.
        - ○ Metastatic tumors.
      - ◇ *Hypogonadism and delayed puberty require CNS evaluation by MRI.*
    - ■ Clinical signs of the non–prolactin-secreting adenoma.
    - ■ Acromegaly.
      - ◇ Amenorrhea and/or galactorrhea may precede full clinical expression.
      - ◇ Measure growth hormone during oral glucose tolerance test; lack of suppression of growth hormone is diagnostic.

Table 11.4.   Dosage relative to risk of sterilization

Ovarian Dose	Sterilization Effect
60 rad	No effect
150 rad	Some risk over age 40
250–500 rad	Ages 15–40: 60% sterilized
500–800 rad	Ages 15–40: 60% to 70% sterilized
over 800 rad	100% permanently sterilized

◇ Measure circulating IGF-I levels in all macroadenomas.
- Cushing disease.
  ◇ Excessive secretion of ACTH occurs.
  ◇ Measure ACTH level and 24-hour urinary levels of free cortisol; perform rapid suppression test.
- TSH-secreting adenoma.
  ◇ Less than 1% to 3% of all pituitary tumors.
  ◇ Unusual cause of secondary hyperthyroidism.
- Nonfunctioning adenomas (null cell).
  ◇ Overview.
    ○ Approximately 30% to 40% of all pituitary tumors are null cell.
    ○ Gonadotrope origin.
      □ Secrete FSH and free α subunit, but rarely LH.
      □ Usually diagnosed in menopausal patient with symptoms of mass effect.
    ○ Fail to down-regulate with GnRH agonist.
    ○ Usually decreased FSH and LH levels secondary to pituitary stalk compression.
      □ Associated with a modest increase in prolactin.
      □ Elevated FSH and LH levels in the presence of a pituitary microadenoma in a patient with amenorrhea are not a consequence of tumor secretion; look for another explanation.
- Nonneoplastic masses.
  ◇ Cysts.
  ◇ Tuberculosis.
  ◇ Sarcoid.
  ◇ Carotid artery aneurism.
  ◇ Lymphocytic hypophysitis—autoimmune infiltration of the pituitary.
    ○ Can mimic pituitary tumor.
    ○ Often occurs in pregnancy or in the first 6 months postpartum.
      □ Initially presents as elevated prolactin.
      □ Eventually leads to hypopituitarism.
        ▲ Potentially lethal.
        ▲ Treat with transsphenoidal resection.
- Treatment of nonfunctioning adenomas.
  ◇ If asymptomatic and <10 mm, follow up every 1 to 2 years.

◇ If asymptomatic and >10 mm, use surgery with possible postoperative radiation therapy.
  ○ Follow up with gonadotropins and α subunit.
  ○ Conduct an imaging study every 6 months for 1 year and then one every year for 3 to 5 years.
  ○ Maintain ongoing surveillance of thyroid and adrenal function.

- Pituitary prolactin-secreting adenomas.
  - Overview.
    ◇ Most common pituitary tumors.
      ○ Approximately 50% of all adenomas at autopsy.
      ○ Nine percent to 27% of patients at autopsy have adenomas; sex distribution is equal.
    ◇ High prolactin is found in one-third of women with amenorrhea; one-third of these will have galactorrhea.
    ◇ Absence of galactorrhea in hyperprolactinemia may be explained by the following:
      ○ Response to low estrogen environment.
      ○ Variation in immunoreactive versus biologically active forms.
        □ Little prolactin is the predominant variant.
        □ Biologic response is the cumulative effect of the circulating family of structural variants.
    ◇ Very high levels of prolactin (>1,000 ng/mL) are often associated with a tumor.
    ◇ Other facts:
      ○ One-third of women with galactorrhea have normal menses.
      ○ One-third of patients with secondary amenorrhea have a pituitary adenoma; if this is associated with galactorrhea, they will have an abnormal sella.
  - Prolactin and amenorrhea.
    ◇ Inhibition of pulsatile GnRH results in the disruption of cyclic menses, probably as a result of the increased opioid activity.
    ◇ Chronic naltrexone treatment does not restore cyclicity; treatment that lowers prolactin restores normal function.
    ◇ Treatment—surgical versus medical.
      ○ Surgical.
        □ Transsphenoidal neurosurgery achieves immediate resolution.
          ▲ Resumption of menses in 30% of patients with macroadenomas;

in 70% of patients with micro-adenomas.
- ▲ Recurrence rate is from 30% to 70%; 10% to 30% develop pan-hypopituitarism.
- □ Complications.
  - ▲ Recurrence.
  - ▲ Cerebrospinal fluid (CSF) leak.
  - ▲ Meningitis.
  - ▲ Transient diabetes insipidus (6 months).
  - ▲ Less than 1% rate of mortality.
- □ Best candidates for transsphenoidal surgery.
  - ▲ Prolactin levels between 150 to 500 ng/mL.
  - ▲ Recurrence of 26% if postoperative prolactin is <20 ng/mL; 50% cure rate.
- □ Surgical failure.
  - ▲ Failure to perform complete resection.
  - ▲ Multifocal tumor.
  - ▲ Hypothalamic dysfunction—unlikely since tumors are unifocal.
- □ Management of surgical cases.
  - ▲ Regular menses—periodic evaluation.
  - ▲ Amenorrhea, oligomenorrhea, or elevated prolactin persisting or recurring—do the following:
    1. Check prolactin every 6 months, and perform an imaging study every year for 2 years.
    2. Follow up with a coned-down view of the sella turcica every few years.
  - ▲ If the tumor regrows, attempt to control with bromocriptine mesylate (Parlodel) or another dopamine agonist if needed.
- ◊ Radiation.
  - ○ Less satisfactory response than surgery.
  - ○ Panhypopituitarism possible.
  - ○ Application of radiation—very limited.
- ◊ Dopamine agonist treatment—bromocriptine.
  - ○ Lysergic acid delivery derivative; bromine at position 2.
  - ○ Dopamine agonist.
    - □ Binds to receptor.
    - □ Directly mimics dopamine inhibition of pituitary prolactin secretion.

- ○ Twenty-eight percent of the bromocriptine is absorbed from the gastrointestinal tract.
  - □ Ninety-four percent metabolized in the first pass.
  - □ Thirty excretory products, mostly biliary.
- ○ 1.25 or 2.5 mg can be effective.
  - □ Also slow release or oral form available.
  - □ Intramuscular preparation also available.
- ○ Ten percent of patients cannot tolerate side effects.
  - □ Include nervousness, headache, and faintness; orthostatic hypotension secondary to splenic–renal bed dilation.
  - □ Neuropsychiatric symptoms seen in less than 1%.
- ○ Avoid symptoms by slowly increasing dose at bedtime; vaginal administration can also be effective.
- ○ Stop in early pregnancy or following ovulation.
- ◇ Results of treatment.
  - ○ Approximately 80% of patients with amenorrhea and/or galactorrhea but no tumor are restored to normal menses.
  - ○ Average time to menses is 5.7 weeks.
  - ○ Complete cessation of galactorrhea is seen in 50% to 60%.
    - □ Seventy-five percent reduction by 6 weeks.
    - □ Complete cessation by 12 weeks.
  - ○ Amenorrhea recurs in 41% within 4.4 weeks of stopping medication.
  - ○ Galactorrhea recurs in 69% within 6 weeks of stopping medication.
- ◇ Tumor regression with bromocriptine.
  - ○ Macroadenomas will regress.
    - □ Doses greater than 10 mg QD are not helpful.
    - □ Visual field improvement will occur within days.
    - □ Usually rapid shrinkage is seen within the first 3 months of treatment.
  - ○ Levels of prolactin >2,000 to 3,000 ng/mL represent probable cavernous sinus invasion; levels >1,000 ng/mL are associated with locally invasive tumors.
    - □ Tumor shrinkage is always preceded by decreased prolactin.

- □ Overall response is difficult to predict.
- □ However, a prolactin level non-responder will be a tumor size non-responder.
- ○ Treatment results in a reduction of cell sizes and cell necrosis; no convincing reports of tumor cure from bromocriptine have been found.
- ◊ Other dopamine agonists.
  - ○ Pergolide.
    - □ Longer lasting.
    - □ Occasionally tolerated better.
    - □ Single daily dose, 50 to 150 mg.
    - □ May be useful in bromocriptine-resistant patients.
  - ○ Cabergoline.
    - □ Oral doses, 0.5 to 3.0 mg Q week.
    - □ Low rate of side effects.
    - □ Can be administered vaginally.
    - □ Limited experience documenting fetal safety.
- ◆ Summary: therapy of pituitary prolactin-secreting adenomas.
  - • Macroadenomas.
    - ■ Use as low a dose of dopamine agonist as possible; may require 5 to 10 mg QD of bromocriptine.
      - ◊ Reduce dose once shrinkage has occurred.
      - ◊ Measure prolactin every 3 months as a marker.
    - ■ Withdrawal of treatment is associated with regrowth; therefore, treatment needs to be long term and indefinite.
    - ■ Repeat the MRI after 1 year to document response.
    - ■ Surgical treatment.
      - ◊ Useful in cases of suprasellar enlargement and for cases of persistent visual impairment after dopamine agonist treatment.
      - ◊ Debulk the largest tumor prior to medical treatment.
    - ■ Defer pregnancy until after shrinkage of the tumor.
    - ■ Ten percent of tumors do not shrink; failure of the tumor to shrink despite normalization of prolactin is consistent with the null cell tumor.
      - ◊ Stalk compression.
      - ◊ Early surgery indicated.
  - • Microadenomas.
    - ■ Treatment indicated in order to alleviate two problems:
      1. Infertility.

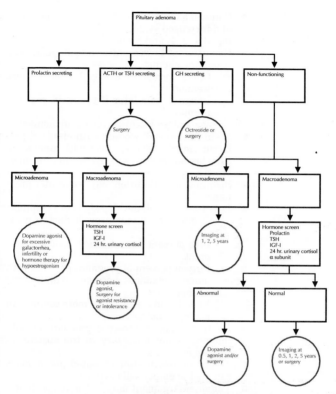

Figure 11.1.   Management of a pituitary adenoma.

    2.   Breast discomfort.
- Indication for treatment in patients not seeking fertility is unclear; monitor closely.
- Look at a coned-down view of the sella every 12 months for 2 years.
  - ◊ If no change is seen, recheck prolactin every year.
  - ◊ If prolactin is elevated, changes in coned-down view are seen, or headache and/or visual symptoms exist, then perform a MRI.
  - ◊ If growth is increasing, it deserves treatment.
  - ◊ Elevated prolactin can occur without tumor growth.
- **A macroadenoma and/or microadenoma should have follow-up every 6 months.** If it is stable, then recheck prolactin every year (Fig 11.1).

- Conduct a CT and MRI for increased prolactin and increased symptoms; also consider imaging at 1, 2, 4, and 8 years.
- Can attempt to wean after 5 to 10 years on a dopamine agonist.
  ◊ Check prolactin every 3 months once weaned.
  ◊ Image 1 year later if prolactin remains normal.

- Pregnancy and prolactin-secreting adenomas.
  - Eighty percent of women with elevated prolactin can achieve pregnancy with bromocriptine; breast-feeding will not stimulate tumor growth.
  - Spontaneous resolution may occur after pregnancy.
  - Less than 2% will develop signs or symptoms consistent with tumor growth during pregnancy.
    ◊ Five percent asymmetric tumor enlargement.
    ◊ Fifteen percent of pregnant patients with macroadenomas become symptomatic during pregnancy.
    ◊ Visual field loss is much more common in macroadenomas.
  - Routine visual field testing, prolactin, or sella imaging is not necessary in the absence of symptoms.
  - Tumor regrowth after repeated pregnancies can lead to empty sella syndrome.
  - Tumor enlargement may be treated with bromocriptine.
    ◊ No adverse effects on the fetus or newborn have been observed.
    ◊ Amniotic fluid prolactin is derived from the decidua.

- Empty sella syndrome: congenital incompleteness of the sellar diaphragm.
  - Subarachnoid space expands into the pituitary fossa.
    ◊ The pituitary gland is separated from the hypothalamus and flattened.
    ◊ Sella floor is demineralized from CSF pressure.
  - This may also occur secondary to surgery, radiation therapy, or infarction of the pituitary tumor.
  - Found in 5% of autopsies (85% female).
    ◊ Four percent to 16% of patients have amenorrhea and/or galactorrhea.
    ◊ Coexisting pituitary-secreting adenoma can be present.
  - Benign condition that does not progress to pituitary failure.

- ◇ Chief hazard is unnecessary surgery.
- ◇ Annual surveillance (prolactin and coned-down view) should be conducted to rule out growth of associated microadenoma.
  - ■ Hormone-replacement therapy or ovulation induction is safe.
- • Sheehan syndrome.
  - ■ Acute infarction and necrosis of the pituitary.
  - ■ Patients usually present with lactational failure and loss of pubic and/or axillary hair.
  - ■ Deficiency in growth hormone and gonadotropins is most common, followed by deficiencies in ACTH and TSH; diabetes insipidus is usually not present.
- ◆ Compartment IV: central nervous system disorders.
  - • Hypothalamic amenorrhea.
    - ■ A deficiency in pulsatile GnRH secretion.
      - ◇ Usually diagnosed by exclusion of pituitary lesion.
      - ◇ Most common category of hypogonadotropic amenorrhea.
        - ○ Frequently associated with stress.
        - ○ High proportion of underweight women.
    - ■ Degree of suppression determines classic presentation.
      - ◇ Mild → inadequate luteal phase.
      - ◇ Moderate → anovulation and menstrual irregularities.
      - ◇ Profound → hypothalamic amenorrhea.
    - ■ Clinical characteristics.
      - ◇ Low or normal gonadotropins.
      - ◇ Normal prolactin levels.
      - ◇ Normal imaging of the sella turcica.
      - ◇ Failure of withdrawal bleeding.
    - ■ Annual surveillance.
      - ◇ Prolactin.
      - ◇ Coned-down view of sella and then every 2 to 3 years after if no change is seen.
    - ■ Spontaneous recovery.
      - ◇ Approximately 72% after 6 years.
      - ◇ In patients with eating disorders, return of menstrual function associated with a gain in body weight.
    - ■ Possible etiology of GnRH and/or gonadotropin dysfunction.
      1. Primate evidence suggests role of corticotropin-releasing hormone (CRH) inhibition of gonadotropin secretion.
      2. Dopaminergic inhibition of GnRH pulse frequency.
    - ■ Future fertility.
      - ◇ Excellent options for ovulation induction.
      - ◇ Ovulation induction with gonadotropins will not stimulate the return of normal menstrual function.

- Weight loss, anorexia, and bulimia.
  - Obesity can be associated with amenorrhea; it is not associated with the hypogonadotropic state.
  - Acute weight loss can result in hypogonadism.
    - ◇ Historic evidence of anorexia leads back to St. Wilgefortis in A.D. 1000.
    - ◇ It stems from an inability to cope with adult sexuality.
    - ◇ Return to a prepubertal state is accomplished by weight loss.
  - Anorexia.
    - ◇ Mortality from 5% to 15%.
      - ○ Diagnosis.
        1. Onset between ages 10 and 30.
        2. Weight loss of 25% or weight 15% below normal for age and height.
        3. Special attitudes are as follows:
           - □ Denial.
           - □ Distorted body image.
           - □ Unusual hoarding and/or handling of food.
        4. One of the following must be present:
           - □ Lanugo.
           - □ Bradycardia.
           - □ Overactivity.
           - □ Episodes of overeating.
           - □ Vomiting.
        5. Amenorrhea.
        6. No known medical illness.
        7. No other psychiatric disorder.
        8. Other characteristics are as follows:
           - □ Constipation.
           - □ Low blood pressure.
           - □ Hypercarotenemia.
           - □ Diabetes insipidus.
    - ◇ Occurs in 1% of young women.
    - ◇ Usually a child who has been placed under undue stress and who perceives a need to be "perfect."
    - ◇ Pubertal weight gain can initiate true anorexia nervosa; excessive physical activity often the earliest sign.
    - ◇ Diuretic and laxative abuse can occur; may be associated with hypokalemia.
    - ◇ Hypercarotenemia—a metabolic marker; not every woman with it will be amenorrheic or anovulatory.
  - Bulimia.
    - ◇ Seen in half of anorexia nervosa patients.
    - ◇ Body weight fluctuates; does not fall to low levels.
    - ◇ High incidence of depressive symptoms.
  - Clinical problems in anorexia.

- ◇ Dysfunction of hypothalamic systems.
- ◇ Appetite.
- ◇ Thirst and water conservation.
- ◇ Temperature.
- ◇ Sleep.
- ◇ Autonomic balance.
- ◇ Endocrine secretion.
  - ○ FSH and LH are low.
  - ○ Cortisol is elevated.
  - ○ Prolactin is normal.
  - ○ TSH and T_4 are normal.
    - □ 3,5,3'-Triodothyronine (T_3) is low.
    - □ Reverse T_3 is high to compensate for state of undernourishment.
- ■ Recovery from anorexia.
  - ◇ GnRH response normalizes at weight that is 15% below ideal body weight.
  - ◇ With weight gain, maturity of GnRH axis occurs.
  - ◇ Neuropeptide Y may provide a further link between food and menstrual dysfunction.
- • Exercise and amenorrhea.
  - ■ As many as two-thirds of runners may have menstrual cycles with short luteal phases or that are anovulatory.
  - ■ Training can delay menarche by 3 years.
  - ■ Two major influences are the following:
    1. Critical level of body fat.
    2. Effect of stress itself (Fig. 11.2).
  - ■ Other methods of detecting body fat are hydrostatic weighing and dual-energy x-ray absorptiometry (DEXA).
  - ■ Critical weight hypothesis.
    - ◇ A drop below the tenth percentile results in abnormal menstrual function.
    - ◇ Considerable variation is seen.
      - ○ Questionable cause and effect and/or correlation exist between these.
      - ○ Leptin suggests a direct relationship.
    - ◇ Running in the dark adds to dysfunction.
    - ◇ Changes with acute exercise include the following:
      - ○ Suppressed gonadotropins.
      - ○ Elevated prolactin (variable, small amplitude).
      - ○ Elevations in growth hormone.
      - ○ Elevated testosterone.
      - ○ Elevated ACTH.
      - ○ Elevated nocturnal increase in melatonin in hypothalamic amenorrhea.
      - ○ Low T_4; amenorrheic athletes have an overall suppression of thyroid hormones.

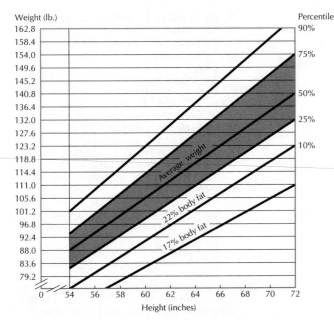

Figure 11.2. A fatness index nomogram.

- ◇ Conversion of estrogen to catecholestrogens occurs.
  - ○ Yields 2-hydroxyestrone, 4-hydroxyestrone.
    - □ Converted to 2-methoxyestrogen, 4-methoxyestrogen.
    - □ Increased by physical exercise.
  - ○ Response to a suboptimal amount of body fat.
- ■ Runner's high.
  - ◇ Possible psychological reaction versus increased endogenous opiates.
  - ◇ Endogenous opiates suppress GnRH; naltrexone can restore menstrual function.
  - ◇ Measurement of circulating β-endorphin is not helpful.
- ■ Athletes and energy balance.
  - ◇ Reproduction is suspended as available energy is directed to exercise; body fat is a marker of the energy state.
  - ◇ Leptin also modulates response to stress.
  - ◇ Elevations in insulin-like growth factor–binding protein–1 (IGFBP-1) increase insulin sensitivity, decrease insulin levels,

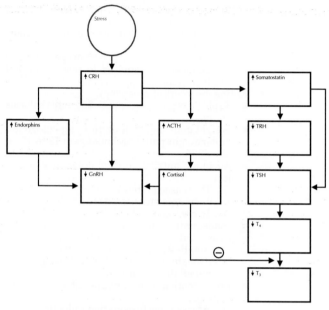

Figure 11.3.   Effect of stress on hormone production.

and increase growth hormone levels; all of these interact to suppress GnRH secretion (Fig. 11.3).

◇ CRH elevations are puzzling; the decrease in leptin and increase in neuropeptide Y may be insufficient to suppress CRH excretion.

◇ Leptin levels.
   ○ The normal diurnal pattern is observed in athletes with cyclic menses; absence of a diurnal pattern is seen in athletes with amenorrhea.
   ○ Both cycling and amenorrheic athletes have decreased leptin levels.
      □ Reduced body fat.
      □ Hypoinsulinism.
      □ Hypercortisolism.
   ○ Low levels signal low fat stores, which should stimulate hyperphagia, reduce energy expenditures, and suppress gonadotropin secretion.

■ Anorexic reaction.
   ◇ Similarities to anorexia nervosa.
      ○ Patients can still respond to criticism with regard to body image.

○ However, progression to true anorexia nervosa can occur.

◇ Simple weight gain can reverse amenorrhea.

◇ Hormone therapy is encouraged; dietary changes are required to restore normal bone density.

- Eating disorders of pregnancy.
  - Typical pregnancy requires 300 extra calories per day.
  - Weight gain should be 10 to 12 kg (22–26 lb); underweight patients should gain 12 to 15 kg (26–33 lb).
  - Adequate nutrition during pregnancy is critical.
    ◇ Decreases preterm delivery.
    ◇ Increases mean birth weight.
    ◇ Decreases late fetal death.
  - Inadequate weight gain before 24 weeks is associated with a significantly increased risk of a small–for–gestational–age baby, even if later weight gain brings the final weight into normal adult standards.
  - Preconception counseling and intervention are appropriate.
    ◇ Assess prior to ovulation induction.
    ◇ Address early in pregnancy.
- Inherited genetic defects.
  - Specific defects causing hypogonadotropic hypogonadism are not commonly recognized.
  - No α subunit mutations have been reported; high FSH, low or normal LH, increased α subunit, and a pituitary mass suggest gonadotroph adenoma.
  - LH-β and FSH-β mutations have been reported; they are present with primary amenorrhea.
  - Amenorrhea, anosmia, and Kallmann syndrome—a deficiency in GnRH associated with anosmia or hyposmia.
    ◇ Primary amenorrhea.
    ◇ Sexual infantilism.
    ◇ Low gonadotropins.
    ◇ Normal 46,XX.
    ◇ Inability to perceive odors.
    ◇ Often unrecognized.
  - The three modes of transmission are as follows:
    1. X-linked.
       ◇ Most common.
       ◇ Can be associated with other disorders.
       ◇ Short stature.
       ◇ Ichthyosis.
       ◇ Sulfatase deficiency.

2. Single gene (KAL) at Xp22.3.
   ◇ Codes for anosmin-1.
   ◇ Renal, bone, and hearing abnormalities and cleft lip and palate are also seen.
3. Autosomal dominant and autosomal recessive are also seen.
- Postpill amenorrhea—pursue investigation if patient is amenorrheic for 6 months after stopping oral contraception or for 12 months after stopping medroxyprogesterone acetate (Depo-Provera).

IX. Hormone Therapy
- Patients who are hypoestrogenic and who are not candidates for ovulation induction warrant hormone replacement therapy.
- Bone density is dependent on normal reproductive age and levels of estrogen and progesterone; strenuous exercise does not balance the consequences of hypoestrogenism.
- The degree of bone loss is dependent on athletic activity.
- A hypoestrogenic state is associated with greater risk of stress fractures.
- Bone loss is most rapid in the first few years.
- Bone density correlates with body weight; the response will be impaired as long as abnormal weight is maintained.
- Bone density changes in the hyperprolactinemic state are secondary to hypoestrogenism; this is not an independent effect of prolactin.
- Treatment.
  - 0.625 mg conjugated equine estrogens, or 1 mg estradiol daily; 5 mg medroxyprogesterone acetate or 0.7 mg norethindrone for 2 weeks/month.
  - Periodic measurements of bone density worthwhile.
  - Supplemental calcium (1,000 to 1,500 mg QD) if the patient refuses estrogen therapy; needs at least normal calcium and vitamin D if on hormone replacement therapy.
  - Low-dose oral contraceptive provides contraception, as well as hormone replacement benefits.

Anovulation and the Polycystic Ovary

I. Pathogenesis of Anovulation
  - The normal cycle.
    - Increased levels of follicle-stimulating hormone (FSH) are noted just before and during menses; estradiol, progesterone, and inhibin are decreased, releasing FSH from negative feedback.
    - The initial increase is necessary for follicular growth and steroidogenesis; an estrogen microenvironment is created.
    - FSH and activin lead to luteinizing hormone (LH)-receptor formation on granulosa cells.
    - Rapid rise in estradiol levels leads to positive feedback at the level of the pituitary and hypothalamus.
    - LH surge is initiated.
    - Fourteen-day luteal phase.
      - Rise in progesterone.
      - Secondary rise in estradiol.
      - FSH and LH levels are low.
  - Early follicular phase.
    - Activin from granulosa cells enhances the FSH effect on P450 aromatase.
    - Activin enhances the FSH effect on both LH- and FSH-receptor formation.
    - Activin inhibits thecal androgen production.
  - Late follicular phase.
    - Inhibin production in granulosa cells promotes androgens in response to LH and insulin-like growth factor–II (IGF-II); estrogen production increased.
    - Activin levels fall, which further enhances androgen production.
  - The dominant follicle.
    - Possesses highest level of aromatase activity; activin serves to prevent premature luteinization and progesterone production.
    - Contains highest level of estradiol—central feedback and LH receptors.
    - Produces greatest level of inhibin—both local and central actions.
    - The key to success—the conversion of inhibin production to LH responsiveness.
  - The coordinated cycle.
    - The concentration of androgens in granulosa cells promotes aromatase activity and inhibin production.
    - Inhibin promotes LH stimulation of thecal androgens; LH stimulation is further enhanced by IGF-II within theca cells.
    - With continued follicular development inhibin comes under control of LH.

- The key to successful ovulation and luteal function is conversion of inhibin production to LH responsiveness.
  - Suppresses FSH centrally.
  - Enhances LH locally.
- Central defects.
  - Hypothalamic dysfunction is a likely explanation for ovulatory failure.
  - Gonadotropin-releasing hormone (GnRH) secretion must fall in a critical range; GnRH suppression via corticotropin-releasing hormone release leads to increased dysfunction and can be caused by the following:
    - Stress.
    - Anxiety.
    - Borderline anorexia.
    - Acute weight loss.
  - Hyperprolactinemia.
    - Measurement of prolactin and a search for galactorrhea are important screenings for all women who are not ovulating normally.
    - The presence of galactorrhea or elevated prolactin levels dictates a choice of dopamine agonist for ovulation induction.
    - Treatment can reduce androgens and restore cyclicity even in women with polycystic ovaries (PCOs) and normal prolactin levels.
  - Abnormal GnRH pulsatility in PCOs.
    - Higher LH (and presumably GnRH) pulse frequency and amplitude.
    - Central opioid tone suppressed; no difference in response to naloxone.
    - Enhanced GnRH secretion possibly due to reduced hypothalamic opioid inhibition because of the absence of progesterone.
    - Interaction at dopamine–endorphin sites possibly altered.
- Abnormal feedback signals—two possible signal failures as follows:
  1. Estradiol may not fall low enough to allow the FSH response needed for initial growth stimulus.
  2. The levels of estradiol may not be high enough to induce the LH surge.
     - Loss of FSH stimulation.
       - The nadir in sex steroid levels must occur to allow a rise in FSH.
       - Persistent elevation suggests abnormal secretion (inappropriate clearance and metabolism or the presence of extragonadal sources).
         - ◊ Persistent estradiol secretion.
           - ○ Pregnancy.
           - ○ Ovarian or adrenal tumor.
         - ◊ Abnormal estrogen clearance—thyroid or hepatic disease (both hyperthyroidism and hypothyroidism can alter clearance and peripheral conversion rates).

◇ Extraglandular estradiol production.
  ○ Psychological or physical stress may increase C-19 androgenic precursors from the adrenal.
  ○ Adipose tissue conversion of androstenedione to estrogens may sustain levels of estrogen.
- Loss of LH stimulation—a relative deficiency in midcycle estradiol in perimenopausal women.

♦ Local ovarian conditions—failure of follicle to grow and ovulate may result from inadequate expression or impaired function of any of the following local ovarian activities:

1. Selection of dominant follicle occurs in cycle days 5 to 7; increased peripheral levels of estradiol are noted by day 7.
2. Estradiol levels increase as a result of the dominant follicle; increased FSH suppression centrally.
3. IGF-II is increased in theca cells.
   - Enhanced by estradiol and growth hormone.
   - Increases LH stimulation of androgen production in theca cells.
4. IGF-II stimulates granulosa cell proliferation and aromatase and progesterone synthesis.
5. FSH inhibits insulin-like growth factor–binding protein (IGFBP) synthesis and maximizes IGF-II availability.
6. FSH stimulates inhibin and activin production by granulosa cells.
7. Activin augments FSH activity.
   - FSH-receptor expression.
   - P450 aromatase activity.
   - Inhibin and activin production.
   - LH-receptor expression.
8. Inhibin enhances LH stimulation of androgen synthesis in theca cells.
9. The midfollicular estradiol rise directs a decline in FSH and gives positive feedback on LH secretion; androgen production in theca cells is further enhanced.
10. The LH molecule is modified by positive action of estradiol—increased bioactivity and increased secretion of LH at midcycle.
11. Inhibin and follistatin suppress pituitary FSH secretion.
12. FSH induces LH-receptor formation on granulosa cells.
    - Perturbations in the above may arise from the following:
      - Infectious process.
      - Endometriosis.
      - Abnormal qualitative or quantitative changes in tropic hormone receptors.
      - Improper molecular constitution of gonadotropins; heterogeneity of glycopeptide hormones.

♦ Critical role for androgens.
  • In low concentration, they enhance aromatization and estrogen production.
  • In high concentration, the 5α-reductase activity is favored—5α-reduced androgens, of which the following is true:
    1. Cannot be converted to estrogen.
    2. Inhibit aromatase activity.
    3. Inhibit FSH induction of the LH receptor.
  • Local androgens can thus inhibit emergence of the dominant follicle and can lead to atresia.
♦ Excess body weight.
  • Frequency of obesity in women with anovulation and PCO is between 35% and 60%.
  • Obesity is associated with the following three alterations that interfere with normal ovulation:
    1. Increased peripheral aromatization of androgens to estrogen.
    2. Decreased sex hormone–binding globulin (SHBG), which results in increased free estradiol and free testosterone.
    3. Increased insulin levels, which lead to increased stromal androgens.
♦ Precise etiology.
  • Often difficult and unnecessary to determine the precise etiology of anovulation.
  • Three categories as follows:
    1. Ovarian failure—hypergonadotropic hypogonadism.
    2. Central failure—hypogonadotropic hypogonadism.
    3. Anovulation dysfunction—asynchronous gonadotropin and estrogen production.

II. The Polycystic Ovary
  ♦ First described by Stein and Leventhal in 1935.
    • Seven patients (four obese) with amenorrhea, hirsutism, and enlarged polycystic ovaries.
    • Performed wedge resections.
      ▪ Seven of seven ovulated.
      ▪ Two of seven became pregnant.
    • Represents a broad spectrum of etiologies and clinical manifestations of persistent anovulation.
  ♦ The characteristic polycystic ovary emerges as an end point of anovulation; 75% of anovulatory women will have polycystic-appearing ovaries (PCO-like) on ultrasound.
  ♦ In normal women, 8% to 25% will have PCO-like ovaries on ultrasound.
  ♦ In women on oral contraceptives, 14% will have PCO-like ovaries on ultrasound; the majority of ovulatory women with PCO-like ovaries on ultrasound are endocrinologically normal.
    • Occasionally an androgen level is elevated.
    • Such subtle changes are unlikely to be clinically important.

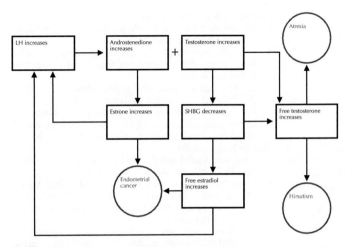

Figure 12.1.   Ovarian and end organ impact of hormonal abnormalities in patients with polycystic ovarian syndrome.

♦ Hormonal changes with anovulation represent a "steady state."
  • Increased estrogens (estrone).
  • Increased androgens.
    ▪ Dehydroepiandrosterone (DHEA).
    ▪ Dehydroepiandrosterone sulfate (DHEAS; adrenal)—elevated in 50% of anovulatory women with PCO.
    ▪ Androstenedione.
    ▪ Testosterone.
  • Increased 17-hydroxyprogesterone (Fig. 12.1).
♦ GnRH agonist treatment yields the following observations:
  1. Increases in androstenedione and testosterone in PCO patients are almost exclusively from the ovary.
  2. The increase in 17-hydroxyprogesterone is also from the ovary.
  3. Secretion of DHEA, DHEAS, and cortisol is not influenced by short-term GnRH agonist therapy.
    • Long-term therapy results in decrease in DHEAS in some women.
    • This decrease suggests that increased adrenal androgens may be due either to P450c17 17,20-lyase hyperactivity or to acquired response due to the anovulatory hormone steady state.
♦ Peripheral conversion of androstenedione to estrone occurs; circulating estrone levels are slightly elevated, but estradiol levels are comparable to the early follicular phase.

- ◆ Gonadotropin levels.
  - • A higher mean LH but low to low-normal levels of FSH are found.
    - ■ Higher LH due to increased pulse amplitude and frequency.
    - ■ LH bioactivity also increased.
  - • An increased frequency of GnRH pulses is observed; the central opioid tone is suppressed because of absence of progesterone.
  - • The above changes are independent of obesity.
    - ■ Obesity attenuates the LH response to GnRH.
    - ■ The LH pulse amplitude is normal, but the frequency is increased.
    - ■ This is possibly a direct effect of hyperandrogenism.
  - • Increased LH secretion positively correlates with increased free estradiol; FSH is under negative feedback from estradiol.
  - • FSH suppression may also be the result of inhibin B production; new follicular growth is continually stimulated. However, these follicles have the following problems:
    - ■ Fail to reach full maturation.
    - ■ Surrounded by hyperplastic theca cells.
      - ◇ Functional increase in stroma leads to increased androstenedione and testosterone production.
      - ◇ Androgens compound the problem via extraglandular conversion and SHBG suppression.
  - • SHBG.
    - ■ Testosterone inhibits SHBG synthesis.
    - ■ Estrogen and thyroxine stimulate its synthesis.
    - ■ In anovulatory women with PCO, SHBG levels are reduced by 50% as a result of androgens and hyperinsulinemia.
    - ■ Free estradiol levels are increased.
- ◆ Other changes.
  - • Increased pituitary and hypothalamic sensitivity; a result of increased estrone levels.
  - • Secondary to decreased SHBG as follows:
    - ■ Increased free estradiol.
    - ■ Increased free estradiol feedback on LH secretion.
  - • Low FSH—secondary to negative feedback from estradiol and estrone.
    - ■ Change in GnRH pulsatility.
    - ■ New follicular growth stimulated by constant low levels of FSH.
      - ◇ Follicles are surrounded by hyperplastic, luteinized theca cells; the polycystic ovary represents a self-sustaining situation.
        - ○ Follicles undergo atresia.
        - ○ Theca cells persist.
        - ○ Androgens remain elevated.

      ○ SHBG levels are reduced.
      ○ Increased androgens block follicular growth; this aspect is reduced by wedge resection, which ultimately leads to normal ovulation.

    ◇ This vicious cycle can be initiated at any point, but one must remember that the polycystic ovary is a sign, not a disease.

    ◇ Anatomy.
      ○ Ovarian surface area doubled in these patients; volume increased by 2.8-fold.
      ○ Same number of primordial follicles.
        ▲ Number of growing and/or atretic follicles is between 20 to 100.
        ▲ This is increased over normal by 100%.

    ◇ Tunica thickened by 50%.

    ◇ A one-third increase in cortical stromal thickness; a fivefold increase in the subcortical stroma.

    ◇ Four times more ovarian hilar cells.

◆ Hyperthecosis.
- Patches of luteinized theca-like cells scattered through the stroma.
- Clinical picture—one of increased androgenization.
- Lower LH levels observed; possibly a result of increased testosterone levels blocking estradiol effect at the hypothalamus or pituitary level.
- Greater insulin resistance; hyperinsulinemia may be an important incitement toward hyperthecosis.

◆ PCOs are a functional derangement.
- No specific pathophysiologic defect is observed.
- Hypothalamic–pituitary response is the appropriate response to elevated estrogen feedback.
    ■ The initial derangement is brought about by accumulated and increased androgens.
    ■ PCO-like ovaries may be associated with extragonadal sources of androgens, ovarian androgen-secreting tumors, or exogenous androgens (e.g., female-to-male transsexuals).
- Functional problems related to the two-cell theory are as follows:
    ■ Follicles are unable to convert to the estrogen microenvironment.
      ◇ IGFBP levels are similar to those of atretic follicles (↑ IGFBP-2 and IGFBP-4).
      ◇ Limitation of IGF-I and IGF-II activity reduces aromatase action and allows androgenic dominance.
      ◇ The granulosa cells from PCO patients are sensitive to FSH, which differs from those obtained from atretic follicles.
    ■ Arrested granulosa and overactive theca cells are observed.
      ◇ Granulosa block—secondary to androgens.

◇ Treatment involves either increasing FSH (clomiphene) or decreasing androgens (wedge resection).

- Genetic considerations.
  - Familial clustering supports an underlying genetic basis.
    - Possibly X-linked dominant.
    - Possibly autosomal dominant.
  - The association with hyperinsulinemia has led to a possible locus on the insulin gene and the gene encoding P450scc (CYP11a) but not P450c17α (CYP17); theoretically, 50% of mothers and sisters within a family may be affected.
- P450c17 dysregulation.
  - Popular hypothesis of dysregulation of 17,20-lyase activity; would explain adrenal and ovary participation.
  - Attractive, but clinical data fall short.
    - Adrenocorticotropic hormone (ACTH) stimulation testing in 92 women was not consistent with disorders of P450c17.
    - Testing of ovarian and adrenal responses has failed to delineate a clear-cut disorder.
    - Genetic screening has not detected sequence variation in promoter or coding regions of P450c17.
  - Enzyme changes probably secondary to the dysfunctional state.

III. Insulin Resistance, Hyperinsulinemia, and Hyperandrogenism
- An association was first recognized in 1921 by Archard and Thiers.
- A clinical association is found throughout the world; this is often associated with acanthosis nigricans.
  - A gray-brown velvety skin discoloration.
    - Usually at the neck, groin, axillae, and below the breasts.
    - Hyperkeratosis and papillomatosis.
    - Dependent on hyperinsulinemia.
  - Presence not an absolute marker for hyperandrogenism and/or hyperinsulinemia; other growth factors may play a role.
- Insulin resistance.
  - Defined as a reduced glucose response to a given amount of insulin; resistance to glucose uptake is sometimes referred to as "syndrome X."
  - Majority of patients with non–insulin-dependent diabetes mellitus (NIDDM) have peripheral insulin resistance; not all women who are insulin-resistant are hyperandrogenic.
  - Hyperinsulinemia represents a compensatory response; if insulin levels are not high enough to suppress free fatty acids, then hepatic glucose production increases → hyperglycemia.
  - Several mechanisms.
    - Peripheral target tissue resistance.

- ■ Decreased hepatic clearance.
- ■ Increased pancreatic sensitivity.
- ◆ Euglycemic clamp technique.
  - Establish steady state of hyperinsulinemia with a normal glucose level; glucose infusion = glucose utilization.
  - Adding insulin will increase the glucose uptake rate → the more insulin required = insulin resistance.
  - Studies in women with hyperandrogenism and hyperinsulinemia indicate these patients have increased peripheral insulin resistance and decreased hepatic insulin extraction.
- ◆ Clinical presentation.
  - Pancreatic compensation is variable.
    - ■ Effective compensation leads to impaired glucose tolerance.
    - ■ Ineffective compensation leads to type II NIDDM.
  - Hyperinsulinemia leads to hypertension, coronary heart disease, increased triglycerides, and decreased high-density lipoprotein (HDL); also, increased levels of plasminogen activator inhibitor–1 (PAI-1) → vascular disease.
- ◆ Causes of hyperinsulinemia.
  - Congenital—type A syndrome.
    - ■ Mutation of insulin-receptor gene.
    - ■ Decreased number of receptors.
    - ■ Leprechaunism—a rare syndrome.
  - Acquired—type B syndrome; autoantibodies to insulin receptors.
  - Functional problems and inhibitors.
- ◆ Insulin-receptor defect involving post–receptor activation has been found in some PCO patients.
  - Reduced tyrosine autophosphorylation; excessive serine phosphorylation.
    - ■ Changes signal transduction.
    - ■ May also affect 17,20-lyase activity (Fig. 12.2).
  - Abnormalities could be associated with normal numbers of receptors and with normal receptor function.
- ◆ Leptin levels and PCO.
  - When controlled for body weight, no difference is seen in leptin levels between women with or without PCO.
  - However, leptin may still be involved, as insulin-sensitizing agents may decrease leptin gene transcription.
- ◆ Hyperinsulinemia, hyperandrogenism, and obesity.
  - Obese, hyperandrogenic, and anovulatory women have android obesity with fat deposited in abdominal wall and visceral mesenteric locations.
    - ■ Fat in these locations is more sensitive to catecholamines, less sensitive to insulin, and more active metabolically.

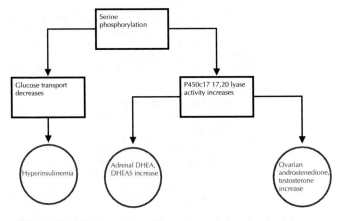

Figure 12.2.   The effects of serine phosphorylation on glucose transport and P450c17 17,20 lyase activity.

- Android obesity is also associated with an increased cardiovascular risk; the waist:hip ratio is >0.85.
- Hyperinsulinemia and hyperandrogenism are not explained solely by obesity; the presence of obesity adds greater hyperinsulinemia and insulin resistance to the PCO patient.
- Six reasons to believe hyperinsulinemia causes hyperandrogenism are as follows:
  1. Insulin increases androgens in women with PCO.
  2. Glucose increases insulin and androgen secretion in hyperandrogenic women.
  3. Weight loss decreases androgens and insulin and increases IGFBP-1.
  4. *In vitro*, insulin increases androgen production by theca cells.
  5. Decreased insulin levels lead to decreased androgens in women with PCO but not in normal women.
  6. Use of GnRH agonist will normalize androgens but will not normalize glucose intolerance.
- How does increased insulin produce hyperandrogenism?
  - Insulin at higher concentrations binds the IGF-I receptor.
    ◊ Increased action of LH upon theca cells.
    ◊ Both IGF-I and IGF-II activity potentially mediated by the IGF-I receptor.
  - Insulin also decreases SHBG synthesis; decreased SHBG levels represent an independent risk factor for NIDDM.
  - Insulin also decreases IGFBP-1 production, thus allowing increased IGF-I levels.

      ◇ Increase in local ovarian action.
      ◇ Possible endometrial action of IGF-I and insulin as well (possible mechanisms for endometrial hyperplasia) (Fig. 12.3).

♦ Treatment with diabetic drugs.
- Best approach—improve peripheral insulin sensitivity.
- Metformin.
  - Improves insulin sensitivity.
  - Primary effect—significant reduction in gluconeogenesis.
  - Treatment (500 mg TID).
    - ◇ Reduces hyperinsulinism.
    - ◇ Reduces basal and stimulated LH levels.
    - ◇ Reduces free testosterone levels.
    - ◇ Reduces PAI-1 levels.
  - Improvements in clomiphene responsiveness seen as well.
  - May be less effective in extremely overweight women.
  - Effectiveness possibly related to decreases in body weight.
  - Nonobese women with hyperinsulinism—will respond to treatment.
- Thiazolidenediones (troglitazone)—no longer available due to hepatotoxicity.
  - Markedly improves insulin sensitivity and secretion.
  - Decreases hyperinsulinemia.
  - Improves metabolic parameters.
    - ◇ Decreases androgens.
    - ◇ Increases SHBG.
    - ◇ Decreases PAI-1.
    - ◇ Decreases LH.
- Extensive research ongoing in this area.

IV. Clinical Consequences
  ♦ Overview.
- Anovulation is the key factor in PCO (50% of women are amenorrheic; dysfunctional uterine bleeding in 30%).
- Hirsutism can be found in 70% of women with PCO.
  - Depends upon androgen concentration and the genetic sensitivity of the hair follicles.
  - Alopecia and acne can be seen as well.
- Obesity is variable (35% to 60%).
- Approximately 20% to 40% may have a normal LH:FSH ratio.
- Diagnosis is made by the clinical presentation given above.

  ♦ Clinical considerations.
1. Infertility.
2. Menstrual irregularities.
3. Hirsutism, acne, and alopecia.
4. Increased risk of endometrial cancer; a questionable increased risk of breast cancer.

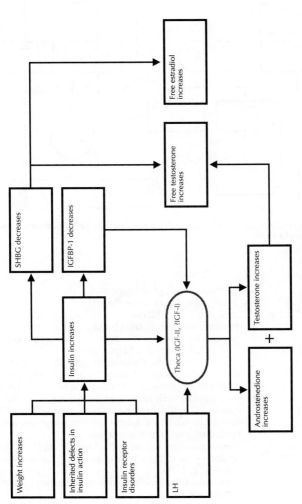

Figure 12.3.   Hormonal derangements in PCO.

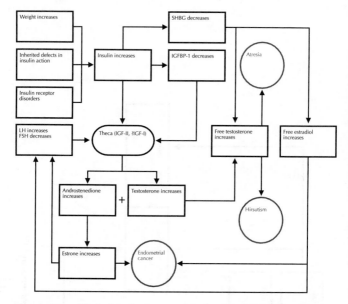

Figure 12.4.   Clinical endpoints as a result of the hormonal derangements in PCO.

      5.   Increased risk of cardiovascular disease.

      6.   Increased risk of overt diabetes.

- Clinical recommendations.
  - Perform an endometrial biopsy to rule out hyperplasia; the duration of unopposed estrogen should determine who has a biopsy done.
  - In patients with no desire for pregnancy, medroxyprogesterone acetate (Depo-Provera), 10 mg, cycle days 1 to 10 per month, is adequate for protection.
  - In patients with increased cardiovascular risk, abnormal lipids, hirsutism, or no desire for pregnancy but who have a need for contraception, oral contraceptives are appropriate.
  - Treatment of hirsutism with glucocorticoids should be done with caution in women with insulin resistance (Fig. 12.4).
  - Spironolactone and flutamide do not affect insulin sensitivity.
  - Weight loss should be recommended to all patients above ideal body weight.
    - A very good idea.
    - Reduces insulin and androgens (free testosterone).
    - No insulin resistance in patients with body mass index (BMI) <27.

- Even a small weight loss (5% to 10%) possibly has a significant beneficial impact.
- ◆ Overall goals of treatment are as follows:
  1. Reduce production/circulatory levels of androgens.
  2. Protect the endometrium.
  3. Support lifestyle changes to achieve normal body weight.
  4. Lower the risk of cardiovascular disease.
  5. Avoid effects of hyperinsulinemia or risk of cardiovascular disease.
  6. Induce ovulation to achieve pregnancy.
- ◆ Testing for hyperinsulinemia—classical recommendations.
  - Consider testing in specific groups as follows:
    - Family members of already-diagnosed patients; both brothers and sisters can be insulin-resistant.
    - Patients with android obesity; waist circumference >100 cm in men and >90 cm in women.
    - Teenagers with persistent anovulation; some teenagers fail to normalize the hyperinsulinemia associated with the increase in growth hormone in early puberty.
    - Cases of premature adrenarche.
    - Unusual cases of hyperandrogenism; high testosterone without an adrenal or ovarian tumor.
  - Results of testing.
    - Fasting insulin in cases of normal glucose tolerance should be from 10 to 20 U/mL.
    - Measurement of the ratio of fasting glucose to fasting insulin may provide credence to assist in counseling.
- ◆ Testing for hyperinsulinemia—new recommendations.
  - All anovulatory women who are hyperandrogenic should be assessed for insulin resistance and glucose tolerance.
    - Fasting glucose:insulin ratio <4.5 suggests insulin resistance.
    - Two-hour glucose following 75-g glucose load:
      - ◊ Normal <140 mg/dL.
      - ◊ Impaired = 140 to 199 mg/dL.
      - ◊ NIDDM >200 mg/dL.
  - Anovulatory women without hyperandrogenism should be evaluated for free testosterone.
    - If elevated, assess for insulin resistance and glucose intolerance.
    - May be more economical to measure fasting glucose/insulin ratio in all anovulatory women.

Hirsutism

I. The Biology of Hair Growth
   - Embryology.
     - Each hair follicle develops at 8 to 10 weeks of gestation.
       - It is a derivative of the epidermis.
       - Column elongates and encounters mesodermal cells (dermal papilla).
       - Column hollows out to form the hair canal.
       - The pilosebaceous apparatus (hair follicle, sebaceous glands, and arrector pili muscles) is laid down.
     - Lanugo hair (hair covering the fetus).
       - Lightly pigmented.
       - Thin in diameter.
       - Short in length.
       - Fragile in attachment.
     - Total endowment of hair follicles is formed by 22 weeks.
     - Racial differences in hair distribution depend upon the following:
       - 5α-Reductase activity.
       - Density of hair follicles.
     - Hair growth pattern is genetically determined.
   - Structure and growth.
     - Anagen—growing phase.
     - Catagen—rapid involution phase.
     - Telogen—quiescent phase.
     - Length of hair determined by duration of growth phase (anagen).
       - Scalp hair is in anagen phase for 3 years; it has a short resting phase.
       - Forearm hair has a short anagen and a long telogen.
       - Scalp hair growth is asynchronous and always seems to be growing; only 10% to 15% is in telogen; in cases of marked synchrony, all hairs may undergo telogen at the same time and shed at once.
         - ◇ This shedding is called telogen effluvium.
         - ◇ Ruling out thyroid disease when this occurs is worthwhile.
     - Hypertrichosis.
       - A general increase in fetal lanugo hair; drugs and malignancy are the most common causes.
       - Vellus hair—downy, prepubertal hair.
       - Terminal hair—coarse hair on various body parts.
     - Hirsutism = conversion of vellus hair to terminal hair.
   - Factors influencing hair growth.

- The dermal papilla is the director of hair growth; if the dermal papilla survives major injury (e.g., freezing, x-rays, and skin graft), the hair follicle will regenerate and regrow hair.
- Sexual hair.
  - Defined as hair responsive to sex steroids.
  - Influenced by androgens. Sensitivity of hair follicle depends on 5α-reductase activity.
    ◇ Initiates growth.
    ◇ Increases diameter and pigmentation of keratin color; probably increases the rate of mature cell of mitosis in all but scalp hair.
  - Estrogen—retards the rate and initiation of growth.
  - Progestins—minimal effect.
  - Pregnancy—can cause synchrony of hair growth and, therefore, periods of growth or shedding.
- Effect of castration.
  - Prior to puberty, no beard will occur.
  - After puberty, normal sexual hair differentiation will be seen, but the hair will have slower growth and a finer caliber.
- Other endocrine problems.
  - Hypopituitarism—marked reduction in hair growth.
  - Acromegaly—associated with hirsutism in 10% to 15% of cases.
  - Hypothyroidism—scalp alopecia; decreased axillary, pubic, and lateral eyebrow hair.
  - Anovulation—leads to increased insulin-like growth factor I (IGF-I); this can increase 5α-reductase activity; hyperinsulinemia can intensify hirsute response.
  - Central nervous system pathology and some drugs—can cause excessive hair growth.

II. Androgen Production
   - Testosterone, 0.2 to 0.3 mg/day.
     - Fifty percent is from peripheral conversion of androstenedione.
     - Fifty percent of production is split equally between the ovary and the adrenal.
       - Eighty percent is bound to sex hormone–binding globulin (SHBG).
       - Nineteen percent is bound to albumin.
       - One percent is free.
       - Increased ovarian contribution is found at midcycle.
   - Dehydroepiandrosterone sulfate (DHEAS) is produced almost exclusively in the adrenal.
   - Ninety percent of dehydroepiandrosterone is from the adrenal.
   - SHBG.
     - Decreased by androgens and insulin.

- Binding capacity decreased in men; levels from 2% to 3% of free testosterone.
- Increased by estrogen and thyroid hormone.
♦ Total testosterone can be normal in hirsute women.
- No clinical need to check free testosterone exists.
- If increased androgen effect is observed, then increased testosterone must be present.
♦ Hirsute women.
- Only 25% of testosterone is from peripheral conversion.
- Most is secondary to direct secretion.
  - The ovary is the major source of testosterone and androstenedione.
  - Adrenal causes are uncommon.
♦ 3α-Androstanediol glucuronide (3α-AG).
- DHT is the major nuclear androgen.
- 3α-AG is the peripheral metabolite.
  - Glucuronide correlates with 5α-reductase activity.
  - No such thing as true idiopathic hirsutism exists.
- Why do we not measure 3α-AG?
  - The normal range overlaps the abnormal by 20%.
  - Ultimately, diagnosis and therapy are unchanged.

III. Evaluation of Hirsutism
♦ A number of factors, including the following, determine the end result of hirsutism:
1. Number of hair follicles.
2. Degree of conversion of vellus hair to terminal hair.
3. Ratio of growth to resting phases in affected hair follicles.
4. Asynchrony.
5. Thickness and pigmentation of individual hairs.
♦ The primary factor is increased androgens.
- Every woman with hirsutism will have an increased rate of testosterone and androgen production.
- In women with anovulation, the most common signs are as follows:
  - Hirsutism.
  - Acne and skin oiliness.
  - Increased libido.
  - Clitoromegaly.
  - Masculinization.
- Alopecia.
  - Usually a temporary period of dyssynchrony of scalp hair.
  - May be a response to an acute and/or stressful event.
  - Can be associated with polycystic ovary syndrome (PCOS) and increased androgens.
  - Reflects increased scalp 5α-reductase activity.

- ■ Thyroid disease; chronic disease.
- ■ Pregnancy and postpartum.
- Acne—60% of women who have normal circulatory androgens again demonstrate increased levels of 5α-reductase.
- Acanthosis nigricans.
  - ■ Associated with hyperinsulinemia.
  - ■ Assessment of glucose metabolism warranted.
- Anovulation and/or irregular menses.
  - ■ Approximately 70% of women will develop hirsutism.
  - ■ The onset is usually at the teenage years or the early 20s.
    - ◊ If later or acute, consider a tumor or, rarely, congenital adrenal hyperplasia (CAH).
    - ◊ Classic CAH.
      - ○ Usually found prior to puberty.
      - ○ Genetic problems may also manifest at puberty.
- Rapidity of development—hirsutism in patients >25 years and with rapid progression of masculinization is usually associated with an androgen-producing tumor.
- Pregnancy.
  - ■ Virilization may be the result of luteoma.
  - ■ Unilateral in 45% and associated with a normal pregnancy; it is not a true tumor but rather an exaggerated reaction of ovarian stroma.
  - ■ Masculinization of female fetuses can occur in about 80% of these cases.
  - ■ Maternal virilization is observed in 35%.
- Bilateral theca lutein cysts.
  - ■ No virilization of female fetus.
  - ■ Maternal virilization possible.

IV. Diagnostic Evaluation
- ◆ Initial laboratory evaluation.
  - Testosterone, 17-hydroxyprogesterone (17-OHP).
  - Prolactin, thyrotropin (TSH).
  - Breast examination, endometrial biopsy.
  - Consider evaluation for hyperinsulinemia.
  - Screen for Cushing syndrome; a common referral diagnosis, but an uncommon final diagnosis.
- ◆ Cushing syndrome.
  - Persistent oversecretion of cortisol.
  - Five possible etiologies include the following:
    1. Pituitary adrenocorticotropic hormone (ACTH) —Cushing disease.
    2. Ectopic ACTH by tumor.
    3. Autonomous adrenal cortisol production.
    4. Autonomous cortisol production by an ovarian tumor (rare).
    5. Corticotropin-releasing hormone (CRH)-producing tumors (extremely rare).

- Useful tests to make a diagnosis of Cushing syndrome (hypercortisolism).
  - Twenty-four–hour urinary free cortisol (10 to 90 μg).
  - Late evening plasma cortisol (>15 μg/dL).
- Single dose overnight dexamethasone suppression test (DST).
  - Dexamethasone, 1 mg orally, at 11:00 P.M.
  - Check A.M. cortisol at 8:00.
    - ◊ If <5 μg/dL, no evidence of Cushing syndrome.
    - ◊ If 5 to 10 μg/dL, Cushing syndrome unlikely.
    - ◊ If >10 μg/dL, diagnostic of adrenal hyperfunction.
  - Obese patients have a 13% false-positive rate.
- If the single-dose overnight test is abnormal, check the 24-hour urinary free cortisol.
- Low-dose DST can provide the final confirmation.
  - Two days of baseline 24-hour urinary 17-hydroxysteroid and free cortisol determination.
  - Dexamethasone, 0.5 mg every 6 hours × 2 days.
  - Collect urine × 2 days.
    - ◊ 17-Hydroxysteroid level should be <2.5 mg/day on the second day.
    - ◊ Serum free cortisol should be <10 μg/dL on the second day.
      - ○ Urinary free cortisol levels >250 μg indicate Cushing syndrome.
      - ○ Levels >200 μg indicate a 90% chance of Cushing syndrome.
- If pseudo-Cushing is a consideration (e.g., alcoholism, anorexia, severe obesity, depression), consider combining a low-dose DST with a CRH stimulation test.
  - Two days of 0.5 mg DST every 6 hours.
  - Check plasma cortisol 15 minutes after 1 μg/kg of CRH; if cortisol >1.4 μg/dL, the condition requires further evaluation.
- Determining etiology.
  - High-dose DST, 2 mg every 6 hours, × 2 days and blood ACTH.
  - Measure basal ACTH, urinary free cortisol, and 17-hydroxysteroid on the second day of suppression.
    - Results.
      - ◊ Basal ACTH <5 pg/mL and urinary steroids that are not suppressed by at least 40% → adrenal tumor.
      - ◊ Basal ACTH >20 pg/mL → ectopic ACTH tumor is unlikely if urinary steroids decrease by 40%.
      - ◊ Basal ACTH >50 pg/mL suggests ectopic ACTH release if poor suppression by steroids.

◊ Normal ACTH, normal chest x-ray, and abnormal sella → Cushing disease.

- Imaging of adrenals—computed tomography (CT) scans are better than magnetic resonance imaging (MRI) and/or ultrasound.
- Confirming a diagnosis of a pituitary source of ACTH.
  ◊ Inferior petrosal sampling before and after CRH stimulation confirms a pituitary origin.
  ◊ Fifteen percent of patients with ACTH-dependent Cushing disease will have an occult ectopic source; most are thoracic sources (small cell carcinoma).

♦ Assessment of insulin secretion.
  - Hyperandrogenism and hyperinsulinemia are commonly associated with one another.
  - Effects of hyperinsulinemia include the following:
    - Augmentation of thecal cell androgen production.
    - Inhibition of SHBG synthesis.
    - Inhibition of insulin-like growth factor–binding protein I (IGFBP-I) synthesis.
  - Hirsutism in an elderly patient may sometimes result from hyperinsulinemia.
  - Recommendations are as follows:
    1. Check the fasting glucose:insulin ratio. A ratio of <4.5 is consistent with insulin resistance.
    2. Perform a 2-hour glucose tolerance test (75-g glucose load).

Normal	<140 mg/dL
Impaired	140 to 199 mg/dL
Non–insulin-dependent diabetes	>200 mg/dL

♦ DHEAS level.
  - Circulates in higher concentration than any other steroid.
  - Correlates clinically with urinary 17-ketosteroids.
  - Random sample okay.
  - Serves as a prehormone in hair follicles.
  - Almost exclusively produced by the adrenal.
  - Decreases with age; accelerated decrease following menopause; almost undetectable after 70 years of age.
  - Decline is 4× greater than the decline in cortisol.
  - Increased prolactin → increased DHEAS and 17-ketosteroids; also, in hyperprolactinemia, free testosterone will increase because of the decrease in SHBG.
  - Moderate increase in DHEAS is normal in anovulation; CAH patients have normal levels.
  - DHEAS >700 µg/dL.
    - Very rare.

- No increased benefit to the patient from screening for this hormone.
- Assessment *not* cost-effective.
  - ◇ Measure only testosterone.
  - ◇ If testosterone is elevated, imaging of the adrenals is appropriate.

♦ Nonclassic CAH.
  - Most common defects are 21-hydroxylase deficiency, 11β-hydroxylase deficiency, and 3β-hydroxysteroid dehydrogenase (3β-HSD).
  - 21-Hydroxylase deficiency.
    - Late-onset CAH patients demonstrate an ACTH response between the classic homozygote response and the mild heterozygote response (see nomogram).
    - 21-Hydroxylase deficiency is the most common autosomal disorder (Fig. 13.1).
    - Three reasons to seek diagnosis are as follows:
      1. Long-term therapy is required.
      2. Prenatal counseling is necessary if the father of the child is a carrier.

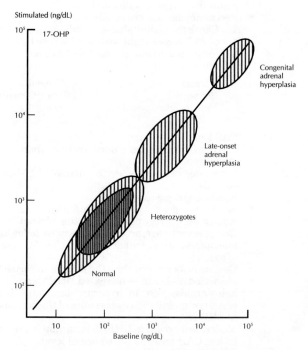

Figure 13.1.   Results of adrenocorticotropic hormone stimulation test. 17-OHP levels in response to the test and their significance.

3. Theoretically, cortisol deficiency can occur, but clinically it is not a problem.
- 3β-HSD deficiency.
  - Enzyme present in both the ovary and adrenals.
  - Deficiency difficult to diagnose.
  - Altered 17α-hydroxypregnenolone to 17-OHP ratio observed with ACTH stimulation test.
  - Response possibly consistent with adrenal hyperactivity, not true enzyme defect; molecular studies have failed to find a gene mutation.
- 11β-Hydroxylase deficiency.
  - Quite rare.
  - Usually detected at an early age.
  - Not usually worth screening for in adults, given its rare nature and the fact that diagnosis is generally made earlier.
- 17-OHP level.
  - Elevated in 1% to 5% of hirsute women.
  - Routine 17-OHP screening in hirsute women is indicated; ACTH stimulation test is not.
  - Enzyme defect usually found in patients who have more severe hirsutism at a younger age and short stature; with normal baseline measurements of 17-OHP the presence of a subtle enzyme defect found by stimulation testing would not alter management.
  - Measure in the morning and interpret as follows:
    - Baseline should be <200 ng/dL.
    - Levels of 200 to 800 ng/dL require the stimulation test.
    - Levels >800 ng/dL are diagnostic.
    - Baseline values are often unimpressive.
- ACTH stimulation test.
  - 21-Hydroxylase deficiency.
    - ACTH (Cortrosyn), 250 µg intravenously at 8:00 A.M.; check 17-OHP at 0 hours and at 1 hour.
    - Response in heterozygotes of up to 1,000 ng/dL.
    - Homozygotes, late onset, >1,200 ng/dL.
    - Normal levels of DHEAS observed.
  - 3β-HSD deficiency and ACTH stimulation test.
    - Ratio of 17-hydroxypregnenolone/17-OHP >6.0.
    - Significant increase in DHEAS noted with normal or only mildly increased testosterone.
  - 11β-Hydroxylase deficiency—level of 11-deoxycortisol will be increased with ACTH stimulation test.

V. The Adrenal Gland and Anovulation
- Is adrenal hyperactivity primary or secondary in an anovulatory patient?
- If women with elevated DHEAS are treated with a gonadotropin-releasing hormone (GnRH) agonist, DHEAS levels will decrease.
  - This indicates a primary ovarian problem.

- Excess adrenal activity occurs in one-half to two-thirds of anovulatory women.
- Hyperinsulinism is found in 70%.
- Women with PCOS and hyperinsulinism have a greater response to ACTH than do anovulatory women with normal cortisol levels.
- Circulating DHEAS serves as a precursor to ovarian testosterone; dexamethasone suppression can initiate an ovulatory response.

♦ The testosterone level is elevated in 70% of women with anovulation and hirsutism.
- The level can be normal, but a decrease in the binding protein results in elevated free testosterone.
- If testosterone >200 ng/dL, an androgen-producing tumor must be suspected; if rapid virilization is present, evaluate for a tumor even in the presence of normal serum testosterone.
- Pregnancy levels of testosterone are elevated.
  - First trimester: >100 ng/dL.
  - At term: 500 to 800 ng/dL.

♦ Androgen-producing tumors.
- Should be suspected in the presence of the following two findings:
  1. Rapid masculinization (months).
  2. Testosterone >200 µg/dL.
- If an androgen-producing tumor is suspected and imaging reveals no adrenal or adnexal mass, consider selective angiography of adrenal and ovarian veins.
- Postmenopausal women with hyperandrogenism should be evaluated for tumor, but this may represent hyperinsulinism.

♦ Incidental adrenal mass.
- Found in 10% of autopsies.
- Bilateral lesions more serious—metastatic cancer, infection, CAH.
- Bilateral lesions <2 cm in diameter usually from metastatic disease.
- Excise unilateral masses >4 cm; fine needle aspiration may be helpful (after excluding pheochromocytoma) for ruling out metastatic disease.
  - If >3 cm, image at 3, 9, and 18 months.
  - If no change by 18 months, no further follow-up is required.
- Screening tests for incidental adrenal masses.
  - Twenty-four–hour urinary catecholamines and free cortisol.
  - Testosterone.
  - Renin activity, aldosterone, and electrolytes.
- Provocative tests for subclinically active incidental adrenal masses.
  - Overnight DST.
  - 17-OHP response to ACTH.

- Clonidine suppression test (clonidine, 0.3 mg orally in a supine position, followed by plasma norepinephrine levels at 0, 2, and 3 hours; a norepinephrine level >500 pg/mL or 50% greater than the 0-hour level is a positive result).

♦ Summary of key recommendations for the evaluation of hirsutism.
1. The laboratory evaluation of hirsutism consists of the measurement of the circulating levels of testosterone and 17-OHP. When alopecia is present, a TSH screen for thyroid function is also indicated.
2. The single-dose overnight DST is used to screen for Cushing disease. Abnormal results are confirmed by measuring the 24-hour urinary free cortisol.
3. A clinician should always consider the possibility of hyperinsulinemia and should emphasize preventive health interventions (as discussed in Chapter 12).
4. Any patient with rapidly progressive virilization must be evaluated for an androgen-secreting tumor regardless of the results of screening laboratory tests.
5. Incidentally discovered adrenal masses require evaluation.

VI. Treatment of Hirsutism
♦ Attempt to interrupt the steady state of persistent anovulation and luteinizing hormone (LH) through the action of progestational agents or to induce ovulation.
♦ Oral contraceptive pills (OCPs).
- Progestins decrease LH and 5α-reductase activity.
- Estrogens increase SHBG.
- Desogestrel, gestodene, and norgestimate may increase levels of SHBG and may significantly decrease free testosterone; theoretically, this is an advantage, but it is clinically unsupported.
- OCPs are helpful even in patients using antiandrogens (Fig. 13.2).
♦ If OCPs are inappropriate or unwanted, consider medroxyprogesterone acetate.
- Regimen: 150 mg intramuscularly every 3 months, or 10 to 20 mg orally QD.
- LH suppressed, but follicular activity continues, resulting in decreased testosterone production and increased testosterone clearance.
- Decreased SHBG observed, but production of androgens is suppressed so greatly that free testosterone decreases.
♦ Slow response can be anticipated.
- Six months needed to suppress new hair growth.
- Need to continue with adjuvant treatments (e.g., electrolysis).
♦ DHEAS levels.
- Suppressed by progestational agents; the mechanism is unknown, but it is possibly due to the

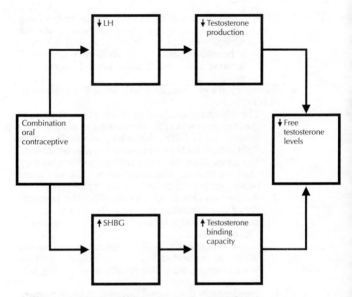

Figure 13.2.   Hormonal changes in response to treatment of hirsutism with a combination oral contraceptive.

change in the endocrine milieu or the alteration in ACTH secretion or response.
- Adrenal suppression.
  - Can result in ovulatory cycles; lower precursor available to stimulate follicular androgen production.
  - Not as effective as clomiphene in inducing ovulation, except in patients with documented adrenal enzyme deficiency.
- Older patients.
  - Consider hysterectomy and bilateral salpingo-oophorectomy.
  - In the presence of hyperinsulinism, consider treatment with metformin.

VII.   Additional Methods of Treatment
- Spironolactone.
  - Aldosterone antagonist diuretic.
  - Multiple actions in hirsutism as follows:
    1. Inhibits steroidogenesis via cytochrome P450 system.
    2. Receptor-blocking activity (most important mechanism).
    3. Direct inhibition of 5α-reductase.
  - Better effect in patients on 200 mg QD; attempt to decrease to 25 to 50 mg QD.
  - Response is slow (about 6 months).

- Combine with OCPs to avoid abnormal bleeding and the theoretic risk of feminization of a male fetus.
- ◆ Cyproterone acetate.
  - Potent progestational agent.
  - Inhibits gonadotropins.
  - Direct effect on androgen receptor in combination with spironolactone.
  - No real benefit over combination OCPs.
- ◆ Dexamethasone.
  - Useful in women with an adrenal enzyme defect.
  - Dosage of 0.5 mg at bedtime; alternatively, use prednisone, 5 to 7.5 mg QD.
  - If plasma cortisol <2 µg/dL, decrease dose to avoid inability to respond to stress.
  - Moderate elevations in DHEAS do **not** identify patients who may benefit from dexamethasone treatment.
- ◆ GnRH agonists.
  - Greater doses are needed to suppress androgens.
  - Monitor testosterone levels (goal <40 ng/dL).
  - Initiate add-back therapy once the maintenance dose is established.
  - This is useful in rare cases of ovarian hyperandrogenism.
    - Hyperthecosis.
    - Patients with marked hyperinsulinism.
- ◆ Flutamide.
  - Nonsteroidal antiandrogen at the receptor level.
  - Hepatotoxicity possible; limits its usefulness.
  - Must use contraception; must combine with OCPs.
- ◆ Finasteride.
  - Inhibits 5α-reductase activity; blocks conversion of testosterone to dihydrotestosterone.
  - Type I enzyme found in the skin.
  - Type II enzyme found in the reproductive tissues.
  - Finasteride (Proscar, Propecia)—inhibits both enzymes.
  - Effective dosage ≤5 mg/day.
  - Must be combined with effective contraception to avoid risk of a urogenital sinus malfunction in the male fetus.
- ◆ Other agents.
  - Cimetidine, 300 mg QID.
  - Ketoconazole, 400 mg QD.
    - Last resort, with frequent monitoring of liver enzymes.
    - Blocks androgen synthesis via cytochrome P450.
- ◆ End-organ hypersensitivity (idiopathic hirsutism).
  - Some patients with hirsutism ovulate regularly; this is more pronounced in certain geographic areas and among certain ethnic groups.

- Hypersensitivity is probably due to increased 5α-reductase activity; normal levels of androgens promote hair growth.
- OCPs are effective; spironolactone, flutamide, and finasteride can be used as well.
- Finasteride may be preferred for this condition, especially for patients with alopecia.

VIII. Summary of Recommendations for the Treatment of Hirsutism

1. The initial treatment of choice for anovulatory women with hirsutism is low-dose (<50 μg estrogen) OCPs.
2. The response is relatively slow, and at least 6 months of treatment is required to demonstrate an impact.
3. When patients do not respond well to OCPs, an antiandrogen should be added, preferably (in order) spironolactone or finasteride.
4. No overwhelming evidence demonstrates that one agent is better than another, and choices should be governed by cost and side effects.
5. The addition of a GnRH agonist should be reserved for patients resistant to initial therapy.
6. Finasteride may be more effective for idiopathic hirsutism and androgenic alopecia.

IX. Limitations and Pitfalls

1. Testosterone >200 mg/dL does not always indicate the existence of a tumor.
2. The appearance of the ovaries is variable.
3. The ovary does not need to be biopsied in the evaluation of hirsutism.
4. Increased testosterone and hirsutism in patients with normal cycles indicates a probable adrenal problem.
5. Suppression of androgens by progestin does not rule out an ovarian tumor.
6. Failure of progestin to suppress testosterone and hair growth after 6 to 12 months raises suspicion of adrenal disease or a small ovarian tumor.
7. Androgen levels in postmenopausal women are lower, so testosterone >100 ng/dL provides suspicion of a tumor.

Menstrual Disorders

I. The Premenstrual Syndrome (PMS)
    ♦ Definition: the cyclic appearance of one or more of a large constellation of symptoms (over 100) just prior to menses occurring to such a degree that lifestyle or work is affected and followed by a period of time that is entirely free of symptoms.
    ♦ Most frequent symptoms.
      • Abdominal bloating.
      • Anxiety or tension.
      • Breast tenderness.
      • Crying spells.
      • Depression.
      • Fatigue.
      • Lack of energy.
      • Unprovoked anger.
      • Difficulty concentrating.
      • Thirst and appetite changes.
      • Edema.
    ♦ Fewer than 50% of women who complain of PMS can be demonstrated to have a pattern of mood changes that is cyclic.
    ♦ Diagnosis: two guidelines—the American Psychiatric Association (APA) and the National Institute of Mental Health (NIMH).
      • APA.
        ■ Premenstrual dysphoric disorder (PMDD).
        ■ Symptoms are temporally related to the menstrual cycle, beginning during the last week of the luteal phase and remitting after the onset of menses.
        ■ The diagnosis requires at least five of the following, and one of the symptoms must be one of the first four:
          ◊ Affective lability (e.g., sudden onset of sadness, tears, irritability, or anger).
          ◊ Persistent and marked anger or irritability.
          ◊ Anxiety or tension.
          ◊ Depressed mood and feelings of hopelessness.
          ◊ Decreased interest in usual activities.
          ◊ Easy fatigability or a marked lack of energy.
          ◊ Subjective sense of difficulty in concentrating.
          ◊ Changes in appetite; overeating or food craving.
          ◊ Hypersomnia or insomnia.
          ◊ Feelings of being overwhelmed or out of control.

        ◇   Physical symptoms, such as breast tenderness, headaches, edema, joint or muscle pain, and weight gain.
- The symptoms must interfere with work or usual activities or relationships.
- The symptoms are not an exacerbation of another psychiatric disorder. Thus, PMDD is, in part, a diagnosis of exclusion.

- NIMH.
  - Definition: a 30% increase in severity of symptoms in the 5 days prior to menses as compared with the 5 days following menses.
  - Epidemiology.
    - ◇ Five percent of women meet the diagnostic criteria.
    - ◇ Forty percent of women report problems related to their cycle.
    - ◇ Two percent to 10% report a degree of impact upon their work or lifestyle.
    - ◇ Are these learned responses? Scientific study has been hampered by the influence of traditions and social and/or cultural beliefs.
  - Etiology—numerous theories.
    - ◇ Low progesterone levels.
    - ◇ High estrogen levels.
    - ◇ Falling estrogen levels.
    - ◇ Changes in estrogen/progesterone ratios.
    - ◇ Increased aldosterone activity.
    - ◇ Increased renin–angiotensin activity.
    - ◇ Increased renal activity.
    - ◇ Endogenous endorphin withdrawal.
    - ◇ Subclinical hypoglycemia.
    - ◇ Central changes in catecholamines.
    - ◇ Response to prostaglandins (PGs).
    - ◇ Vitamin deficiencies.
    - ◇ Excess prolactin secretion.
  - Studies prior to 1983 did not incorporate the appropriate diagnostic criteria.
  - Studies since 1983 reveal no apparent hormonal differences.
    - ◇ The NIMH study used RU486 and human chorionic gonadotropin (hCG) to alter the cycle.
    - ◇ No effect has been noted in alterations of the luteal phase.
  - Ten percent of women with PMS have abnormal thyroid function; no difference is seen between the follicular and luteal phase responses.
  - Treatment.
    - ◇ The following failed to demonstrate a benefit over a placebo:

- ○ Oral contraceptive pills (OCPs).
- ○ Vitamin B_6.
- ○ Bromocriptine.
- ○ Monoamine oxidase inhibitors.
- ○ Progesterone.
- ○ Evening primrose oil.
- ◇ The following demonstrated a proven benefit:
  - ○ Surgical therapy—hysterectomy and oophorectomy.
  - ○ Medical therapy—gonadotropin-releasing hormone (GnRH) agonist with add back; the response indicates that PMS represents an abnormal response to normal hormonal changes.
- ■ Problems and questions.
  - ◇ Clinical symptoms are variable.
  - ◇ Discrepancy between retrospective and prospective symptom reporting.
  - ◇ PMS research has often lumped everything (e.g., behavioral changes, somatic complaints, psychological problems) into the PMS category.
  - ◇ Experimenter expectancy effect.
  - ◇ High placebo response rate.
    - ○ Not a pill, but a process.
    - ○ A response to care and gain in control.
- ■ Evaluation.
  - ◇ Menstrual calendar.
  - ◇ Three months of prospective reporting.
- ■ Broad involvement of the clinician.
- ■ If the symptoms are cyclic, tailor treatment to the patient as follows:
  - ◇ Fluid retention → spironolactone.
  - ◇ Dysmenorrhea → OCPs or PG synthetase inhibitor.
  - ◇ Calcium supplementation, 1,200 mg QD.
  - ◇ Lack of specific symptoms.
    - ○ Daily OCPs.
    - ○ Daily medroxyprogesterone.
    - ○ Medroxyprogesterone (Depo-Provera)—intramuscularly every 3 months.
    - ○ GnRH agonist with add back—60% to 70% success.
  - ◇ Serotonin reuptake inhibitors—begin with luteal phase therapy only.

II. Dysmenorrhea
  - ◆ Pain with menstruation that is centered in the lower abdomen.
  - ◆ Prevalence studies are limited.
    - • Approximately 45% to 72% of females experience dysmenorrhea during adolescence; 14% to 25% report missing school.
    - • Most symptoms are related to PG release; prostaglandin $F_{2\alpha}$ ($PGF_{2\alpha}$) is the likely agent.

- Treatment.
  - OCPs.
  - Nonsteroidal antiinflammatory drugs (NSAIDs)—80% of women report relief.
  - Propionic acid derivatives.
    - ◊ Ibuprofen.
    - ◊ Naproxen.
    - ◊ Ketoprofen.
  - Fenamates → more effective.
    - ◊ Mefenamic acid.
    - ◊ Meclofenamate.
    - ◊ Flufenamic acid.
  - Begin treatment at the time of bleeding.
  - Failure to respond may imply other conditions.
    - ◊ Müllerian duct abnormalities.
    - ◊ Endometriosis.
    - ◊ Pelvic inflammatory disease.

III. Menstrual Headache
  - ♦ This can be part of the constellation of PMS symptoms.
  - ♦ Migraines have a peak incidence of first occurrence between the ages 15 to 19.
    - Most prevalent in women between the ages of 30 to 40.
    - Menstrual association in 60%; 7% to 14% exclusively associated with menses.
  - ♦ Definition of migraines.
    - Classic—associated with visual aura.
    - Common—no neurologic auras.
    - Complicated—associated with dramatic neurologic features.
    - Other types of headaches.
      - Vascular—can be precipitated by stress, alcohol, or tyramine and/or tryptophan-rich foods.
      - Tension.
      - Secondary, due to an underlying organic disease.
  - ♦ Evaluation and management.
    - The acute onset of a severe headache deserves attention.
    - Treatment of the menstrual migraine requires oral or subcutaneous sumatriptan.
      - NSAIDs are also helpful.
      - Daily OCPs can be dramatic in inducing a response but are contraindicated in true, severe vascular headaches, such as migraine with aura.
      - Daily progestin can be used in patients with these headache concerns.

IV. Catamenial Seizures
  - ♦ Epileptic seizures increase during menstruation but decrease in the luteal phase.
    - Fifty percent of epileptic women note an exacerbation.

- Treatment with progesterone may be beneficial; use parenteral forms secondary to ↑ in hepatic enzyme activity from antiepileptic drugs.

V. Premenstrual Asthma
  ♦ Thirty percent to 40% of asthmatics note an increase in symptoms.
  ♦ It is impaired by estrogen administration and other hormonal manipulations.

VI. Catamenial Pneumothorax
  ♦ Requires long-term suppression.
  ♦ Treatment.
    • OCPs.
    • GnRH agonist with add back.

15

Dysfunctional Uterine Bleeding

I. Introduction
   ♦ Definition: a variety of bleeding manifestations of anovulatory cycles in the absence of pathology or medical illness.
   ♦ Types of dysfunctional uterine bleeding:
     • Estrogen withdrawal bleeding.
     • Estrogen breakthrough bleeding.
     • Progestin breakthrough bleeding.
   ♦ Usually easily managed with the appropriate sex steroids; failure to control the bleeding in spite of this therapy suggests a reproductive tract abnormality.
II. Normal Menstrual Bleeding
   ♦ Overview.
     • Postovulatory estrogen–progesterone withdrawal bleeding is the most reproducible, but minor variability may induce undue worry and concern.
     • Menarche is usually followed by 5 to 7 years of relatively long cycles.
       ■ These shorten and then lengthen again in the 40s.
       ■ At age 25, 40% of cycles are from 25 to 28 days.
       ■ Between 25 and 35, >60% of cycles are 25 to 28 days.
     • Fifteen percent of cycles are 28 days in length.
     • The usual duration is 4 to 6 days; some women flow as little as 2 or as many as 7 days.
     • The normal blood loss is 30 mL; >80 mL is abnormal.
     • The proliferative phase is more variable; however, cycles <24 days or >35 days deserve evaluation.
   ♦ Self-limiting nature of menstrual bleeding.
     • It is a universal endometrial event.
     • Random breakdown is avoided.
     • Events that correlate with the start of the next cycle limit bleeding in the prior cycle.
   ♦ Vascular sequence of events in the endometrium.
     1. Tissue height shrinks secondary to hormone withdrawal.
     2. Spiral arteriole blood flow decreases.
     3. Venous drainage decreases.
     4. Vasodilation ensues.
     5. Spiral arterioles undergo rhythmic vasoconstriction and relaxation.
     6. Endometrial blanching occurs.
     7. Endometrial ischemia and stasis occur.
     8. White blood cells and red blood cells escape the vessels and enter the stroma.
     9. Thrombin plugs appear in superficial vessels.

10. Prostaglandin $F_{2\alpha}$ ($PGF_{2\alpha}$) and prostaglandin E_2 (PGE_2) content reaches high levels, leading to continued vasoconstriction and myometrial contractions.
11. Lysosomes release enzymes.
12. Matrix metalloproteinase secretion increases; it is suppressed in early pregnancy by continued progesterone secretion.
13. Interstitial hemorrhage occurs.
14. Bleeding is controlled by tissue factor.
15. Cell necrosis and vessel defects add to menstrual effluvium.
16. Cleavage plane develops between the basalis and spongiosum.
17. Platelets and fibrin play a direct part in the bleeding menstrual endometrium.
18. Healing endometrium is pale, collapsed, and disorderly.

Traditional definitions

Oligomenorrhea	Intervals >35 days
Polymenorrhea	Intervals <24 days
Menorrhagia	Regular normal intervals; excessive flow and duration
Metrorrhagia	Irregular intervals; excessive flow and duration

III. Why Is Anovulatory Bleeding Excessive?
   ♦ In absence of growth-limiting progesterone, the endometrium attains an abnormal height.
      • Densely vascular.
      • Poor stromal support matrix.
   ♦ The usual control mechanisms are absent.
      • Not a universal event.
      • Well-developed stroma absent.
      • Not an orderly collapse with rhythmic vasoconstrictive events.
   ♦ It must rely on the local healing effects of estrogen, but this begins a vicious cycle.
   ♦ Alternative hypothesis: bleeding occurs because the tissue loss is insufficient stimulus for binding surface restoration to occur.
IV. Differential Diagnosis
   ♦ Dysfunctional uterine bleeding is a diagnosis of exclusion.
   ♦ Other causes of abnormal bleeding are as follows:
      1. Pregnancy.
      2. Exogenous hormones and/or herbs (e.g., ginseng).
      3. Neoplasms.
         • Cervical.
         • Uterine.
         • Polyps.
         • Fibroids.
      4. Infection.

5. Thyroid disease.
6. Hepatic or renal disease.
7. Foreign body.
8. Coagulation defect.
   - Includes 20% of adolescents with dysfunctional uterine bleeding.
   - May be the only sign of a bleeding disorder.
9. Possibly tubal sterilization—inconsistent data.

♦ Appropriate, but not always necessary, tests include the following:
   - Prothrombin time, partial thromboplastin time, and bleeding time.
   - Platelet count.
   - Complete blood cell count.
   - Ristocetin cofactor assay (von Willebrand factor).
   - β-Human chorionic gonadotropin (hCG).
   - Prolactin.
   - Thyroid function tests.
   - Renal and liver function tests.
   - Cervical cultures.

V. Treatment
   ♦ Progestin therapy.
      - Usually, this will successfully control the bleeding once a uterine pathology is excluded.
      - Progestins are powerful antiestrogens.
         ■ Stimulate 17β-hydroxysteroid dehydrogenase.
         ■ Inhibit replenishment of estrogen receptors.
         ■ Suppress estrogen-mediated oncogene transcription.
         ■ Usually requires 5 to 10 mg of medroxyprogesterone acetate for at least 10 days per month.
         ■ Use of oral contraceptive pills (OCPs) better if contraception is desired.
   ♦ OCP therapy.
      - Any of the low-dose monophasics are useful.
         ■ Begin with one pill BID × 5 to 7 days.
            ◊ Continue therapy despite cessation of flow.
            ◊ Anticipate heavy flow 7 days after discontinuation.
         ■ Begin on the fifth day of flow or in the usual Sunday start.
      - After 3 months, consider monthly progestin therapy; rule out pregnancy each month.
      - Medroxyprogesterone acetate (Depo-Provera) can also be used (150 mg every 3 months).
   ♦ Estrogen therapy.
      - Intermittent spotting is frequently associated with low estrogen stimulation; the beneficial effect of progestin is not achieved.
      - This may also be true in the young patient with prolonged hemorrhagic desquamation.
      - Acute therapy is as follows:
         ■ Give a dose of 25 mg intravenous conjugated equine estrogens (CEEs) every 4 hours until bleeding abates or for 24 hours.

- Start concurrent progestin therapy.
- Oral doses of estrogen can be substituted for intravenous doses.
    ◇ Less bleeding: CEE, 1.25 mg/day; estradiol, 2.0 mg/day.
    ◇ Heaviest bleeding: CEE, 1.25 mg every 4 hours; estradiol, 2.0 mg every 4 hours for 24 hours, then QD.
- Clinician must provide progestin withdrawal bleeding following estrogen therapy.
    - In cases of progestin breakthrough bleeding, consider the following:
        - Pharmacologically induced pseudoatrophy may be responsible.
        - Can use CEE, 1.25 mg, or estradiol, 2 mg, QD for 7 days.
    - Risks of high-dose estrogen therapy are as follows:
        - Could precipitate a thromboembolic event.
        - Should be avoided in patients with a prior episode or a family history of idiopathic thromboembolism.

◆ Antiprostaglandins.
   - Prostaglandins clearly have important actions on the endometrial vasculature.
   - Nonsteroidal antiinflammatory drugs (NSAIDs) may alter the balance between thromboxane A_2 and prostaglandin I_2 (PGI_2).
       - Can reduce bleeding by 40% to 50%.
       - Occasionally can cause an anomalous response with ↑ bleeding.
   - These may be useful first-line therapy.

◆ Progestin intrauterine device (IUD).
   - Studies have shown that the levonorgestrel IUD is better than NSAIDs.
       - Reduction in flow of 96% after 12 months.
       - Comparable to endometrial ablation.
   - It is useful in patients with chronic illness.

◆ Gonadotropin-releasing hormone (GnRH) agonists.
   - May be useful for short-term therapy in transplant patients.
   - Consider add-back therapy if long-term use desired.

◆ Desmopressin.
   - A synthetic analog of arginine vasopressin.
   - Helpful in von Willebrand disease.
   - Administration: 0.3 µg/kg in 50 mL saline intravenously over 15 to 30 minutes.
   - Causes rapid increase in coagulation factor VIII and von Willebrand factor that lasts 6 hours.

◆ Endometrial ablation.
   - An alternative to a hysterectomy.
   - Technical aspects now easier with new thermal balloon therapy.
   - Ninety percent of cases demonstrate improvement; 40% to 50% become amenorrheic.

- Not recommended for patients at high risk for endometrial cancer.

VI. Hyperplasia versus Neoplasia
  ♦ Endometrial hyperplasia.
    - No atypia.
    - Not usually a precursor to cancer.
  ♦ Endometrial intraepithelial neoplasia (EIN).
    - Cytologic atypia.
    - Present in 75% of cases after multiple curettage or high-dose progestins.
  ♦ EIN is best treated surgically.
    - If future fertility is desired, treat with progestin—30 mg medroxyprogesterone (Provera) QD × 3 to 4 months.
    - If EIN persists, surgery or additional progestin therapy is warranted.
      - Two hundred milligrams medroxyprogesterone acetate **OR**
      - Five hundred milligrams megestrol acetate twice weekly **OR**
      - Medroxyprogesterone, 1,000 mg weekly.
  ♦ Benign lesions can be treated hormonally; a failure to respond raises the question of the accuracy of the initial diagnosis.
  ♦ Evaluate by biopsy; it is not the age of the patient but the duration of exposure to unopposed estrogen that determines the risk of cancer.
  ♦ Estrogen therapy versus progestin therapy versus curettage.
    - Estrogen is initial choice in the following:
      1. Cases with many days of heavy bleeding and likely a raw basalis layer.
      2. Cases with minimal tissue on curettage.
      3. Cases where the patient has been on progestin therapy.
      4. Cases where follow-up is uncertain as it will arrest bleeding in all categories.
    - Curettage is *not* the first line of defense but the last.
    - Consider imaging with saline infusion sonography in cases where medical therapy fails.

The Breast

I. Growth and Development
- Each alveolus is lined by a single layer of milk-secreting cells.
  - This layer is derived from the ingrowth of epidermis into the underlying mesenchyme at 10 to 12 weeks of gestation.
  - The mantle of myoepithelial cells encases each alveolus.
  - The lumen of the alveolus connects to the interlobular duct.
  - The ducts terminate in 15 to 20 collecting ducts in a radial arrangement corresponding to 15 to 20 distinct lobules.
- Nearly half of all newborns have breast secretions (Fig. 16.1).
- The growth of the alveolus is estrogen-dependent.
  - The first change in the alveolus is an increase in size and pigmentation and the formation of breast tissue beneath.
  - Breast tissue expresses both estrogen receptor–α (ER-α) and ER-β.
  - The development of ERs is prolactin-dependent.
  - Estrogen stimulates ductal growth.
  - Progesterone stimulates growth of the alveolus.
  - Full differentiation of breast tissue requires the following:
    - Insulin.
    - Cortisol.
    - Thyroxin.
    - Prolactin.
    - Growth hormone (GH).
  - Maximum breast size occurs during the luteal phase; fluid secretion, mitotic activity, DNA production of nonglandular tissue, and glandular epithelium peak during the luteal phase.
  - The final differentiation into a mature milk cell is dependent on the gestational increase in estrogen and progesterone.
- Abnormal shapes and sizes.
  - Early differentiation is under fetal hormonal control.
  - Abnormalities may reflect the impact of hormones.
  - Inequalities in size usually resolve by the completion of development; significant asymmetry requires surgical correction.
  - Accessory nipples are found in 1% of women; no therapy is required.
II. Pregnancy and Lactation
- Prolactin secretion.

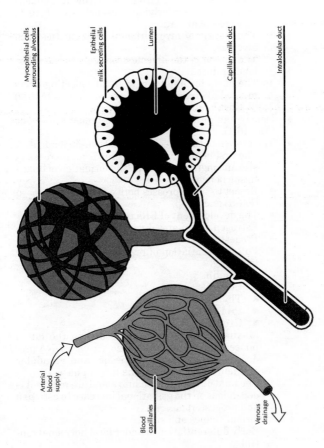

Figure 16.1. Structure of the breast lobule.

- A single chain polypeptide of 199 amino acids; 40% homology with GH and human placental lactogen.
- Encoded by a single gene on the short arm of chromosome 6.
- Protein maintained in three loops.
- Heterogeneity at many levels.
    - Transcription.
    - Translation.
    - Posttranslation.
    - Peripheral metabolism.
    - Glycosylation.
    - Phosphorylation.
- Other forms.
    - Little prolactin—proteolytic deletion of amino acids.
    - Big prolactin—failure to remove introns.
    - Big big prolactin—examples of prolactin molecules binding to each other.
- Bioactivity and immunoactivity may not correlate.

◆ Pit-1.
- A transcription factor required for normal development of lactotrophs, somatotrophs, and thyrotrophs.
- Also binds the prolactin gene in multiple sites both in the promoter region and in the distal enhancer region.
    - Pit-1 binding is a requirement for prolactin promoter activity and gene transcription.
    - Estrogen response element may explain the estrogen effect on prolactin secretion (Fig. 16.2).

◆ Prolactin and pregnancy.
- Surfactant synthesis is dependent upon prolactin.
- Decidual prolactin modulates prostaglandin (PG)-mediated uterine contractility.
- Prolactin also suppresses the maternal immune response.

◆ The prolactin-inhibiting factor (PIF) is believed to be dopamine.
- Secreted by the basal hypothalamus and conducted to the anterior pituitary.
- Binds to lactotrophs and suppresses the secretion of prolactin.
    - G protein–coupled receptor.
    - Long form (D_2) present on lactotrophs.

◆ Prolactin-releasing factor.
- Clearly present in fowl.
- Possibly thyrotropin-releasing hormone (TRH) in humans, but normal and abnormal prolactin secretion is more likely related to dopamine.

◆ The prolactin receptor.
- Encoded by a gene on 5p13-14 that is located near the GH receptor gene.

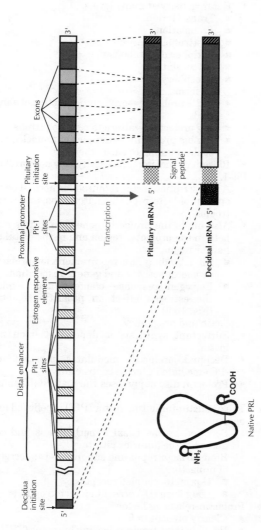

Figure 16.2.   Structure of the prolactin gene and transcription variations.

- Receptors exist in more than one form but all contain the following:
  - Extracellular region.
  - Single transmembrane region.
  - Relatively long cytoplasmic domain.
- Thirty percent homology with GH receptor.
- Expressed in many tissues.
♦ Amniotic fluid prolactin.
  - It parallels maternal serum levels until week 10.
  - It rises markedly until week 20, then decreases.
  - Maternal prolactin does not pass to fetus in significant amounts.
  - Amniotic fluid prolactin is from the decidua; it has a slightly larger RNA transcript, but the proteins are identical.
  - It probably plays a role in the control of salt and water transport across the amnion.
♦ Lactation.
  - During pregnancy, prolactin levels rise from normal levels of 10 to 25 ng/mL to between 200 to 400 ng/mL at term; this is probably related to the estrogen suppression of dopamine and the direct stimulation of prolactin gene transcription.
  - Human placental lactogen rises to 6,000 ng/mL at term → exerts a lactogenic effect.
  - Only colostrum is produced during gestation.
    - Full lactation is inhibited by progesterone.
    - Pharmacologic amounts of estrogen also block prolactin.
  - Without prolactin, synthesis of the primary milk protein (casein) will not occur.
  - Breast engorgement begins once the steroids are cleared.
  - Prolactin levels decline by 50% in first postpartum week.
    - Suckling elicits increases in prolactin; it releases both prolactin and oxytocin.
    - Optimal quantity and quality of milk are dependent upon the thyroid, insulin, insulin-like growth factors (IGFs), cortisol, and dietary intake.
  - Calcium.
    - Daily losses of calcium double.
    - Bone loss occurs even in the presence of high calcium intake.
    - Recovery requires adequate calcium intake (1,500 mg/day); rapidly restored after weaning.
  - Antibodies and viruses.
    - Immunoglobulins provide passive immunity.
    - Human immunodeficiency virus (HIV), cytomegalovirus, and hepatitis B virus can be transmitted via breast-feeding.
  - Mechanism of lactation.
    - Tactile sensors in the areola activate via thoracic sensory nerve roots 4, 5, 6—an afferent sensory neural arc.

■ Stimulates oxytocin synthesis and transport.
- Adoptive mothers—can treat to induce lactation.
  ■ Requires several months.
  ■ Twenty-five milligrams chlorpromazine TID with vigorous nipple stimulation every 1 to 3 hours.
- Cessation of lactation.
  ■ Lactation is terminated by discontinuing suckling.
  ■ The swollen breast diminishes in size over a few days.
  ■ Dopamine production is reactivated.
  ■ The routine use of dopamine agonists is not recommended; cases of hypertension, seizure, myocardial infarctions, and strokes have been reported.
- Contraceptive effect of lactation.
  ■ Depends upon level of maternal nutrition, intensity of suckling, and extent of supplemental feedings.
  ■ Fully breast-feeding women have 92% contraceptive efficacy at 1 year; supplemental feeding markedly reduces this efficacy.
  ■ Follicle-stimulating hormone (FSH) and luteinizing hormone (LH) concentrations are in the low-to-normal range.
  ■ Some ovarian effect but mainly a central action.
    ◊ Pulsatile gonadotropin-releasing hormone (GnRH) is inhibited.
    ◊ Exact mechanism is unknown.

III. Inappropriate Lactation—Galactorrheic Syndromes
  ♦ Nonphysiologic secretion of a milky fluid.
    - Hormonal secretions are usually from multiple duct openings.
    - Bloody discharge is more typical of cancer.
  ♦ Differential diagnosis of galactorrhea.
    - Difficult and complex clinical challenge.
    - Important considerations include the following:
      1. It may be a consequence of prolactin elaboration and secretion from pituitary tumors, which function independently; it may interfere with secretion of other tropic hormones.
      2. A variety of drugs can inhibit hypothalamic PIF.
         ■ Usually function in manner similar to estrogens.
         ■ Phenothiazine treatment never associated with prolactin levels as high as 100 ng/mL.
      3. Hypothyroidism can be associated with galactorrhea; TRH serves as a prolactin-releasing factor.
      4. Excessive estrogen could cause galactorrhea; prolactin secretion in users of low-dose oral contraceptive pills (OCPs) is not out of the normal range.

5. Prolonged intensive suckling can cause prolactin release, as can thoracotomy scars, cervical spinal lesions, and herpes zoster.
6. Stress from trauma, surgical procedures, or anesthesia can inhibit PIF.
7. Hypothalamic lesions, stalk lesions, or stalk compression can be a factor.
8. Nonpituitary sources can also be involved.
   - Lung and renal tumors.
   - Renal disease with decreased glomerular filtration rate.

IV. Clinical Problem of Galactorrhea
- ♦ Hyperprolactinemia may be associated with a variety of menstrual disturbances; one-third of women with secondary amenorrhea will have elevated prolactin levels.
- ♦ Mild hirsutism can accompany ovulatory dysfunction caused by hyperprolactinemia.
  - Possibly from direct prolactin effect on adrenal cortex.
  - Or from increased ovarian androgen secretion (Fig. 16.3).
- ♦ Not all hyperprolactinemic patients have galactorrhea.
  - Usually one-third of patients.
  - Absence probably related to hypoestrogenic state or due to the heterogeneity of prolactin molecules.
- ♦ Not all galactorrhea patients have elevated prolactin; in these, it is possibly from episodic or nighttime fluctuations or nonimmunoreactive prolactin (Fig. 16.4).

V. Mastalgia
- ♦ A very common problem.
- ♦ A bewildering array of treatment options.
- ♦ Five milligrams methyltestosterone every other day—effective.
- ♦ One hundred to 200 mg/day of danazol; requires method of effective contraception to avoid teratogenic effects.
- ♦ Six hundred units/day of vitamin E; mechanism of action unknown.
- ♦ Bromocriptine, 2.5 mg/day.
- ♦ Abstinence from methylxanthines; significant placebo response.

VI. Cancer of the Breast
- ♦ Scope of the problem.
  - Female American newborns have a 12.5% lifetime risk of developing breast cancer (double the 1940 risk).
  - This has increased over the past 4 decades but plateaued in 1987; 180,000 new cases of invasive breast cancer annually.
  - Survival rates have improved.
    - Five-year survival is 97% for localized disease.
    - Five-year survival is 76% for regional spread and 21% for distant metastases.

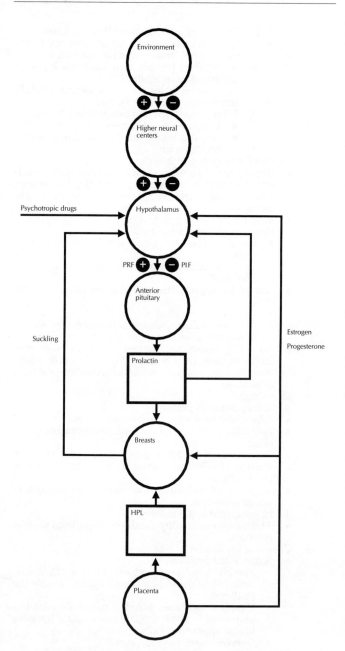

Figure 16.3.   Factors influencing prolactin secretion.

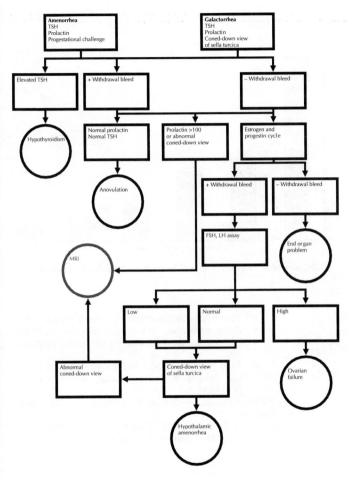

Figure 16.4.   Algorithm detailing investigations of amenorrhea and/or galactorrhea.

- All stages combined have the following survival rates:
    ◇ Eighty-four percent at 5 years.
    ◇ Sixty-seven percent at 10 years.
    ◇ Fifty-six percent at 15 years.
- The increase in incidence cannot be explained solely by increased screening; it can probably be attributed to lifestyle and reproductive changes.
- Breast cancer is the leading type of cancer in U.S. women and is second in deaths to lung cancer (Figs. 16.5–16.7).
- Age and rate of cancer.

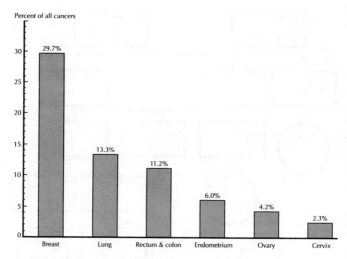

Figure 16.5. **Cancer site incidence in United States women.**

- Seventy-seven percent in women over age 50.
- Sixty-six percent in women under the age of 70.
- Fifteen percent in women under 50 years of age.
- Five-year survival = 79% for women <45 years old versus 87% for women >65 years old (Table 16.1).
  ◆ Pathophysiology—should be viewed as a systemic disease.
  • Occultly metastatic at time of presentation.
  • Axillary node status predictive of survival.

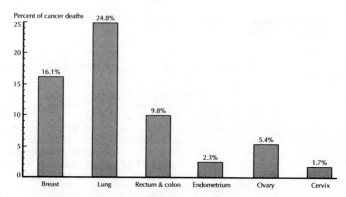

Figure 16.6. **Cancer deaths in United States women.**

Mortality rate per 100,000 female population

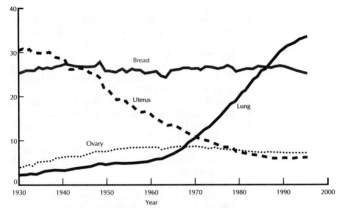

Figure 16.7. Mortality rate, by cancer site, of specific cancers in the female population of the United States.

- ♦ Risk factors.
  - • Eighty-five percent of women who develop breast cancer have no identifiable risk factors other than age.
  - • Reproductive experience.
    - ■ Risk increases with the increase in age at which a woman bears her first full-term child; pregnancy over the age of 30 results in a greater risk than for the nulliparous patient.
    - ■ Increasing risk is seen with age at last child's birth but it decreases with increasing parity.

**Table 16.1.   The chances of
developing breast cancer according to age**

By age 25	1 in 19,608
By age 30	1 in 2,525
By age 35	1 in 622
By age 40	1 in 217
By age 45	1 in 93
By age 50	1 in 50
By age 55	1 in 33
By age 60	1 in 24
By age 65	1 in 17
By age 70	1 in 14
By age 75	1 in 11
By age 80	1 in 10
By age 85	1 in 9
Lifetime	1 in 8

- Strong family history results in enhanced risk with pregnancy.
- Recent pregnancy may worsen the prognosis.
- Abortions are unlikely to alter risk of breast cancer; the initial studies were flawed by relying on patient recall.
- Changes in the hormonal milieu or anatomic changes in breast tissue may explain the protective effect of pregnancy.
- Lactation may provide a weak protective effect.
- Breast augmentation does not alter the risk.
- Oophorectomy prior to the age of 35 results in a 70% risk reduction.
- A small decreased risk exists with late menorrhea and a moderate increased risk with late menopause.

- Benign breast disease.
  - Most important variable on biopsy is the degree and character of epithelial proliferation.
  - **Classification of breast biopsy tissue according to risk for breast cancer.**
    No increased risk:
      Adenosis
      Duct ectasia
      Fibroadenoma
      Fibrosis
      Mild hyperplasia (three to four cells deep)
      Mastitis
      Periductal mastitis
      Squamous metaplasia
    Slightly increased risk (1.5 to 2.0×):
      Moderate or florid hyperplasia
      Papilloma
    Risk increased by 3 to 5×:
      Atypical hyperplasia

- Familial tendency.
  - Most breast cancers are sporadic.
  - Female relatives of breast cancer patients have a 2× increased risk.

Affected mother or sister:	2.3 relative risk
Affected aunt or grandmother:	1.5 relative risk
Affected mother and sister:	14.0 relative risk

- BRCA1 (breast and ovarian cancer gene).
  - Associated with familial cancer.
  - Long arm of chromosome 17 (17q12-q21).
  - Mutations believed to be responsible for 45% of familial breast cancer; accounts for 80% of families with early onset breast and ovarian cancer.
  - Five percent to 10% of women with ovarian cancer.

- Male carriers have an increased risk of colon or prostate cancer.
- Gene encodes 1,863-amino acid protein with zinc finger domain.
  - ◇ Probably a tumor suppressor important in DNA transcription.
  - ◇ Loss of function mutations may result in cancer.
- BRCA2 on chromosome 13 (13q12-q13).
  - Accounts for 45% of families with early onset breast cancer; lower rates of ovarian cancer.
  - Male carriers are at risk for prostate, pancreatic, and male breast cancer.
- BRCA1 and BRCA2.
  - These account for 5% of breast cancer in general population.
  - Approximately 0.04% to 0.2% of U.S. women carry BRCA1.
  - About 2% to 3% of Ashkenazi Jews carry BRCA1 and BRCA2.
  - **Family history characteristics associated with the presence of BRCA1.**
    Early age of onset of breast cancer within a family
    Relatives with ovarian cancer
    Three or more relatives with breast cancer
    Ashkenazi ancestry (Table 16.2)
  - Not all families carry BRCA1 or BRCA2.
    - ◇ When three or more closely related individuals within a family have been diagnosed with breast cancer, then the likelihood of an inherited dominant mutation is high.
    - ◇ Identification and counseling should be the same as if the mutation were present.

Table 16.2.   Breast cancer risk as predicted by family history

Affected Relative	Age of Affected Relative	Cumulative Breast Cancer Risk by Age 80
One first-degree relative	<50 yr old	13% to 21%
	≥50 yr old	9% to 11%
One second-degree relative	<50 yr old	10% to 14%
	≥50 yr old	8% to 9%
Two first-degree relatives	Both <50 yr old	35% to 48%
	Both ≥50 yr old	11% to 24%
Two second-degree relatives but both parental or maternal	Both <50 yr old	21% to 26%
	Both ≥50 yr old	9% to 16%

♦ With information about higher risk, what should one do with the information? A prophylactic mastectomy lowers, but does not eliminate, the risk.
- Recommendations.
  - Conduct a clinical breast examination and mammogram every 6 to 12 months starting at age 25 to 35.
  - Offer a prophylactic mastectomy.
  - Perform a pelvic examination, serum Ca-125, and endovaginal sonogram with Doppler studies every 6 to 12 months for women >40.
  - Offer prophylactic oophorectomy to women at the completion of child bearing, preferably before the age of 35.
  - OCP use reduces the risk of ovarian cancer by up to 60% with ≥6 years of use.
- Dietary factors.
  - Dietary fat may be a risk factor for postmenopausal breast cancer.
  - Android obesity is definitely associated with an increased risk.
  - Peripheral insulin resistance may increase the risk.
    - ◇ A decrease in sex hormone–binding globulin (SHBG).
    - ◇ An increase in free estradiol.
  - Soy intake may reduce the risk, but this may also reflect other lifestyle or dietary issues.
  - Premenopausal obese patients actually have lower risk, while postmenopausal obese women are at an increased risk.
- Alcohol.
  - Modest increase with ≥ one drink/day; two drinks/day increases risk by 30% to 40%.
  - May result in increased estradiol levels.

VII. Specific Endocrine Factors
  ♦ Adrenal steroids.
  - Subnormal excretion of etiocholanolone increases risk; a urinary excretion product of androstenedione.
  - Could be a useful screening tool.
  ♦ Endogenous estrogen.
  - Clear suggestion of estrogen-related promoter function is as follows:
    1. Breast cancer is 100× more common in women.
    2. It invariably occurs after puberty.
    3. Untreated gonadal dysgenesis and breast cancer are virtually exclusive.
    4. Sixty-five percent excess rate is seen in women who have had endometrial cancer.
    5. Breast tumors contain ERs.
  - Estriol may be protective.
    - Women with pregnancies at an early age excrete more estriol.

- - Asian women also excrete higher levels of estriol; the amount changes when Asian women migrate to the United States.
    - Estriol has 20% to 30% affinity for ER; however, if the effective concentration is high enough, it can produce a similar biologic response.
  - The Korenman "open window" hypothesis proposed the following:
    - Suggested that endocrine status influences a patient's susceptibility to environmental carcinogens.
    - Two major open window periods:
      ◇ Pubertal years prior to establishment of regular menses.
      ◇ Perimenopausal years.
    - Thesis not confirmed by all studies; anovulatory women in the Nurses Health Study had reduced rates of breast cancer.
    - Studies seeking correlation between circulating levels of sex hormones and breast cancer yield conflicting results.
    - Women with higher bone density = greater risk of breast cancer.
    - Decreased risk in women born to mothers with preeclampsia (associated with lower estrogen levels).
- ◆ Endogenous progesterone.
  - Mitotic activity in the breast is higher in the luteal phase.
  - However, no reliable data suggesting an influence of progesterone on the risk of breast cancer exists.
- ◆ Exogenous estrogen and progestin—currently no conclusive evidence that estrogen in doses that are protective against osteoporosis and cardiac disease increases the risk of breast cancer.
  - Some epidemiologic case-control and cohort studies conclude that long-term (5 or more years) use of postmenopausal hormone therapy is associated with a slight increase in the risk of breast cancer. This conclusion might be due to confounding biases, particularly detection and surveillance bias.
  - All epidemiologic studies have failed to find an increased risk of breast cancer associated with short-term (less than 5 years) current use or prior use of postmenopausal hormone therapy.
  - The epidemiologic data agree that the addition of a progestin to the treatment regimen neither increases nor decreases the risk observed in individual studies.
  - The epidemiologic data indicate that a positive family history of breast cancer should not be a contraindication to the use of postmenopausal hormone therapy.

- Women who develop breast cancer while using postmenopausal hormone therapy have a reduced risk of dying from breast cancer. This is due to the following two factors: (a) increased surveillance and early detection and (b) acceleration of tumor growth so that tumors appear at a less virulent and aggressive stage.
- ♦ Thyroid, prolactin, and various nonestrogen drugs—hypothyroidism, reserpine, and prolactin excess are not related to an increased risk of breast cancer.
- ♦ OCPs and breast cancer.
  - This has been a source of concern for many years.
  - Several large studies have failed to show any significant differences between users and nonusers.
  - Long-term use during the reproductive years is not associated with a risk after the age of 45.
  - Slightly increased risk (1.2) in a subgroup of young users with >4 years of use of developing cancer prior to 45 years of age; this could represent a surveillance or detection bias given the rarity of this situation.
  - OCPs may reduce the risk of metastatic breast cancer.
  - They have no adverse impact on women with positive family histories.
  - Low-dose formulations may not be protective with regard to benign breast disease.
- ♦ Breast cancer in diethylstilbestrol (DES)-exposed women.
  - A small but significant increase in breast cancer has been seen in women exposed to DES during pregnancy.
  - DES-exposed women should adhere religiously to screening guidelines.
- ♦ Receptors and clinical prognosis.
  - Receptor-positive patients survive longer and have longer disease-free intervals; this correlates with increased survival regardless of node status.
  - ER-positive tumors are more likely to respond to endocrine treatment.
  - Progesterone receptors are dependent upon estrogen.
    - This correlates as well with disease-free survival.
    - Loss of progesterone receptors in recurrent disease is an ominous sign.
- ♦ Tamoxifen and breast cancer.
  - Tamoxifen binds to the ER.
    - Competitively inhibits estrogen binding.
    - Must be present in concentration that is 100 to 1,000 times greater than estrogen.
  - No change in activity in doses higher than 20 mg/day.
  - The mechanism of action is reviewed in Chapter 2.
  - Adjuvant therapy reduces recurrences and increases survival for all patients.

- It has an impact on recurrence in the first 5 years, but the effect is greater with longer treatment; a 20% increase in survival is seen at 5 years.
- Response rates are 30% to 35% in advanced disease.
- Extending therapy >5 years is not supported by the results; tamoxifen-resistant tumors may emerge.
- Tamoxifen results in increased hot flushes.
- It may result in slight reductions in bone mineral density.
- An increased risk of venous (and possibly arterial) thromboembolic events is seen.
- Levels decreased by tamoxifen include the following:
  - Antithrombin III.
  - Cholesterol.
  - Low-density lipoprotein (LDL) cholesterol.
  - Free estrogen.
- Those increased by tamoxifen are as follows:
  - High-density lipoprotein (HDL) cholesterol.
  - SHBG.
  - Circulating estrogens.
- Tamoxifen breast cancer prevention trials.
  - The study was unblinded after 4 years of followup.
  - Forty-nine percent fewer cases of invasive breast cancer and 50% fewer cases of noninvasive breast cancer were seen in the treatment arm.
  - The increased risk of endometrial cancer was 2.4.
    - ◇ Pulmonary embolism—2.8.
    - ◇ Venous thrombosis—1.6.
    - ◇ Cataracts—1.6.
  - This protective effect failed to be demonstrated in the Italian and UK studies; possibly, this was the effect of having younger women enrolled.
  - Also possible is the fact that longer treatment leads to the emergence of tamoxifen-resistant and more aggressive tumors.
  - European results suggest that tamoxifen functions through a deceleration effect.
- **These results lead us to recommend tamoxifen prophylaxis (20 mg/day for 5 years) for those women who are diagnosed with ductal carcinoma *in situ* of the breast or who have atypical hyperplasia in a breast biopsy (especially if a positive family history of breast cancer is also present). For others who seek tamoxifen preventive treatment, we advise that the final answers are not in and that clinical trial results from long-term follow-up will be necessary before fully informed decision-making is possible.**
- Gynecologic problems with tamoxifen.

- Incidence of endometrial cancer in tamoxifen-treated women is 6.3/1,000 patients after 5 years; similar to unopposed estrogen treatment.
- Not a surprising finding, because the duration of exposure is more important than the dose.
- Other gynecologic problems.
  ◇ Growth of fibroids.
  ◇ Adenomyosis.
  ◇ Endometriosis.
  ◇ Uterine polyps.
- Progesterone treatment inappropriate for these polyps.
  ◇ Progestin challenge test may allow detection.
  ◇ Use of sonohysterography may be best choice; identifies subendometrial sonolucent changes unique for tamoxifen.
- Hot flushes possibly helped by transdermal clonidine, 100 mg once weekly.
- Other options for hot flushes.
  ◇ Veralipride, 100 mg QD—may induce mastodynia, galactorrhea.
  ◇ Medroxyprogesterone acetate, megestrol—concern over exogenous steroids.
  ◇ Methyldopa, 500 to 1,000 mg QD.
  ◇ Venlafaxine hydrochloride, 25 mg QD.

We recommend the following program for monitoring women during long-term tamoxifen treatment:

All women: Careful pelvic examination every 6 months to detect the emergence of endometriosis, ovarian cysts, and/or uterine leiomyomata

Postmenopausal women: Annual measurement of endometrial thickness by transvaginal ultrasonography. Endometrial biopsy of all women with a two-layer thickness of 5 mm or greater. Saline instillation (sonohysterography) when the appearance is not totally benign

Premenopausal women: Periodic assessment for ovulation; if ovulatory, no further intervention is necessary; however, contraceptive counseling should not be ignored. If anovulatory, an annual endometrial aspiration biopsy is indicated since the interpretation of endometrial thickness measurements by ultrasonography is uncertain in premenopausal women. Consider the use of the progestin-releasing intrauterine device for both contraception and protection against endometrial change.

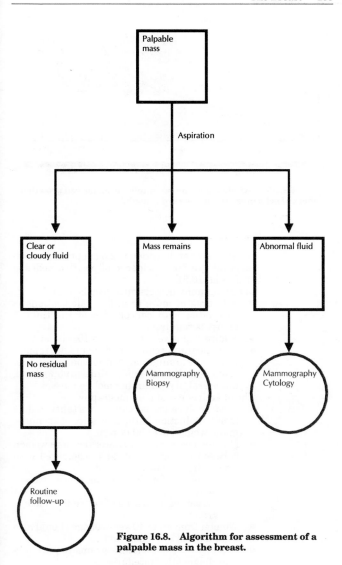

Figure 16.8.   Algorithm for assessment of a palpable mass in the breast.

- ◆ Needle aspiration.
  - • A cost-effective and easy method of assessment.
  - • When aspiration yields clear, cloudy, green-gray, or yellow fluid and the mass resolves, then the procedure is diagnostic and therapeutic (Fig. 16.8).
- ◆ Screening mammography.
  - • Means of detecting a nonpalpable cancer.
  - • In general, a tumor doubles in size every 100 days.

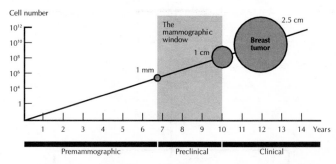

Figure 16.9.   The window for mammography in tumor cell growth by numbers of cells present and years of growth.

- Average size at detection is 2.5 cm prior to mammography; a 50% incidence of positive nodes is seen (Fig. 16.9).
- Mammography detects microcalcifications.
  - A finding of more than five calcifications is associated with cancer 25% of the time; a biopsy is required.
  - A false-negative rate of 5% to 10% is seen.
  - Mammography cannot and should not replace physical examination; cancer commonly presents as a solitary, solid, painless (90%), hard, unilateral, irregular, nonmobile mass.
- The effectiveness of mammography.
  - It can reduce breast cancer mortality; a 30% to 40% reduction in the mortality of asymptomatic women over 50 is seen.
  - Nineteen percent more cancers occur in women between the ages of 40 to 49 compared with women from 50 to 59 years of age.
    - ◇ Accounts for 20% of all breast cancer deaths.
    - ◇ Screening is just as effective for this age group.
  - Women from 40 to 49 years of age should also have annual mammograms.
  - Roughly 50/1,000 mammograms require further diagnostic procedures.
  - Small nonpalpable lesions have <5% rate of malignancy; overall, 20% to 30% of biopsies reveal cancer.
  - An analysis of the increased costs suggests the overall benefit is worthwhile.
  - Older women should still be screened.
- ◆ Screening for breast cancer.
  All women should be taught self-examination of the breast by age 20. Because of the changes that occur routinely in response to the hormonal sequence of

a normal menstrual cycle, breast examination is most effective during the follicular phase of the cycle; it should be performed monthly.

All women over the age of 35 should have an annual breast examination.

Women with a first-degree relative with premenopausal breast cancer should begin annual mammography 5 years before the age when the relative was diagnosed.

Annual mammography should be performed in all women over the age of 39.

Menopause and the Perimenopausal Transition

I. Introduction
   ◆ Scientific study of menopause is hampered by the overpowering influence of social and cultural beliefs.
      • The variability in menopausal reactions necessitates longitudinal rather than cross-sectional studies.
      • Massachusetts Women's Health study revealed that menopause is not viewed as a negative experience by the vast majority of women.
   ◆ Women who expect to have difficulty experience greater symptoms and higher levels of depression.
   ◆ Menopause is not a disease.
   ◆ Medical issues revolve around preventative care.
      • Body weight.
      • Alcohol consumption.
      • Prevention of cardiovascular disease and osteoporosis.
      • Maintenance of mental and sexual well-being.
      • Cancer screening.
      • Treatment of urologic problems.
II. Growth of the Older Population
   ◆ A relatively new phenomenon.
      • 1000 B.C. life expectancy—18 years.
      • 100 B.C. life expectancy—25 years.
      • A.D. 1900 life expectancy—49 years.
      • A.D. 2000 life expectancy—79.7 years (72.9 for men).
   ◆ Eventually, two-thirds of the population will survive to the age of 85 or more (Fig. 17.1).
   ◆ An elderly population is the largest contributor in the United States to illness and human need.
      • By 2030, the elderly population (>65) will reach 57×10^6 (17% of the total population).
      • Influenced by the Baby Boom and the declining death rate (Fig. 17.2).
   ◆ World population.
      • Predicted to stabilize at 11 billion in 2150.
      • Poorest countries account for 87% of world's population; by 2025, more than 70% of people >60 years of age will live in developing countries.
   ◆ Sex ratio—gender difference is pronounced in those older than 85 (Fig. 17.3).
   ◆ Possibly the result of sex hormone–induced differences in cardiovascular disease.
      • Use of postmenopausal estrogen replacement therapy may exaggerate the sex differential.
      • Lifestyle differences very important in tobacco and/or alcohol use.

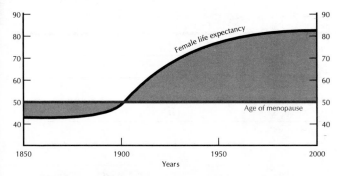

Figure 17.1. Female life expectancy changes in the last 150 years.

- ♦ Rectangularization of life.
  - • Lifespan is the biologic limit to life.
    - ■ This number is fixed.
    - ■ Death converges at the same maximal age.
  - • Life expectancy is increasing, but it cannot exceed the lifespan.
  - • Premature death has almost been eliminated as a result of success in treating infectious diseases.
  - • The new era of medicine will deal with nonfatal age-dependent conditions.
- ♦ Concept of compression of morbidity.
  - • Chronic diseases are incremental; if the rate of development is changed, then the disease is effectively prevented.

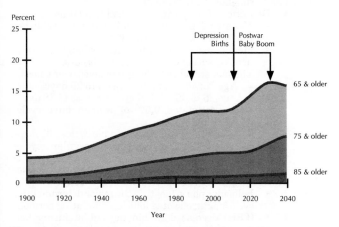

Figure 17.2. The percentage of elderly in the United States population.

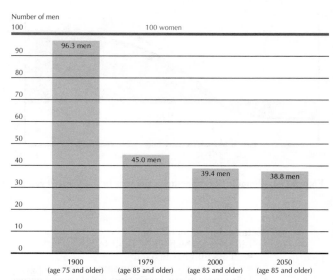

Number of men

Figure 17.3.   The number of men per 100 women in the United States, age 85 or older.

- Smoking has seen some significant declines.
    - It remains the single most preventable cause of premature death in the United States.
    - The effects of smoking are reversible within 1 to 5 years.
- Cardiovascular disease mortality has declined.

III.   The Perimenopausal Transition
- Definition of the perimenopausal transition.
    - Menstrual irregularity defines and establishes the perimenopausal transition.
    - Menopause is the point in time when the permanent cessation of menstruation occurs.
    - The menstrual cycle length evolves over time.
        - Age 25: 40% of cycles are 25 to 28 days.
        - Age 25 to 35: 60% of cycles are 25 to 28 days.
        - An estimated 0.5% of women have cycles <21 days.
        - Roughly 0.9% of women have cycles >35 days.
        - About 20% experience irregular cycles (Fig. 17.4).
    - Anovulation is more prevalent in the 40s; cycles lengthen 2 to 8 years prior to menopause.
    - Follicular phase length is the major determinant of cycle length; elevated follicle-stimulating hormone (FSH), decreased inhibin, normal luteinizing hormone (LH), and slightly increased estradiol.
- Estradiol levels.

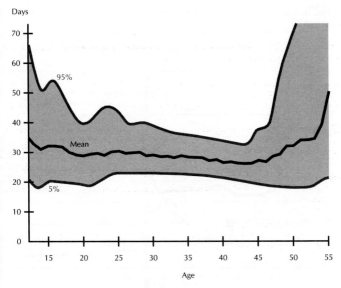

Figure 17.4.   The length of the menstrual cycle by age.

- • Contrary to previous belief, estradiol levels do not gradually wane.
- • They remain in the normal to slightly elevated range until 6 months to 1 year prior to cessation of follicular growth.
♦ Follicular atresia.
  - • Women experience from 2 to 8 years of increasingly prevalent anovulatory cycles.
  - • An accelerated rate of follicular loss occurs; it begins when 25,000 follicles remain.
  - • This correlates with a rise in FSH and a decline in inhibin levels.
    - ■ Inhibin B—follicular phase.
    - ■ Inhibin A—luteal phase.
  - • The loss of inhibin explains the inability of estrogen alone to suppress gonadotropins.
    - ■ Pregnancy can occur until both FSH and LH are elevated (FSH >20 and LH >30).
    - ■ The oldest reported spontaneous pregnancy was 57 years 120 days.
  - • Demographics of perimenopause.
    - ■ Age of onset is 46 years (95% confidence interval [CI], 39–51).
    - ■ Average duration is 5 years (95% CI, 2–8).
    - ■ Ten percent cease abruptly (Fig. 17.5).
♦ Preventive health screening.

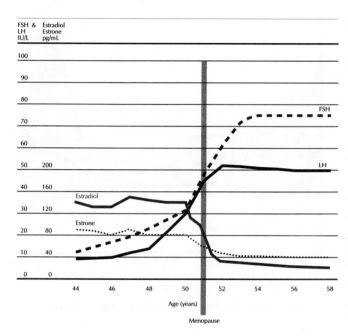

Figure 17.5. The perimenopausal transition and mean ciculating hormone levels.

- The three major goals of screening are as follows:
  1. To prolong the period of maximal physical energy.
  2. To detect the major chronic diseases early.
  3. To help the patient smoothly traverse the menopausal period of life.
- Suggested schedule.
  - Complete medical history and physical examination every 5 years, beginning at 40 years of age.
  - On annual visits, conduct breast/pelvic examination and Pap test, and screen for sexually transmitted diseases (STDs) as appropriate.
  - Assess thyrotropin (TSH) in the 40s and every 2 years after the age of 60.
  - Hemoccult after the age of 50 (yearly).
  - Annual screening mammogram starting at age 40.
- The age of menopause.
  - The median age is 51.3; 1% prior to age 40.
  - Smoking causes a shift to earlier menopause of 1.5 years.
  - Mothers and daughters have similar experiences.

- Earlier menopause is seen in undernourished patients and vegetarians.
- Later menopause occurs with alcohol consumption.
- It has no correlation with the age of menarche.
♦ Sexuality and menopause.
  - Fifty percent to 60% of women >50 years old are interested in sex or are sexually active.
    - Influenced most by culture and attitudes.
    - Most significant determinant—the unavailability of a partner.
  - Illness and sex.
    - Sexual problems are not limited to surgical procedures or genital illnesses.
    - Hysterectomy does not seem to have a detrimental impact.
    - Sexual counseling before and after surgery is often ignored.
    - Medications may also interfere with normal sexual experiences.

IV. Hormone Production after Menopause
  ♦ Shortly after menopause, no follicles remain.
    - Eventually, FSH increases 10 to 20×, and LH increases 3×.
    - Maximal rise occurs at 1 to 3 years after menopause.
  ♦ Postmenopausal ovary secretes primarily androstenedione and testosterone.
    - Most androstenedione is from the adrenal.
    - Dehydroepiandrosterone and dehydroepiandrosterone sulfate also decline markedly (70% and 74%, respectively).
  ♦ Testosterone production from the ovary increases, but the overall circulatory levels decline because of a lack of conversion of androstenedione to testosterone.
    - Testosterone that is decreased with gonadotropin-releasing hormone (GnRH) agonist therapy indicates an ovarian source (Tables 17.1 and 17.2).
    - The onset of mild hirsutism can occur because of the change in the androgen:estrogen ratio.
    - The extraglandular conversion of androgens represents the major source of estrogens.
      - This varies with body weight.
      - Sex hormone–binding globulin (SHBG) levels decrease with weight, allowing for greater free estrogen concentrations and an increased risk of endometrial cancer.
    - With increasing age, the adrenal contribution of precursors proves inadequate; the ovarian stroma becomes exhausted.
    - Symptoms of estrogen loss and decreasing follicular competence include the following:
      1. Disturbed menstrual pattern.
      2. Vasomotor instability.
      3. Atrophic conditions.
      4. Osteoporosis and cardiovascular disease.

Table 17.1. Blood production rates of steroids

	Reproductive age	Postmenopausal	Oophorectomized
Androstenedione	2 to 3 mg/d	0.5 to 1.5 mg/d	0.4 to 1.2 mg/d
Dehydroepiandrosterone	6 to 8 mg/d	1.5 to 4.0 mg/d	1.5 to 4.0 mg/d
Dehydroepiandrosterone sulfate	8 to 16 mg/d	4 to 9 mg/d	4 to 9 mg/d
Testosterone	0.2 to 0.25 mg/d	0.05 to 0.18 mg/d	0.02 to 0.12 mg/d
Estrogen	0.350 mg/d	0.045 mg/d	0.045 mg/d

**Table 17.2.   Changes in circulating
hormone levels at menopause**

	Premenopause	Postmenopause
Estradiol	40 to 400 pg/mL	10 to 20 pg/mL
Estrone	30 to 200 pg/mL	30 to 70 pg/mL
Testosterone	20 to 80 ng/dL	15 to 70 ng/dL
Androstenedione	60 to 300 ng/dL	30 to 150 ng/dL

V.   Problems of Estrogen Excess
   ♦   Exposure to unopposed estrogen.
   •   The greatest concern is neoplasia; the usual find-
        ing is nonneoplastic tissue.
   •   Four mechanisms that could result in increased
        endogenous estrogens are as follows:
        1.   Increased precursor androgen.
        2.   Increased aromatization.
        3.   Increased direct secretion (ovarian tissue).
        4.   Decreased levels of SHBG.
   •   Dysfunctional uterine bleeding requires evalua-
        tion.
        ■   Endometrial biopsy.
             ◊   Postmenopausal women with an ultra-
                  sound-measured endometrium <4 mm do
                  not require biopsy.
             ◊   Biopsy can be done in the office.
                  ○   Try without tenaculum.
                  ○   Curette in all directions.
                  ○   Consider a prostaglandin (PG) synthe-
                       sis inhibitor prior to biopsy.
             ◊   A biopsy is adequate in >90% of post-
                  menopausal patients; consider dilation
                  and curettage and/or hysteroscopy if the
                  uterus is NOT normal on examination.
        ■   Examine the vulva, vagina, and cervix.
        ■   Other procedures include the following:
             ◊   Colposcopy.
             ◊   Endocervical curettage.
             ◊   Hysterosalpingography, hysteroscopy, and
                  saline infusion sonography.
        ■   Persistent bleeding demands repeat evalua-
             tion.
        ■   Treat the cause.
             ◊   Progestin therapy for endometrial hyper-
                  plasia without atypia.
             ◊   Oral   contraceptives   in   nonsmoking
                  healthy premenopausal patient.
             ◊   Switch from low-dose oral contraceptive
                  pills to traditional hormone-replacement
                  therapy (HRT) when FSH is high on day
                  6 to 7 of pill-free week.

VI. The Impact of Postmenopausal Estrogen Deprivation
   ♦ Vasomotor symptoms—hot flush is the hallmark of female climacteric.
      • This is experienced by most women.
      • Duration varies from a few seconds to several minutes.
      • Frequency is from rare to recurrent.
      • It is more frequent and/or severe at night (Table 17.3).
      • The physiology is poorly understood; it seems to originate in the hypothalamus and is brought about by the decline in estrogen.
      • Document estrogen deficiency as the cause by the presence of elevated FSH levels.
      • Flushes are absent in hypogonadal women until estrogen is administered and subsequently withdrawn.
      • It coincides with an LH surge.
         ■ It is preceded by a subjective prodrome.
         ■ The body surface experiences an increase in temperature and changes in skin conductance, which are followed by a fall in core temperature.
      • Flushes persist after hypophysectomy.
      • Premenopausal causes include the following:
         ■ Psychoneurotic.
         ■ Stress.
         ■ Thyroid disease.
         ■ Pheochromocytoma.
         ■ Carcinoid.
         ■ Leukemia.
         ■ Cancer.
   ♦ Atrophic changes.
      • Genitourinary atrophy can affect the quality of life.
         ■ Urethritis.
         ■ Urgency incontinence.
         ■ Urinary frequency.

Table 17.3.   The hot flush

Premenopausal	10% to 25% of women
Postmenopausal:	
No flushes	15% to 25%
Daily flushing	15% to 20%
Duration	1 to 2 yr average; 5 plus yr., 25%
Other causes:	
Psychosomatic	
Stress	
Thyroid disease	
Pheochromocytoma	
Carcinoid	
Leukemia	
Cancer	

- Genuine stress urinary incontinence may or may not improve with estrogen.
- The full restoration of the genitourinary tract requires 6 to 12 months; sexual activity itself will aid in this effect.
- The decline in collagen content and skin thickness can be improved.

♦ Psychophysiologic effects.
- Depression is less common, not more common, among middle-aged women.
- Multiple studies show no link between menopause and depression.
- Studies are hampered by the subjectivity of complaints and the high placebo effect.
- Patients who seek medical assistance may not be representative of the population.
- Quality of sleep may be improved in patients with hot flushes by estrogen therapy.

♦ Cognition and Alzheimer disease.
- Evidence for beneficial effects on cognition can be found but may be of little clinical value; the Rancho Bernardo study failed to support a significant impact.
- Protection against Alzheimer disease may be from several mechanisms.
  - Protection against oxidation.
  - Reduces serum levels of amyloid P.
  - Increases synapses and neuronal growth—dendritic spine density.

VII. Cardiovascular Disease
- ♦ Diseases of the heart are the leading cause of death for U.S. women; the death rate is 3× greater than for breast or lung cancer.
- ♦ Most result from atherosclerosis in major vessels.
  - Risk factors.
    - Hypertension.
    - Smoking.
    - Diabetes.
    - Obesity.
  - Women have an advantage over men, but this decreases with advancing age.
- ♦ Etiology of cardiovascular disease.
  1. Adverse changes in circulating lipid–lipoprotein profile.
  2. Oxidation of low-density lipoprotein (LDL) that eventually results in trapped macrophages and endothelial cell injury.
  3. Endothelial cell injury affecting nitric oxide and prostacyclin production.
  4. Macrophage migration and function.
  5. Proliferation and migration of smooth muscle cells.
  6. Vasoconstriction and thrombogenic events.
  7. Remodeling of coronary arteries (Fig. 17.6).
     - Mechanism of gender-based protection.

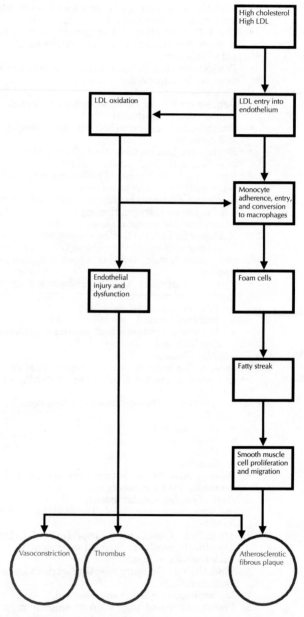

Figure 17.6. Mechanism of plaque formation in atherosclerosis.

Table 17.4. The optimal cholesterol lipoprotein profile

Total cholesterol	Less than 200 mg/dL
HDL cholesterol	Greater than 50 mg/dL
LDL cholesterol	Less than 130 mg/dL
Triglycerides	Less than 250 mg/dL

Abbreviations: HDL, high-density lipoprotein; LDL, low-density lipoprotein.

- Women have higher high-density lipoprotein (HDL) levels at all ages.
- Premenopausal women have lower total cholesterol and LDL levels.
♦ Cholesterol levels.
  • HDL cholesterol is the strongest predictor of heart disease in women.
    - A decrease of 10 mg/dL increases the risk by 40% to 50%.
    - Even if total and LDL levels are normal, treatment of patients with low HDL reduces their risk.
    - Women with very high HDL (>55 to 60 mg/dL) have no increased risk even in the presence of elevated total cholesterol.
  • Concern if HDL cholesterol is <50 mg/dL is appropriate (Table 17.4).
  • Triglycerides (TGs) represent an increased risk when associated with low HDL (i.e., TG >400 mg/dL and HDL <50 mg/dL).
  • TGs can be lowered by weight loss (Table 17.5).
♦ Determinants of blood lipid levels.
  • Diet: high in saturated fats and dietary cholesterol.
  • Excess caloric intake/obesity: ↓ HDL; ↑ total cholesterol, LDL cholesterol, and TGs.
  • Smoking: ↓ HDL cholesterol, ↓ estrogen, early menopause.
  • Genetic defects: only a small percentage.
  • Impaired fetal growth.
    - Perhaps, changes occur *in utero* that result in permanent adverse change.

Table 17.5. Heart disease risk based on cholesterol/HDL ratio

Lowest risk	Less than 2.5
Below average risk	2.5 to 3.7
Average risk	3.8 to 5.6
High risk	5.7 to 8.3
Dangerous	Greater than 8.3

Abbreviation: HDL, high-density lipoprotein.

- These also lead to insulin resistance and lower HDL levels.
  - Central fat distribution.
    - Truncal obesity.
    - Interplay with estrogens and insulin.
- ◆ The evidence for protection against cardiovascular disease.
  - Overwhelming support for a 50% reduced risk of coronary heart disease in estrogen users; "healthy user" effect has been examined, but benefit is still apparent.
  - Data on stroke more confusing but consistent with the possibility that hormone use decreases the severity of strokes and the incidence of fatal strokes.
  - No relationship between hypertension and post-menopausal therapy.
- ◆ Mechanisms of action. See Table 17.6 and Fig. 17.7.

Table 17.6.   Summary—estrogen and the cardiovascular system

The possible beneficial actions of estrogens on cardiovascular disease include all of the following. A study in mice lacking the estrogen receptor–α (ER-α) suggests that some (perhaps many or all) of these actions are mediated by the ER-β or by nongenomic actions of estrogen. ER-α and ER-β are both prevalent in coronary and aortic smooth muscle cells from monkeys. Only ER-β is expressed in umbilical vein endothelial cells.

1. A favorable impact on the circulating lipid and lipoprotein profile, especially a decrease in total cholesterol and LDL cholesterol and an increase in HDL cholesterol.
2. A direct antiatherosclerotic effect in arteries.
3. Augmentation of vasodilating and antiplatelet aggregation factors, specifically nitric oxide and prostacyclin (endothelium-dependent mechanisms).
4. Vasodilation by means of endothelium-independent mechanisms.
5. Direct inotropic actions on the heart and large blood vessels.
6. Improvement of peripheral glucose metabolism with a subsequent decrease in circulating insulin levels.
7. Antioxidant activity.
8. Favorable impact on fibrinolysis, at least partially mediated by endothelial nitric oxide and prostacyclin synthesis.
9. Inhibition of vascular smooth muscle growth and migration—intimal thickening.
10. Protection of endothelial cells from injury.
11. Inhibition of macrophage foam cell formation.
12. Reduced levels of angiotensin-converting enzyme and renin.
13. Reduction of P-selectin levels.
14. Reduction of homocysteine levels.

Abbreviations: HDL, high-density lipoprotein; LDL, low-density lipoprotein.

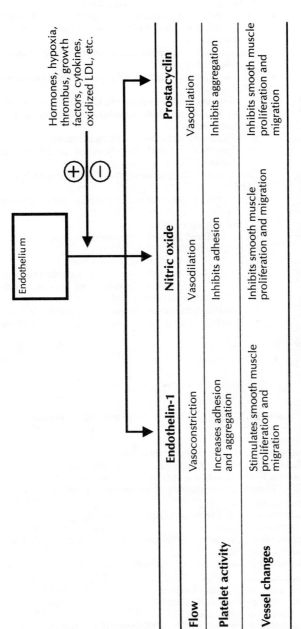

Figure 17.7. Formation of endothelial lesions and effects on blood flow, platelet activity, and vessel changes.

VIII. Cardiovascular Disease and Progestins
- ◆ Very much influenced by the progestin and the dose.
  - • No effect on lipids is seen with oral micronized progesterone.
  - • Continuous regimen also seems to maintain favorable profile.
- ◆ Postmenopausal Estrogen/Progestin Interventions (PEPI) trial.
  - • HDL levels were greatest in the unopposed estrogen group and the sequential estrogen oral micronized group.
  - • LDL levels were decreased in all groups.
  - • Favorable insulin was observed in all groups (Table 17.7).
- ◆ Heart and Estrogen/progestin Replacement Study (HERS).
  - • Increase in adverse cardiovascular events during the first year of use.
  - • Surprising results.
    - ▪ Differed from observational studies.
    - ▪ Explanation of the difference:
      1. Possibly a healthy user bias.
      2. May be that observational studies were in women without preexisting disease, which was not true in fact.
  - • Pretrial assumptions versus outcomes (Table 17.8).
  - • Possibility that continuous progestin could be worse.

IX. Osteoporosis
- ◆ Introduction.

Table 17.7.   Progestin effects on estrogen actions

Attenuation
1. Increase in HDL and triglyceride levels.
2. Measure of acute reactivity (e.g., acute vasodilation).
3. Cardiac inotropic activity; compliance responses.
4. Effect of estrogen on coronary atherosclerosis in the monkey.

No attenuation
1. Decrease in cholesterol and LDL.
2. Increase in fibrinolysis.
3. Inhibition of atherosclerosis (intimal thickening and remodeling).
4. Antioxidant activity.
5. Reduction in angiotensin-converting enzyme activity.

Uncertain
1. Reduction in hyperinsulinemia.
2. Favorable changes in P-selectin.
3. Protection of endothelial cells.
4. Inhibition of macrophage foam cell formation.

Abbreviations: HDL, high-density lipoprotein; LDL, low-density lipoprotein.

Table 17.8. Outcomes of the HERS trial

	Assumption	Actual
Clinical event rate in the placebo group	5%/yr	3.3%/yr
Dropout rate	5% in yr 1	18% in yr 1
Conversion of placebo to treatment rate	1%/yr	1.7%/yr
Average follow-up	4.75 yr	4.1 yr
Recruitment	Paced	Late

- Bone remodeling involves constant resorption (osteoclastic activity) and bone formation (osteoblastic activity).
  - Osteoblasts are derived from mesenchymal stem cells.
  - Osteoclasts are from hematopoietic white cell lineage.
- The amount of bone represents a balance.
- Responsiveness is governed by serum levels of calcium, parathyroid hormone (PTH) secretion, estrogen levels, and vitamin D levels.
- Osteoporosis—decreased bone mass with a normal ratio of mineral to matrix, leading to an increase in fractures; 20 million affected individuals in the United States.
- Osteopenia—low bone mass.
- Pathophysiology.
  - Characterized by a microarchitectural deterioration of bone tissue.
  - Results in increased fragility and an increase in fractures.
- Bone types.
  - Cortical bone.
    - Bone of the peripheral skeleton.
    - Responsible for 80% of bone mass.
  - Trabecular bone.
    - Bone of the axial skeleton; a honeycomb structure filled with red marrow.
    - Faster turnover in comparison to cortical bone.
- Fracture risk.
  - Depends on the following two features:
    1. Bone mass at the time of menopause.
    2. Rate of bone loss following menopause.
  - Almost all bone mass is acquired by late adolescence; after age 30, a slow decline occurs (0.7%/year).
  - Onset of spinal bone loss becomes important in menopause.
    - Loss of trabecular, 5% per year.
    - Loss of total bone mass, 1.5% per year.

- In the first 20 years after menopause:
    ◇ Reduction in trabecular bone, 50%.
    ◇ Reduction in cortical bone, 30%.
- ♦ Estrogen and bone remodeling.
    - Bone remodeling increases when estrogen declines.
    - Estrogen exerts a tonic suppression of remodeling.
        - It maintains the osteoclast:osteoblast balance.
        - In the absence of estrogen, osteoclast becomes dominant.
    - Mechanism of protection.
        - Increased efficiency of calcium absorption probably secondary to vitamin D.
        - Direct effect on osteoblasts.
        - Estrogenic effect on growth factors.
            ◇ Lowers interleukin (IL)-1, IL-6.
            ◇ Increases insulin-like growth factor I (IGF-I), IGF-II, and transforming growth factor–β.
            ◇ Increases vitamin D receptors.
        - No major effect on calcitropic hormones.
    - Estrogen is a critical hormone in both sexes.
        - Males who lack estrogen receptor–α or aromatase are characterized by the following.
            ◇ Slow growth.
            ◇ Markedly reduced bone density.
        - Optimal bone mass requires the presence of estrogen.
    - Other factors.
        - Race.
        - Weight.
        - Smoking.
        - Sedentary lifestyle.
        - Genetic predisposition.
            ◇ Twin studies → 70% of the variation in bone density is hereditary.
            ◇ Variations in vitamin D receptor gene.
            ◇ Collagen synthesis genes (COLIA1) (Fig. 17.8).
- ♦ Timing of bone loss and estrogen deficiency.
    - An estimated 75% of bone loss in first 15 years after menopause is attributable to estrogen deficiency.
    - Vertebral bone mass decreases in perimenopause.
    - Bone loss in radius is not evident until 1 year after menopause.
- ♦ Signs and symptoms.
    1. Spinal (vertebral) compression fractures.
        - Symptomatic spinal osteoporosis is 5× more common in white women than in men.
        - Approximately 50% of women over 65 years of age have spinal compression fractures; two-thirds are clinically unrecognized.
        - Each fracture is equal to a 1 cm of loss in height.
        - Most common sites are the 12th thoracic and the first three lumbars.

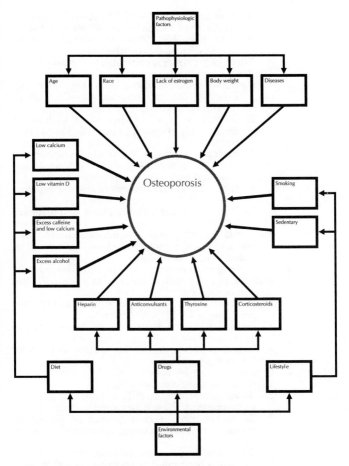

Figure 17.8.   Pathophysiologic and environmental factors contributing to osteoporosis.

2. Colles' fracture.
    - An increase of roughly 10× in white women as they age from 35 to 60 years.
    - Lifetime risk is 15%.
    - This is the most common fracture until the age of 75; then the hip fracture is more common.
3. Femoral head.
    - Incidence increases with age.
      - Age 45: 0.3/1000.
      - Age 85: 20/1000.
    - About 80% are associated with osteoporosis.

- Approximately 15% to 20% mortality is seen in the first 3 months; only 50% survive 1 year.
- This affects 300,000 women/year and is associated with 40,000 deaths/year.

4. Tooth loss is strongly correlated with osteoporosis.

♦ Diagnostic tests.
- Screen for other conditions, such as the following:
  1. Primary hyperparathyroidism—Ca^{+2}, PO_4^{-3}, alkaline phosphatase, and serum PTH.
  2. Secondary hyperparathyroidism with renal failure—blood urea nitrogen (BUN) and creatinine.
  3. Multiple myeloma, leukemia, lymphoma—blood count, peripheral smear, sedimentation rate, and protein electrophoresis.
  4. Hyperthyroidism, excessive thyroid replacement—TSH, and free thyroxin (T_4).
  5. Hypercortisolism, alcohol abuse, and metastatic cancer.
- Serum calcium, phosphorus, alkaline phosphatase, and 1,25-dihydroxyvitamin D levels are normal in osteoporosis (Table 17.9).

♦ Measuring bone density: 50% to 100% increase in fracture risk for each standard deviation (SD) decline in bone mass.
- Measurement in hip bone mass is an even better predictor → ↓ 1 SD = 3× ↑ in risk.
- Increases in bone density do not demonstrate a direct correlation with risk reduction.
- Bone loss at heel and radius accurately predicts future fracture risk.

♦ Reasons to measure bone mass.
1. To aid in decisions about HRT.
2. To assess response to HRT in high-risk patients (e.g., smokers, those with eating disorders).
3. To assess bone mass in women on long-term steroids, thyroid hormone, anticonvulsants, or heparin.
4. To confirm the diagnosis and to assess the severity.
5. To assess bone mass in postmenopausal women who present with fractures, who have more than one risk factor, or who are >65 years.

Table 17.9. Specific causes of bone disease

Drugs	Heparin, anticonvulsants, high intake of alcohol
Chronic disease	Renal and hepatic
Endocrine diseases	Excess glucocorticoids
	Hyperthyroidism
	Estrogen deficiency
	Hyperparathyroidism
Nutritional	Calcium, phosphorous, vitamin D deficiencies

- ◆ Measurements.
  - Single photon absorptiometry uses ^{125}I or miniature x-ray tubes.
  - Dual energy x-ray absorptiometry (DEXA) uses photons from two sources.
    - Good precision.
    - Radiation dose less than chest x-ray dose.
    - Can calculate lean body mass and fat.
  - High precision with DEXA.
    - Measure three sites: radius, hip, and spine.
    - For screening, measure at radius or calcaneus.
  - Quantitative computed tomography (CT).
    - Very accurate at spinal measurements.
    - Higher radiation dose.
    - Cannot measure femur.
  - Ultrasound of the calcaneus may be as accurate as femoral head DEXA measurements for predicting fracture risk.
  - Scoring system.
    - T score—standard deviation between patient and the average peak young adult; more negative = a greater fracture risk.
    - Z score—standard deviation between the patient and the population average for age/weight. A Z score lower than −2.0 requires evaluation for causes other than postmenopausal bone loss.
- ◆ Biochemical markers of bone turnover.
  - Bone formation—serum osteocalcin, total and bone alkaline phosphatase, and procollagen peptide.
  - Bone resorption—urinary calcium, hydroxyproline, pyridinoline and deoxypyridinoline crosslinking of collagen, telopeptides of collagen, and serum cross-linked telopeptides.
  - Markers correlate poorly with bone density but can be used to assess response to therapy.
- ◆ Treatment.
  - Estrogen.
    - Estrogen therapy will stabilize or prevent osteoporosis.
      - ◊ Inhibits osteoclasts.
      - ◊ Increases intestinal calcium absorption.
      - ◊ Increases 1,25-dihydroxyvitamin D.
      - ◊ Increases renal conservation of calcium.
      - ◊ Supports osteoblast survival.
    - Estrogen will result in a 50% to 60% decrease in fractures of the arm and hip and an 80% decrease in vertebral fractures when combined with calcium.
      - ◊ The benefit is seen primarily in women taking estrogen for >5 years.
      - ◊ Rapid bone loss follows the cessation of estrogen therapy.

- Estrogen use actually increases bone density; the PEPI study demonstrated a 5% gain in the spine and 2% in the hip.
- Any incremental increase in estrogen will exert a positive effect → levels as low as 10 pg/mL are better than <5 pg/mL; doses less than the standard 0.625 mg of conjugated equine estrogen or 1.00 mg of 17β-estradiol may be nearly as good.
- Synergistic benefit of progestin and estrogens may be limited to the 19-nortestosterone family.
- Addition of testosterone may not add any benefit.

- Selective estrogen receptor modulators (SERM).
  - Raloxifene—no proliferative effect on endometrium; favorable response on lipids and bone.
  - Favorable effects on the following:
    ◇ LDL cholesterol.
    ◇ Fibrinogen.
    ◇ α-Lipoprotein.
    ◇ Bone density.
  - No effect on HDL cholesterol and plasminogen activator inhibitor–1.
  - Multiple Outcomes of Raloxifene Evaluation (MORE) study demonstrated a 44% reduction in spinal fractures.
  - An option for the prevention of osteoporosis.
- Calcium.
  - In early menopause, calcium cannot abate the rapid bone loss phase; later in menopause, it can provide a positive impact.
  - Absorption decreases with age.
  - Supplementation helps maintain a positive balance.
    ◇ Regimen of 1,000 mg for women on estrogen.
    ◇ Increase to 1,500 mg for women not on estrogen.
  - Calcium is much more important during adolescence → 1,500 mg/day in women <25 years of age.
    ◇ Most efficient absorption occurs with single dose ≤500 mg that is taken with a meal.
    ◇ Calcium carbonate antacids = an excellent source.
- Vitamin D.
  - Age-related decrease in skin and kidney synthesis of 1,25-dihydroxyvitamin D is observed.
  - Also lowered intestinal absorption of vitamin D occurs.
  - People over 70 years of age should add 800 IU of vitamin D to calcium supplementation.
  - Women in cloudy winter areas should add 400 IU of vitamin D daily.
    ◇ High doses can cause stress.

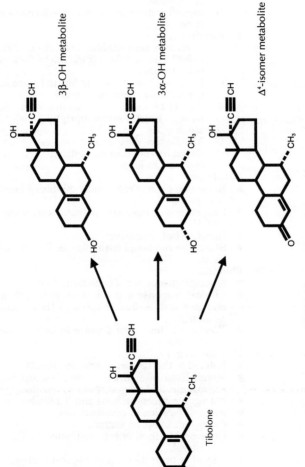

Figure 17.9.   The metabolization of tibolone into its three isomers.

- ◊ Serum levels can be measured.
- ◊ Less than 15 ng/L is abnormal.
- Biphosphonates.
  - Effective in preventing bone loss by inhibiting bone resorption; bind to bone mineral, making bone resistant to osteoclastic resorption.
    - ◊ First generation also inhibited bone mineralization.
    - ◊ Second generation allows bone formation to occur.
  - Alendronate.
    - ◊ Decreases nonvertebral fractures by 30% to 50% and vertebral fractures by 90% in first 3 years.
    - ◊ Increases bone density in hip and spine in normal postmenopausal women.
    - ◊ Should be taken on an empty stomach; patient must remain upright to avoid esophagitis.
    - ◊ An effective means to prevent osteoporosis but has no effect on cardiovascular disease and so forth.
- Calcitonin.
  - Regulates plasma calcium by inhibiting bone resorption.
  - Subcutaneous injection or intranasal spray (200 IU/day).
  - Effective but expensive.
  - Should be combined with vitamin D and calcium.
- Fluoride.
  - A potent stimulator of bone formation.
  - Clinical response dependent on formulation and dose; sodium fluoride, 25 mg BID for 12 to 14 months.
  - Treatment limited to 4 years to avoid toxic accumulation.
- Tibolone (Fig. 17.9).
  - Related to the 19-nortestosterone family.
  - Metabolized into three isomers: estrogenic, androgenic, and progestogenic properties.
  - Estrogenic effects on bone and hot flushes.
  - Nonproliferation in endometrium.
  - Estrogenic effect on vagina.
  - Unfavorable lipid effect—reduction in HDL cholesterol.
  - May offer protection against breast cancer.
  - May offer benefit on insulin resistance.
- Thiazides.
  - Reduced urinary calcium loss.
  - Synergistic effect with estrogen.
- Lifestyle.
  - Load-bearing physical activity.
  - Additive to hormone therapy.
  - Smoking cessation.
  - Limited exposure to steroids.

Postmenopausal Hormone-Replacement Therapy

I. Introduction
   - Treatment is suggested for all women disturbed by the symptoms of hormone deprivation.
   - Prophylaxis against osteoporosis and cardiovascular disease is advocated.

II. History
   - Use of ovarian extracts was first suggested by Charles Edouard Brown-Sequard in 1889.
   - 1897—Ovarian extract is reported to be effective for hot flushes.
   - 1923—Allen and Doisy report isolation of an "ovarian hormone" from pig ovaries.
   - 1926—Parkes and Bellerby coin the word "estrin" to designate the hormone that induces estrus.
   - 1929—Sevringhaus and Evans attempt to treat menopausal signs.
   - 1929—Doisy reports isolation of estrone from urine of pregnant women.
   - 1932—Girard isolates similar hormone from mare's urine.
   - 1934—Crystalline progestin isolated in ovaries from 50,000 pigs yields a few milligrams.
   - 1942—Conjugated estrogens (Premarin) are approved for use in the United States (Table 18.1).

III. Selection of Patients
   - Women under the age of 40.
     - Usually this represents surgically induced menopause or gonadal dysgenesis patients.
     - A daily dose of 0.625 mg conjugated estrogens is usually sufficient.
     - A sequential program is utilized.
     - Its implementation reduces vasomotor symptoms and provides long-term prophylaxis against cardiovascular disease, osteoporosis, and target organ atrophy.
     - Use an estrogen–progestin combination rather than estrogen alone in women with a history of endometriosis to avoid recurrence and development of endometrial cancer in endometriosis implants.
   - Perimenopausal transition years.
     - Vasomotor symptoms despite normal menses suggest thyroid or psychosocial etiology.
     - Bone loss in perimenopause is limited to those women with fluctuating hormonal and/or menstrual function.
   - Early postmenopause.
     - This is the appropriate time to discuss issues pertaining to hormone-replacement therapy (HRT).

Table 18.1.   Composition of conjugated estrogens (Premarin)

Sodium estrone sulfate	49.3%
Sodium equilin sulfate	22.4%
Sodium 17α-dihydroequilin sulfate	13.8%
Sodium 17α-estradiol sulfate	4.5%
Sodium Δ8,9-dehydroestrone sulfate	3.5%
Sodium equilenin sulfate	2.2%
Sodium 17β-dihydroequilin sulfate	1.7%
Sodium 17α-dihydroequilenin sulfate	1.2%
Sodium 17β-estradiol sulfate	0.9%
Sodium 17β-dihydroequilenin sulfate	0.5%

- Women are generally confident at this stage in life and are able to discuss these concerns.
♦ The late postmenopause.
  - Atrophic conditions can be treated.
  - Even very elderly women may benefit from HRT in regard to bone mass.
IV. Hormonal Agents (Table 18.2).
  ♦ Oral administration.
    - The 17α-ethinyl group appears to enhance hepatic effects; the liver is affected regardless of the route of administration.
    - The route of administration influences metabolic response only in the case of specific estrogens.
    - Different potencies depend upon the length of time that the estrogen receptor (ER) complex occupies the nucleus.
      ▪ Estriol has 20% to 30% affinity for the receptor when compared with estradiol.
      ▪ This can have an impact on the biologic response if the concentration is high enough.

Table 18.2.   Relative estrogen potencies

Estrogen	FSH Levels	Liver Proteins	Bone Density
Conjugated estrogens	1.0 mg	0.625 mg	0.625 mg
Micronized estradiol	1.0 mg	1.0 mg	1.0 mg
Estropipate (piperazine estrone sulfate)	1.0 mg	1.25 mg	1.25 mg
Ethinyl estradiol	5.0 μg	2 to 10 μg	5.0 μg
Estradiol valerate	—	—	1.0 mg
Esterified estrogens	—	—	0.625 mg
Transdermal estradiol	—	—	50 μg

Abbreviation: FSH, follicle-stimulating hormone.

- Esterified estrogens are prepared from plant pre-cursors.
  - Mainly sodium estrone sulfate.
  - Six percent to 15% sodium equilin sulfate.
- Estradiol valerate is hydrolyzed to estradiol.
- ◆ Transdermal administration.
  - The first patches contained an alcohol reservoir.
  - Current patches have hormone that is dissolved and distributed with adhesive.
    - Contact dermatitis is less common.
    - Doses: 50 μg, 100 μg.
  - The effect of steroids upon lipids is route-dependent.
    - Transdermal route may initially fail to provide cardiovascular protection.
    - Other studies show no difference with increased duration of use.
    - Perhaps sticking with the oral program is more prudent, given the epidemiologic data.
- ◆ Estradiol implants.
  - Pellets are available in 25-, 50-, and 75-mg doses for subcutaneous administration every 6 months.
  - A cumulative increase in blood levels is observed.
  - This requires the routine use of a progestational agent to protect the endometrium (14 days/month).
  - It has no advantage over oral administration.
  - Keep levels <200 pg/mL (preferably <100 pg/mL).
- ◆ Percutaneous estrogen.
  - Skin gel.
  - High, variable blood levels.
- ◆ The narrow therapeutic window.
  - The dose of estrogen is important in achieving maximal cardiovascular benefit.
    - Relatively normal levels are associated with better left ventricular function; very high levels are detrimental.
      - ◇ Lose insulin benefit.
      - ◇ Possible increase in arterial thrombosis.
    - Measuring levels in those women demanding ever-increasing doses is helpful; keep levels <200 pg/mL (preferably <100 pg/mL).
    - Lower doses may still provide benefit, but the lipid effects with 0.3 mg esterified estrogens may not differ from a placebo.
  - A daily dosage of 0.625 mg conjugated estrogens is needed for bone density.
    - Lower doses provide protection as well; estradiol levels as low as 10 pg/mL are better than those <5 pg/mL.
    - If the 0.3-mg dose is chosen, consider follow-up assessment with either bone density studies or urinary biochemical markers; consider a move up to standard dose after 1 year.
- ◆ Monitoring estrogen dosage with estradiol blood levels.
  - Clinical assays differ significantly.

- Highly specific assays for estradiol will detect only low levels at routine evaluation.
- A clinical assay would report 40 to 100 pg/mL.
- Follicle-stimulating hormone (FSH) levels are not helpful.
  - Only a 10% to 20% reduction in FSH and luteinizing hormone (LH) levels is produced.
  - Great variability in the response occurs.
- Sequential and continuous regimens.
  - Sequential.
    - Regimen of daily 0.625 mg conjugated estrogens with 14 days of 5 mg medroxyprogesterone acetate added each month.
    - Withdrawal bleeding in 80% to 90% of women.
    - Can cause breast tenderness, bloating, fluid retention, depression; switching to norethindrone may improve these complaints.

The sequential program for oral postmenopausal HRT

Daily estrogen:	0.625 mg conjugated estrogens or 1.25 mg estropipate or 1.0 mg micronized estradiol or equivalent doses of other estrogens
Monthly progestin:	5 mg medroxyprogesterone acetate or 0.7 mg norethindrone or 200 mg micronized progesterone or equivalent doses of other progestins given daily for 2 weeks every month

Combined with daily calcium supplementation (500 mg with a meal) and vitamin D (400 IU in winter months and 800 IU for women over age 70).

- Continuous regimen.
  - Allows use of lower progestin doses.
  - Improves compliance.
  - Roughly 80% of patients have amenorrhea; 40% to 60% have breakthrough bleeding for first 6 months.

The continuous combination program for oral postmenopausal HRT

Daily estrogen:	0.625 mg conjugated estrogens or 1.25 mg estropipate or 1.0 mg micronized estradiol or equivalent doses of other estrogens

Daily progestin: 0.35 mg norethindrone or 100 mg micronized progesterone or 2.5 mg medroxyprogesterone acetate or equivalent doses of other progestins

Combined with daily calcium supplementation (500 mg with a meal) and vitamin D (400 IU in winter months and 800 IU for women over age 70).

V. Managing Bleeding During Postmenopausal Hormone-Replacement Therapy
   ♦ Overview.
     • Breakthrough bleeding in patients on continuous therapy is the single most aggravating problem.
     • It originates from an endometrium that is dominated by progestational influence and that has decreased vascular strength and integrity.
     • Bleeding usually disappears with time.
     • No effective method of drug alteration or substitution has been proposed to manage the bleeding.
     • Options available include the following:
       ▪ Sequential therapy.
       ▪ Vaginal hysterectomy.
       ▪ Endometrial ablation.
       ▪ Progestin intrauterine device (IUD).
     • It is most likely to occur in those patients having recently entered the menopause.
   ♦ Endometrial biopsy.
     Indications for pretreatment biopsy
       Characteristics associated with a high risk of pathology
       Previous unopposed estrogen therapy
     Indications for endometrial biopsy during treatment
       Clinician anxiety
       Patient anxiety
       Treatment with unopposed estrogen
       Endometrial thickness greater than 4 mm
       History of unopposed estrogen therapy
     • No need to perform biopsy prior to therapy routinely; endometrial abnormalities in low-risk asymptomatic patients are rare.
     • High-risk patients.
       ▪ Obesity.
       ▪ History of dysfunctional uterine bleeding.
       ▪ Anovulation and infertility.
       ▪ High alcohol intake.
       ▪ Hepatic disease.
       ▪ Metabolic problems.
         ◊ Diabetes.
         ◊ Hypothyroidism.
       ▪ Unopposed estrogen therapy—biopsy annually.

- In the presence of persistent bleeding but normal biopsy, consider office hysteroscopy or saline infusion sonography.
- A day of bleeding on progestin therapy does not predict endometrial safety; another reason to consider the continuous regimen.

♦ Measurement of endometrial thickness by sonogram.
  - Correlates with presence or absence of pathology.
  - Less than 5 mm is reassuring; conservative management.
  - More than 4 mm in a bleeding patient requires biopsy; probably 50% to 75% of bleeding patients.
  - Assess thickness at the end of the progestin phase or at the beginning of the cycle.
  - Other options to evaluate are as follows:
    - Saline infusion sonography.
    - Hysteroscopy.

♦ Progestin challenge test.
  - The test was developed by R. Don Gambrell, Jr.; give 10 mg medroxyprogesterone acetate × 14 days.
  - Withdrawal bleeding in a postmenopausal patient not on HRT indicates the need for endometrial assessment.
  - Several studies support the efficacy and validity of this method.
  - Most patients with an abnormal endometrium will bleed.

VI. Progestational Side Effects

♦ Typical side effects.
  - Breast tenderness.
  - Bloating.
  - Depression.

♦ Placebo-controlled studies fail to demonstrate adverse physical and/or psychological effects.

♦ Less frequent administration.
  - Monthly estrogen–progestin sequential and daily continuous methods are proven.
  - Progestin every 3 months results in longer, heavier bleeding and a 1.5% incidence of hyperplasia after 1 year; the Scandinavian Long Cycle study was canceled after 3 years → 12% hyperplasia.
  - An annual endometrial biopsy is required if treatment deviates from the accepted practice.

♦ Use of norethindrone may reduce the side effects.
  - Dosage of 0.7 mg in sequential regimen.
  - Dosage of 0.35 mg in continuous combined.

♦ Use of progesterone vaginal gel.
  - Dosage of 90 mg every 2 days induces secretory changes, so this could be used in continuous regimen.
  - In sequential regimen, use daily × 10 days.
  - No long-term studies on safety are available (Table 18.3).

♦ Progestin IUD.
  - The levonorgestrel device is now reconfigured.

Table 18.3. Progestins available worldwide

	Estimated Comparable Doses
21-Carbon derivatives	
Medroxyprogesterone acetate	5.0 mg
Megestrol acetate	5.0 mg
Cyproterone acetate	1.0 mg
Dydrogesterone	10.0 mg
Chlormadinone acetate	
Medrogestone	
Demegestone	
Promegestone	
Trimegestone	
Nomegestrol acetate	
19-Nortestosterone family	
Norethindrone	0.7 mg
Norethindrone acetate	1.0 mg
Levonorgestrel	0.75 mg
Desogestrel	0.15 mg
Nomegestrol	
Norethynodrel	
Lynestrenol	
Ethynodiol diacetate	
Gestodene	
Norgestimate	
Dienogest	

- ■ Smaller model.
- ■ Releases 5 µg levonorgestrel per 24 hours.
- ■ Protects against hyperplasia/cancer.
- ■ Does not alter estrogen effects on lipids.
- ■ Breakthrough bleeding in the first 6 months; 60% to 70% amenorrhea after 1 year.
- ■ Good for 10 years.
- Progesterone-releasing device.
  - ■ Must be replaced every 18 months.
  - ■ Larger in size.
  - ■ Few studies in postmenopausal patients.
VII. Progestins in Women after Hysterectomy
  - ♦ Appropriate in a few cases as follows:
    1. Past history of endometriosis.
       - Avoids the development of adenocarcinoma.
       - Limits the growth of endometriosis.
    2. Patients who have had a supracervical hysterectomy or an endometrial ablation.
    3. History of stage I or II adenocarcinoma of the endometrium.
    4. History of an endometrial ovarian tumor.
    5. Women with or at risk for osteoporosis; benefit may be limited to norethindrone.
    6. Women with elevated triglycerides (TGs); norethindrone may attenuate a further increase.

VIII. The Addition of Androgens
  ♦ After menopause, androstenedione levels fall by 50%; most is derived from the adrenal.
  ♦ Testosterone levels do not fall.
    • The postmenopausal ovary secretes more testosterone than the premenopausal ovary.
    • Total testosterone production is lower due to decreased androstenedione.
  ♦ Potential benefits.
    • Psychological well-being.
    • Increase in sexually motivated behavior.
  ♦ Potential adverse effects.
    • Virilization—acne, alopecia, hirsutism.
    • Adverse lipid changes.
      ▪ Apparent within 3 months.
      ▪ Unknown clinical impact.
    • Possible aromatization to estrogen could increase the effective estrogen dose.
      ▪ Could also explain some studies demonstrating increased bone effect.
      ▪ Also, free estrogen levels possibly higher because of ↓ sex hormone–binding globulin.

IX. Selective Estrogen Agonists and Antagonists
  ♦ Raloxifene.
    • No proliferation effect on the endometrium.
    • Favorable effects on bone and lipids.
    • Possible reduction in breast cancer; could reflect the growth deceleration of a preexisting tumor.
    • Increases hot flushing.
    • Decreased vertebral fractures in Multiple Outcomes of Raloxifene Evaluation (MORE) study; a 44% reduction at 2 years.
    • Unknown effect on cardiovascular disease.
      ▪ Will likely be beneficial.
      ▪ Raloxifene Use for The Heart (RUTH) study was started in 1998.
    • A reported 3× ↑ in leg cramping.
    • An alternative therapy for osteoporosis prevention, not an estrogen substitute.

X. Hormone-Replacement Therapy and Fibroids
  ♦ Most studies indicate little effect on growth; high-dose progestin therapy may be an exception.
  ♦ Surveillance is a wise course.
  ♦ No increased risk of uterine sarcoma is observed.

XI. Other Medical Conditions
  ♦ Sleep apnea.
    • Increased frequency after menopause.
    • HRT: no significant impact.
  ♦ Rheumatic diseases.
    • No clear conclusion is evident.
      ▪ Some studies demonstrate a protective role.
      ▪ Others show no effect.
    • No aggravation of the disease is seen.
    • A small increase in systemic lupus erythematosus (SLE) development is possible.

- ■ Substantial cardiovascular benefit in SLE patients.
- ■ Reduced risk of osteoporosis in SLE patients on corticosteroids.
- ■ Okay in SLE patients with stable and/or inactive disease and no renal involvement or high antiphospholipid antibodies.
- ■ Good candidates for biphosphonate therapy; also for calcium and vitamin D supplementation.
- ◆ Osteoarthritis.
  - • Prevalence increases rapidly in women after menopause.
  - • Osteoporosis protects against arthritis.
  - • HRT has been associated with a worsening severity of osteoarthritis of the knee; possibly a reduced prevalence of osteoarthritis of the hip.
- ◆ Asthma.
  - • Estrogen may have an adverse effect; the clinical impact is unclear.
  - • Estrogen may increase the risk of developing adult-onset asthma; consider a continuous regimen in these patients.
- ◆ Oral health.
  - • Estrogen has several positive impacts.
    - ■ Relief from oral discomfort.
    - ■ Reduced gingival inflammation.
    - ■ Reduced tooth loss.
  - • Estrogen may instigate unwanted menopausal voice changes in professional singers.
- ◆ Vision.
  - • May improve visual acuity; reduced incidence of dry eyes.
  - • May protect against lens opacities.
  - • Lowers intraocular pressure in normal women and in those with glaucoma.
- ◆ Hearing loss—demineralization of the cochlear capsule correlates with femoral neck bone loss.

XII. Clinical Questions
- ◆ Should estrogen be used in very elderly patients?
  - • Clear evidence of positive impact on bone in women >65 years old; protects against hip fractures.
  - • Cardiovascular benefit uncertain.
  - • Impact on Alzheimer disease possibly important.
  - • When starting an older patient on estrogen, begin with low doses to avoid side effects (especially breast tenderness).
    - ■ Dosage of 0.3 mg conjugated estrogen.
    - ■ Dosage of 0.5 mg estradiol.
    - ■ Transdermal low dose.
  - • Increase dose after 6 months.
- ◆ How long should treatment be continued?
  - • A woman should continue as long as she wants the benefits.
  - • Cardiovascular benefit is probably lost after 5 years.

♦ Can diet produce variations in estrogen levels? Oral estrogens have an extensive first-pass metabolism.
  • Sulfation and hydroxylation can be inhibited by antioxidants.
  • Flavanoids can produce an increase in bioavailability.
  • Taking HRT at bedtime is probably best.
  • Alcohol may raise the circulating levels of estrogen.

XIII.   Alternative Treatments for Hot Flushes

♦ Clonidine.
  • Taken transdermally, 100 μg weekly; minimal side effects and modest impact.
  • Oral clonidine, bromocriptine, and naloxone are not effective and require a high dose.

♦ Belladonna–Ergotamine–Phenobarbital (Bellergal).
  • Slightly better than a placebo.
  • Very sedating.

♦ Veralipride.
  • Dopamine antagonist.
  • Dosage of 100 mg/day.
  • Relatively effective.
  • Side effects.
    ■ Mastodynia.
    ■ Galactorrhea.

♦ Progestins.
  • Medroxyprogesterone acetate, 10 to 20 mg/day.
  • Megestrol (Megace), 20 mg BID.
  • May be an unwise choice in patients with a history of breast cancer.

♦ Methyldopa.
  • Dosage of 500 to 1,000 mg/day is twice as effective as a placebo.
  • Its effectiveness suggests the role of adrenoreceptors in the hot flush mechanism.

♦ Venlafaxine hydrochloride.
  • Serotonin reuptake inhibitor.
  • Effectively reduces hot flushes at 25-mg dose.

♦ Tibolone.
  • Steroid related to the 19-nortestosterone family.
  • Effective at dose of 2.5 mg/day.
  • Metabolized into three isomers.
    ■ Provides estrogenic activity on bone and hot flushes.
    ■ Induces endometrial atrophy.
    ■ Increases sexual enjoyment and libido.
  • Long-term impact on cardiovascular disease unknown.
  • Short-term benefit to diabetics.
  • Could potentially have beneficial impact on breast cancer.

♦ "Natural" therapies.
  • Dosage and purity are unknown.
  • No substantial studies document either harmful or beneficial effects.

- Herbs can be contaminated with heavy metals.
- ◆ Phytoestrogens.
  - The three groups are isoflavones, coumestans, and lignans.
  - They are present in many plants.
  - They bind to the ER.
  - They have a mixed estrogenic and antiestrogenic effect, depending on the tissue; also soy phyto-estrogens have a greater affinity for ER-β.
  - Monkey studies demonstrate favorable lipid, atherosclerosis effects, and vasomotor effects.
  - Human clinical trials are inconsistent with regard to the lipid effect.
  - Dietary soy reduces hot flushes in women.
    - Significant variability in response.
    - May displace estradiol, producing a benefit with regard to estrogen-sensitive cancer.
  - However, appropriate clinical studies do not exist.
    - Dose unknown (most use 60 mg/day).
    - Efficacy.
    - Safety.
  - Synthetic product—ipriflavone is similar to naturally occurring isoflavones; it prevents postmeno-pausal bone loss.
- ◆ Dehydroepiandrosterone (DHEA).
  - Androgen production decreases with aging; the mechanism is unknown.
  - An approximate 75% to 85% decline in circulating DHEA is seen.
  - Short-term studies indicate an adverse effect on lipids.
  - Must await further clinical trials.
- XIV. Problems of Estrogen–Progestin Therapy
  - ◆ Metabolic.
    - Contraindications.
      - Chronically impaired liver function.
      - Acute vascular thrombosis.
      - Neurophthalmologic vascular disease.
      - Seizure disorders.
      - Familial hyperlipidemia (TGs).
      - Migraine headaches.
    - Pancreatitis and severe hypertriglyceridemia can be precipitated by oral estrogen.
      - Use great caution if TGs are 250 to 750 mg/dL; a nonoral route is preferred.
      - Repeat in 2 to 4 weeks to check levels.
      - A level >750 mg/dL is an ABSOLUTE CONTRAINDICATION.
      - Consider daily continuous combined therapy to mitigate the effect of estrogen; consider 19-nortestosterone progestin.
    - Gallbladder disease is increased, but the overall impact is not great (relative risk [RR] 1.5–2.0).
    - Monitor based upon symptoms.

- New oral routes may offer no improvement.
- Weight gain.
  - Menopausal weight gain is not due to hormonal changes.
  - No changes in the Rancho Bernardo or Postmenopausal Estrogen/Progestin Intervention (PEPI) trial were seen.
  - Estrogen prevents central body fat deposition.
- Venous thrombosis.
  - The conventional wisdom was that HRT did not increase the risk; this was recently challenged by one cohort and four case-control studies.
  - The risk is confined to early use.
    - This lowers to a nonsignificant level after 1 year.
    - The addition of progestin did not alter the risk.
  - HRT has a favorable impact in fibrinolysis; it may result in arterial thrombogenic benefit.
  - Heart and Estrogen/progestin Replacement Study (HERS) represents the clinching argument, a 2.89 RR of venous thrombosis.
  - What should be done?
    - Do not change in women currently on HRT.
    - The actual risk is very low.
      - ◇ One case per 5000 woman-years of use; ↑ threefold over the baseline.
      - ◇ Low mortality risk (1%); most are associated with trauma, surgery, or major illness.
    - However, if the patient has a family history of idiopathic thromboembolism, evaluate as below and consult a hematologist.

Hypercoaguable Conditions	Thrombophilia Screening
Antithrombin III deficiency	Antithrombin III
Protein C deficiency	Protein C
Protein S deficiency	Protein S
Factor V Leiden mutation	Activated protein C resistance ratio
Prothrombin gene mutation	Activated partial thromboplastin time (PTT)
Antiphospholipid syndrome	Hexagonal activated PTT
	Anticardiolipin antibodies
	Lupus anticoagulant
	Fibrinogen
	Prothrombin G mutation (DNA test)
	Thrombin time
	Homocysteine level
	Complete blood cell count

- ■ Consider prophylactic anticoagulant therapy in a patient on hormones who is anticipating immobility with hospitalization, or discontinue therapy 4 weeks prior to major surgery.
- ◆ Endometrial neoplasia.
  - • Two different types of endometrial cancer occur as follows:
    1. Papillary serous—20%.
       - ◊ Develops in atrophic endometrium.
       - ◊ Behaves like ovarian cancer.
    2. Endometrioid—80%.
       - ◊ Develops slowly from precursor lesion.
       - ◊ Less aggressive and better differentiated.
  - • Unopposed estrogen will cause progression.
    - ■ One year → 20% hyperplasia.
    - ■ Three years → 30% adenomatous or atypical hyperplasia (PEPI data).
    - ■ Roughly 10% of complex hyperplasia → cancer.
    - ■ Approximately 25% of complex hyperplasia with atypia → cancer.
  - • The risk of developing endometrial cancer with unopposed estrogen is as follows:
    - ■ Estimated 2 to 10× increase.
    - ■ Increased risk with increased duration of exposure and dose.
    - ■ Lingers for 10 years.
    - ■ Increased risk of extrauterine spread.
    - ■ Unopposed use of 0.3 mg—requires annual surveillance.
  - • Progestin therapy reduces the risk.
    - ■ Reduces cellular ERs.
    - ■ Induces the conversion of estradiol to estrone.
    - ■ Increased retention of receptor complexes in the nucleus.
    - ■ Suppression of estrogen-mediated oncogene transcription.
    - ■ Duration of exposure critical.
      - ◊ Ten days minimal; 2% to 3% hyperplasia.
      - ◊ Twelve to 14 days preferred by most.
    - ■ Extended period of prior exposure to unopposed estrogen will mitigate protective benefit; close surveillance needed in high risk patients.
    - ■ Dose required.
      - ◊ Sequential—5 to 10 mg medroxyprogesterone acetate; combined—2.5 mg.
      - ◊ Sequential—0.7 mg norethindrone; combined—0.35 mg.
- ◆ Ovarian cancer.
  - • Individual studies have been hampered by small numbers.
  - • Metaanalysis suggests an increase in "ever users" of HRT.
  - • Larger case-control study found no association.
  - • No detrimental impact on patients taking HRT after surgery for ovarian cancer has been noted.

- ◆ Cervical cancer.
  - • No adverse effect.
  - • Possible protection but may represent detection bias.
- ◆ Colorectal cancer.
  - • Most but not all studies note a significantly reduced risk.
    - ■ Greatest in current users.
    - ■ Also reduces risk of polyps.
  - • The mechanism is uncertain.
    - ■ Possibly bile changes.
    - ■ May be mucosal cell growth alterations.
- ◆ Malignant melanoma.
  - • No associated risk.
  - • Same as for oral contraceptive pills (OCPs).
- ◆ Breast cancer and HRT.
  - • Some of the problems include the following:
    - ■ One-eighth of women will develop breast cancer in their lifetime (among 85-year life expectancy).
    - ■ This represents the leading type of cancer in U.S. women (29%).
    - ■ It is second to lung cancer as the leading cause of cancer death (16%).
    - ■ Sufficient evidence exists to indicate a slightly increased risk associated with 25 years of postmenopausal estrogen use; the data are neither consistent nor uniform.
  - • Nurses Health study.
    - ■ The study had a sixteen-year follow-up.
    - ■ It examined a total of 1,935 cases of breast cancer.
    - ■ RR for current users is 1.46 (confidence interval [CI], 1.22–1.74) for 5 to 9 years.
    - ■ RR for current users is 1.46 (CI, 1.20–1.76) for >10 years.
    - ■ Some issues about the compounding variables are as follows:
      - ◊ Detection bias? Current users had 14% more mammograms.
      - ◊ Differences between current versus "never users."
        - ○ Benign breast disease.
        - ○ Number of births.
        - ○ Menarche.
        - ○ Body mass index (BMI).
        - ○ Alcohol consumption.
    - ■ Risk of dying was as follows:
      - ◊ Past users—0.80 (CI, 0.6–1.07).
      - ◊ Current users <5 years—0.99 (CI, 0.66–1.48).
      - ◊ Current users ≥ 5 years—1.45 (CI, 1.01–2.09).
    - ■ Could the "never users" be dying of cardiovascular disease?

♦ Metaanalyses.
  • Heterogeneic studies.
    ■ Different doses.
    ■ Different methods of diagnosis.
    ■ Different comparison and central groups.
  • Collaborative Group study (*Lancet*, 1997).
    ■ Fifty-one studies in a combined reanalysis.
    ■ Conclusions are as follows:
      1. "Ever users" had an overall increased RR of breast cancer of 1.14.
      2. Current users ≥5 years had a RR of 1.35 (CI, 1.21–1.49); increased risk with duration.
      3. Current and recent users had evidence of only localized decrease; no metastasis.
      4. No effect of a family history was seen.
      5. No increase in RR was observed in past users.
      6. The increase in RR was greatest in women with lower body weights.
    ■ The issue of localized disease suggests a detection and surveillance bias; it explains increased survival rates for those with breast cancer diagnosed on HRT.
♦ Why has no definitive answer been found despite 50 studies? A large impact is relatively easy to demonstrate with observational studies, but in this situation possible explanations are as follows:
  1. The inability to overcome recognized and unrecognized biases unless the effect is large; ergo, the effect is unlikely to be great.
  2. Heterogeneity of doses, schedules, study design, controls, geographic locations, populations, and drugs.
  3. Metaanalysis was developed to compare small randomized trials.
     • It has been extended to contradictory observational studies; this is where metaanalysis is weakest.
     • Even when used correctly, it may be incorrect by 35% when predicting the outcome of large randomized trials.
     • Metaanalysis has not overcome the problem of statistical power.
     • Metaanalysis of observational studies is not free of selection bias, detection bias, or subgroup overanalysis.
     • Metaanalysis does not correct for heterogeneity and design flaws.
XV. Where Does All This Leave Us?
  ♦ The lack of agreement indicates that the use of HRT cannot be associated with a major impact on the risk of breast cancer.
  ♦ The answer may lie in the Women's Health Initiative and the U.K. Women's International Study of long-

Duration Oestrogen use after Menopause (WISDOM) trial.

- ♦ Wouldn't an increased risk of breast cancer be expected to translate into an increase in mortality?
  - The Leisure World study showed a 19% reduction.
  - A similar reduction was seen in the Nurses Health study and the American Cancer Society cohort.
- ♦ The appropriate approach is to emphasize the benefits of HRT and to point out the continuing concerns about breast cancer.
- ♦ Estrogen–progestin therapy and breast cancer.
  - Obvious need exists to protect from endometrial hyperplasia.
  - Current information suggests a neutral effect.

XVI. Summary: Hormone-Replacement Therapy and Breast Cancer
1. Some case-control and cohort studies conclude that ≥5 years of HRT (current users) is associated with a slight increased risk.
   - ♦ The magnitude is lower than is the risk associated with obesity or alcohol consumption.
   - ♦ This may be due to confounding biases, particularly detection and/or surveillance bias and growth of a preexisting malignancy.
2. Many observational studies have failed to develop much evidence.
3. All studies have failed to find an increased risk associated with short-term (<5 years) or past use.
4. The addition of a progestin has no effect.
5. A family history of breast cancer should not be a contraindication.
6. Women who develop breast cancer while on HRT have a reduced risk of dying from breast cancer.

XVII. Contraindications to Hormone-Replacement Therapy
- ♦ Endometrial cancer, endometrial tumors, and endometriosis.
  - HRT can be used in women with stage I or II endometrial cancer.
    - ■ Uncertain in more advanced disease.
    - ■ Immediate use in ER-negative and progesterone receptor (PR)-negative tumors.
    - ■ Delay use for 5 years in women with high-risk ER-positive tumors.
    - ■ Combined therapy appropriate.
  - Combined therapy is also appropriate for patients with endometriosis or an endometrial tumor.
- ♦ Previous breast cancer and HRT.
  - We currently have no data.
  - The status of axillary nodes is most predictive.
    - ■ Ten years out.
      - ◊ Only 25% with positive nodes are disease-free.
      - ◊ Seventy-five percent of patients with negative nodes are disease-free.

- ■ With more than three nodes positive, the 10-year survival rate is 13%.
- Breast cancer is never viewed as occultly metastatic at time of presentation.
- Is estrogen or progesterone the more important hormonal influence?
- ◆ Estrogen.
  - Korenman proposed the "estrogen window" hypothesis.
  - The open window influences susceptibility to carcinogens; the window is closed by exposure to progesterone.
  - Obesity, anovulation, early menarche, and late menopause would all maintain the estrogen window.
- ◆ Progesterone.
  - Breast mitotic activity is higher in the luteal phase.
  - However, progestins inhibit growth and stimulate differentiation in human breast cancer cell lines.
- ◆ Pregnancy and breast cancer.
  - No difference in survival.
  - Higher risk of metastatic disease; a delay in diagnosis.
  - Termination of pregnancy is not associated with improved survival.
  - Most tumors are receptor-negative.
  - Acceleration of tumor growth possibly from a concurrent or recent (3 to 4 years previously) pregnancy.
- ◆ Breast cancer and subsequent pregnancy.
  - No negative impact on prognosis is seen.
  - However, cell studies are retrospective with small numbers.
- ◆ OCPs and breast cancer—no definitive evidence of increased or decreased risk.
- ◆ Medroxyprogesterone acetate (Depo-Provera) and breast cancer.
  - Very slight increase in the first 4 years of use; no evidence for increased risk with an increased duration of use.
  - Confounding variables present.
  - Suggests pharmacologic doses of progestin are not a risk factor.
- ◆ HRT and recurrent breast cancer.
  - Estrogen deficiency symptoms are the most common complaints associated with the treatment of breast cancer.
  - Several small studies are reassuring. This could represent biases in clinician and patient decision-making.
  - An estimated 50% to 70% of women diagnosed with breast cancer are now cured.
  - At this time, the risks of HRT without treatment for breast cancer are unknown.

♦ Women with cardiovascular disease.
  • Previous history of a cardiovascular event would seem to be an indication for HRT; this is supported by several studies.
    ▪ Leisure World study—50% mortality reduction.
    ▪ Lipids Research Clinics study—85% mortality reduction.
    ▪ Improves survival in severe coronary artery disease.
    ▪ Reduces restenosis following angioplasty.
    ▪ Better survival after coronary artery bypass graft.
    ▪ Reduced intestinal thickening.
  • The HERS study raised significant concerns.
    ▪ Doses >0.625 mg may be problematic.
    ▪ Progestins other than medroxyprogesterone acetate may be preferred.
♦ Women with diabetes.
  • Estrogen has been shown to improve all glucose metabolic parameters in women with non–insulin-dependent diabetes mellitus.
  • Tibolone also has a beneficial impact.
♦ Women with liver disease.
  • These patients are at risk for osteoporosis.
  • Evaluate after 1 month and then every 6 months.
♦ Vaginal estrogen.
  • Estrogen is rapidly absorbed with relatively high circulatory levels; this is especially true with atrophic mucosa.
  • Absorption decreases with cornification; it takes 3 to 4 months.
  • The vaginal ring releases minute doses of estrogen that have a low level of systemic absorption.
XVIII. Other Medical Conditions
  ♦ Close observation for the following patients:
    • Seizure disorders.
    • Familial hyperlipidemia ($\uparrow$ TGs).
    • Migraine headaches; consider continuous combined regimen to avoid menstrual migraine.
    • The following conditions that are not contraindications:
      ▪ Controlled hypertension.
      ▪ Diabetes.
      ▪ Smoking.
      ▪ Varicose veins.
      ▪ Cervical, vulvar, and ovarian malignancies.

19

Obesity

I. Introduction
- Twenty-five percent of U.S. women are overweight (Fig. 19.1).
- Twenty-five percent of U.S. women are obese.
- Obesity has been increasing in the United States and Europe over the past 100 years.
- A clear relationship exists between mortality and weight.
  - An estimated 23% of all deaths in nonsmoking middle-aged women are attributable to being overweight.
  - These women have an increased frequency of the following:
    - Hypertension.
    - Heart disease.
    - Non–insulin-dependent diabetes mellitus.
    - Gout.
    - Gallbladder disease.
    - Colorectal cancer.
    - Endometrial cancer.
    - Postmenopausal breast cancer.
    - Osteoarthritis.
- Modern studies of obesity suggest it is a multifactorial problem.

II. Definition
- Obesity is an excess storage of triglycerides (TGs) in adipose cells.
- Overweight refers to a body weight in excess of some standard or ideal weight.
- Ideal weight.
  - Women: 100 lb + (4 × [height in inches minus 60]).
  - Men: 120 lb + (4 × [height in inches minus 60]).
- At a weight close to the ideal, an individual may be overweight but not overfat.
- The most accurate means of measuring body fat is hydrodensitometry.
  - This is not practical, so skinfold measurements are utilized.
  - The body mass nomogram corresponds closely to densitometry measurements.
- Body mass index (BMI).
  - BMI = kg/m^2.
  - Overweight: BMI = 25 to 29.9.
  - Obesity: BMI = 30 and higher.
- Women versus men.
  - Women have greater prevalence of obesity.
    - Possibly due to a lower metabolic rate.
    - The metabolic rate declines with age.
  - Middle-aged spread is both a biologic and a psycho-sociologic phenomenon.

Percent of population

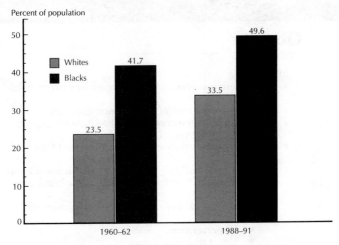

Figure 19.1. The percentage of overweight women in the United States.

III. Physiology of Adipose Tissue
- Adipose tissue serves three general functions as follows:
  1. Storehouse of energy.
  2. Cushion from trauma.
  3. Regulation of body heat.
- Energy storage.
  - Eight calories per gram of TG versus 1 cal/g of glycogen; total tissue store of carbohydrates (300 cal) is inadequate for between-meal energy demands.
  - Mechanism for energy mobilization from fat involves enzymes and neurohormonal agents.
    Fat is ingested,
    ↓
    broken down by gastric and pancreatic lipases,
    ↓
    absorbed in the small bowel.
    ↓
    Chylomicrons are transferred via the lymph into venous circulation,
    ↓
    removed by hepatic parenchymal cells, where new lipoprotein is released into circulation.
    ↓
    Lipoprotein is exposed to adipose tissue,
    ↓
    lipolysis occurs via lipoprotein lipase,
    ↓
    fatty acids are released and enter fat cells and are reesterified into TGs.

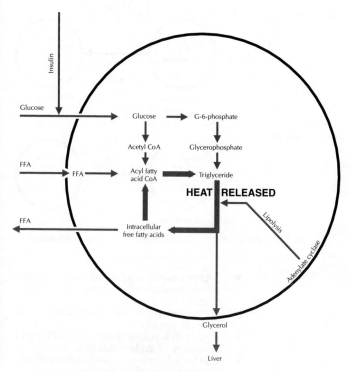

Figure 19.2.   The mechanism for releasing energy from fat.

- ♦ Glucose function.
  1. Supplies carbon atoms in the form of acetyl CoA.
  2. Provides hydrogen for reductive steps.
  3. Main source of glycerophosphate.
     - Required for reesterification of fatty acids → rate-limiting step in lipogenesis (Fig. 19.2).
     - Free fatty acids released by lipolysis.
       - ▪ This varies by anatomic site; omental, mesenteric, and subcutaneous fat is more labile.
       - ▪ Lipase is stimulated by the following:
         - ◊ Epinephrine and norepinephrine.
         - ◊ Adrenocorticotropic hormone (ACTH).
         - ◊ Thyrotropin (TSH).
         - ◊ Growth hormone.
         - ◊ Thyroxin (T_4).
         - ◊ 3,5,3'-Triiodothyronine (T_3).
         - ◊ Cortisol.
         - ◊ Glucagon.
         - ◊ Vasopressin.
         - ◊ Human placental lactogen.

Glucose abundant

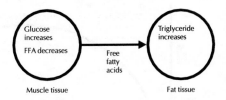

Glucose reduced

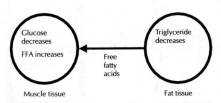

Figure 19.3. Effect of glucose concentrations on fat production.

- Lipase activity is inhibited by insulin; has a relationship with glycose availability (Fig. 19.3).
- If glucose is available → insulin is created → fat is stored.
- If glucose is scarce (starvation) → insulin decreases → fat is mobilized.
- The body learns to convert carbohydrates to fat quickly; therefore, fewer meals → more obesity.

IV. Clinical Obesity
- Leptin and the OB gene (Lep gene in humans).
  - Rat experiments placed the satiety center at the ventromedial hypothalamus; this is actually due to the nearby ventral noradrenergic bundle.
  - Signals arrive at the central nervous system (CNS) centers from the periphery.
    - Opiates.
    - Substance P.
    - Cholecystokinin.
    - Corticotropin-releasing hormone (CRH).
    - Neurotensin.
    - Cyclo (HisPro) → derived from thyrotropin-releasing hormone.
- Leptin.
  - A 167-amino acid peptide secreted in adipose tissue.
  - Acts on CNS neurons that regulate eating behavior and energy balance.
  - OB gene identified in women in 1994.
- Mouse mutations (Table 19.1).
  - The OB/OB mutation was spontaneous in 1949 in Jackson Laboratory mouse colony.

Table 19.1. Genetic rodent models of obesity

	Single Gene Mutations	Gene Product	Rodent Chromosome	Human Chromosome
Mice	ob/ob	Leptin	6	7
	db/db	Leptin receptor	4	1
	fat/fat	Carboxypeptidase E	8	11
	tub/tub	Phosphodiesterase	7	4
	Ay/Ay	Agouti protein	2	20
Rats	fa/fa	Leptin receptor	5	1

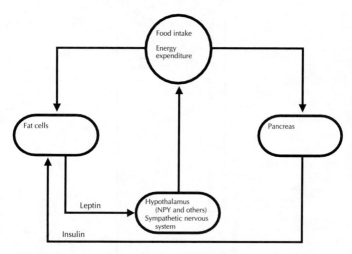

Figure 19.4.   The physiologic feedback loop for energy expenditure and food intake.

- A DB/DB mouse was discovered in 1966—leptin receptor mutation.
♦ Leptin receptor.
  - Belongs to the cytokine receptor family.
  - Two major forms as follows:
    1. OB-RS (short).
    2. OB-RL (long) → likely the signaling receptor.
  - Mode of action.
    ■ The proteins phosphorylate the receptor after binding.
      ◊ The signal transducer and activator of transcription (STAT) proteins are activated after receptor phosphorylation.
      ◊ They translocate to the nucleus.
      ◊ Gene transcription is stimulated.
    ■ DB mutation converts the long form to the short form.
      ◊ Single G for T substitution.
      ◊ Creates new splice site.
      ◊ Truncates intracellular domain.
♦ Physiologic feedback loop.
  - Leptin induces weight loss via decreased appetite and increased activity and heat production; this decreases neuropeptide Y (NPY) (Fig. 19.4).
  - The AY/AY rodent becomes obese late in life.
    ■ Gene knockout ultimately leads to high NPY via blockage of melanocyte action.
    ■ The importance of this pathway is evident in proopiomelanocortin mutations.
    ■ It is deficient in melanocyte-stimulating hormone and ACTH (Fig. 19.5).

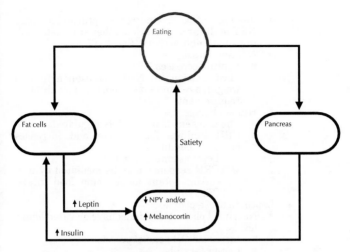

Figure 19.5. The effect of eating on the physiologic feedback loop.

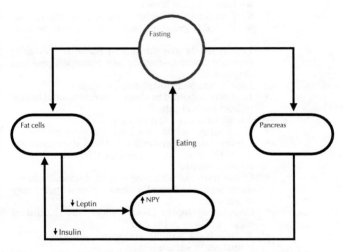

Figure 19.6. The effect of fasting on the physiologic feedback loop.

- Fasting and exercise decrease leptin and increase NPY in the arcuate nucleus; they stimulate feeding and inhibit activity (Fig. 19.6).
- Normal mice.
  - Leptin decreases NPY.
  - Mice deficient in NPY maintain a normal weight; a redundant system is not an absolute requirement.
- Human beings.
  - The Lep gene is not acutely regulated.
  - CRH inhibits food intake and increases energy expenditure.
    - ◇ Leptin stimulates CRH.
    - ◇ CRH response may be mediated by urocortin; potent at reducing food intake (Fig. 19.7).

♦ Leptin in obese people.
  - Nearly all obese individuals have elevated leptin levels.
    - Increased OB gene expression.
    - Larger fat cells.
  - In women, leptin levels increase 3× more rapidly with increases in weight; this suggests greater leptin resistance.
  - In black women, obesity is more common.
    - Lower leptin levels.
    - Correlates with a lower resting metabolic rate.
    - Probably greater sensitivity to leptin mechanism.
  - Leptin levels are normal in obese individuals; possibly leptin resistance or a transport problem (Fig. 19.8).
  - Leptin receptor mutations are rare.
  - Leptin is unbound in obese individuals and bound in lean individuals.

♦ Why is weight loss hard to maintain?
  - The average adult eats 1 million cal/year.
  - Leptin-defective individuals could store more fat when life was tougher, but they became obese in times of plenty.
  - Obese patients who lose weight demonstrate reduced leptin and insulin; their leptin set point may be altered.
  - Circulatory leptin levels reflect the amount of adipose tissue in the body.
  - A 10% body weight reduction induces a 53% reduction in serum leptin.
  - The basal metabolic rate falls when caloric intake falls, which makes maintenance of weight loss difficult.

♦ Congenital leptin deficiency—mutation of the Lep gene plus leptin receptor—is rare.

♦ Leptin and reproduction.
  - Several lines of evidence suggest a role in reproduction as follows:
    1. Leptin administration accelerates the onset of puberty in rodents.

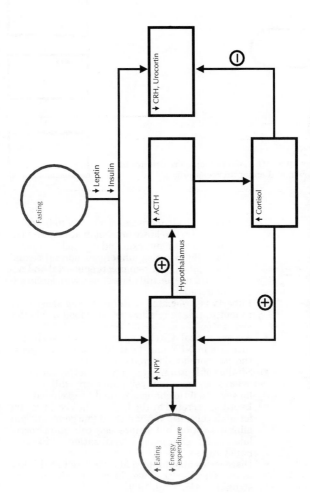

Figure 19.7.   The effect of fasting on eating and energy expenditure.

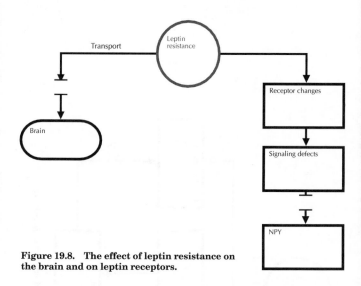

Figure 19.8. The effect of leptin resistance on the brain and on leptin receptors.

   2. Leptin levels increase at puberty in boys.
   3. Low leptin levels are present in athletes and in patients with anorexia and delayed puberty.
   4. The OB/OB mouse undergoes normal sexual development but remains prepubertal and never ovulates; fertility is restored with leptin administration.
- Puberty is associated with increasing sensitivity to leptin; this may allow greater food intake for growth.
- A paradoxical CRH response also is seen; the increase in NPY may be inadequate to suppress the stress-related increase in CRH.
- Studies of leptin in women with polycystic ovary syndrome have not yet noted any differences; however, subtle changes cannot be excluded.
- Leptin is secreted by the follicle; the rise in serum leptin levels after human chorionic gonadotropin administration but before egg collection correlates with higher *in vitro* fertilization (IVF) pregnancy rates.
- Discoveries about leptin also restored credibility to the Frisch critical weight hypothesis for menstrual function (Fig. 19.9).
♦ Leptin summary.
- The purpose of leptin function may be limited to effects at low levels.
- Leptin therapy is not "just around the corner."
- Genetic defects in the OB gene are uncommon.
- A leptin agonist could be therapeutic, but appropriate dietary choices and adequate exercise remain important.

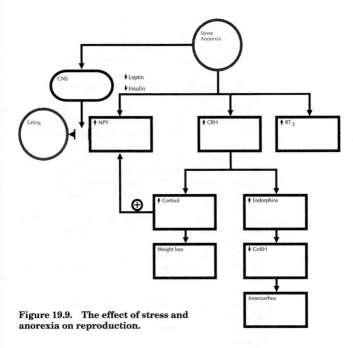

Figure 19.9.   The effect of stress and anorexia on reproduction.

- ♦ Inherited aspects of obesity.
  - • Mean fat cell volume is increased by 3× in obese people, but an increase in fat cells is seen only in the grossly obese; hypercellular obesity may be difficult to overcome.
  - • Hyperplastic obesity may be associated with childhood and with a poor prognosis.
  - • Genetic impairment is seen.
    - ■ The weight of adoptive children correlates with their biologic, not adoptive, parents.
    - ■ Twin studies suggest 70% of the variance is genetic, and 30% is environmental.
  - • Socioeconomic and behavioral factors are important determinants.
- ♦ Endocrine changes.
  - • The most important change is the elevation of basal blood insulin.
    - ■ This is proportional to the volume of body fat.
    - ■ Insulin acts to reduce food intake via NPY signaling.
  - • Insulin resistance is affected by the following:
    - ■ Amount of fat tissue in the body.
    - ■ Caloric intake/day.
    - ■ Amount of dietary carbohydrates.
    - ■ Amount of daily exercise.

- Insulin resistance leads to the following:
  - Increased circulatory free fatty acids.
  - Decreased TG catabolism.
    - ◇ Decrease in high-density lipoprotein (HDL).
    - ◇ Increase in low-density lipoprotein (LDL).
- Assess insulin resistance via fasting glucose–to–insulin ratio (<4.5).
- Measuring insulin response to 1 g/kg glucose is more reliable; the maximum response should not be greater than 150 mU/mL.
- Genetics play a greater role in mature-onset diabetes compared with that of juvenile onset.
- Hypothyroidism does not cause obesity; the weight gain is due to myxedema fluid accumulation.
- Obese people are unable to excrete normal amounts of salt and water renally (especially while dieting); this is mediated via an increased output of aldosterone and vasopressin.
- Weight loss will allow the normalization of insulin and glucose responses.

♦ Anatomic obesity.
  - Gynoid obesity (pear shape)—fat distribution in the lower body (femoral and gluteal regions).
  - Android obesity (apple shape)—central body distribution of fat.
  - Gynoid fat principally is stored fat.
    - Fat accumulates more rapidly in the thighs and buttocks.
    - This is associated with less risk of diabetes and coronary artery disease.
  - Androidal obesity refers to fat in the abdominal wall and visceral–mesenteric locations.
    - More sensitive to catecholamines.
    - Less sensitive to insulin.
    - More active metabolically.
    - Associated with the following:
      - ◇ Hyperinsulinism.
      - ◇ Impaired glucose tolerance.
      - ◇ Diabetes mellitus.
      - ◇ Increased androgens.
      - ◇ Decreased sex hormone–binding globulin.
      - ◇ Increased free testosterone and estradiol.
  - Leptin expression and circulatory levels are not influenced by androidal, central obesity.
  - The waist:hip ratio estimates the degree of upper–to–lower body obesity and the amount of intra-abdominal fat.

V. Management of Obesity
  ♦ This is the most important health measure available for reducing risk of cardiovascular disease; 40% of coronary events are attributed to excess body weight in mildly or moderately obese women.

- ◆ Weight loss reduces mortality.
- ◆ Diet programs.
  - • Set a reasonable goal.
    - ■ Four to 5 lb in the first months.
    - ■ Twenty to 30 lb in 4 to 5 months.
  - • Intake must be 500 to 1,000 cal below energy expenditure.
  - • The best diet limits calories to between 900 and 1,200/day.
    - ■ Fifty percent carbohydrates.
    - ■ Fifteen percent to 20% protein.
    - ■ Less than 30% fat.
  - • One needs to expend the equivalent of 3,500-cal intake to lose 1 lb of fat.
  - • Behavior modification is crucial.
  - • Restriction of caloric intake is the important principle.
  - • Semistarvation diets can be dangerous, and they do not guarantee long-term weight maintenance.
- ◆ Success rates.
  - • Thirty percent lose 20 lb or more.
  - • Four percent lose 40 lb or more.
  - • Ninety percent to 95% of people who lose weight regain it.
- ◆ Pharmacologic therapy.
  - • Catecholamine congeners affect only noradrenergic neurotransmission.
  - • Fenfluramine and dexfenfluramine increase serotonin release and partially inhibit reuptake.
    - ■ CNS levels are depleted.
    - ■ Circulating levels are elevated.
    - ■ The risk of pulmonary hypertension and valvular disease caused their removal from the U.S. market.
  - • Sibutramine, 10 to 15 mg/day, blocks both norepinephrine and serotonin uptake.
  - • Orlistat, 120 mg TID, with meals.
    - ■ Inhibits pancreatic lipase.
    - ■ Annoying gastrointestinal side effects.
  - • Long-term use may allow sustained weight loss, but the attainment of a normal body weight is unlikely.
  - • Surgical therapy is reserved for those who are morbidly obese.
- ◆ Physical exercise.
  - • It reduces the risk of myocardial infarction in all people.
    - ■ Lowers LDL and increases HDL.
    - ■ Increases the resting metabolic rate.
  - • The best time to exercise is either before meals or about 2 hours after eating (Table 19.2).
  - • The dietary maintenance requirement for a sedentary adult is about 1.5× resting metabolic rate (about 1,000-1,500 calories per day); increasing physical activity remains the key to success.

Table 19.2.   Calories burned by various activities

Activity	Calories per Hour
Sleeping	90
Office work	240
Walking	240
Golf	300
Housework	300
Bicycling	360
Swimming	360
Tennis	480
Bowling	510
Running slowly	750 (120/mile)
Cross-country skiing	840
Running fast	960 (160/mile)

- Emotional support is important in breaking the vicious circle of failed diets, resignation to fate, guilt, and shame.

Reproduction and the Thyroid

I. Introduction
   ♦ The thyroid gland was named in 1656 by Thomas Wharton.
   ♦ Thyroid disease is more common in women than in men.
   ♦ The clinical objective is to detect and treat thyroid disease before symptoms and signs are significant and intense; subtle thyroid disease is easily diagnosed by sensitive laboratory assessments now available.
II. Normal Thyroid Physiology
   ♦ Thyroid hormone synthesis depends on an adequate supply of dietary iodine, which is absorbed as iodide in small intestine.
   ♦ Plasma iodide enters the thyroid gland under the influence of thyrotropin (TSH).
      • Iodide $\rightarrow$ elemental iodine $\rightarrow$ bound to tyrosine.
      • Monoiodotyrosine and diiodotyrosine combine to form thyroxine (T_4) and triiodothyronine (T_3).
         ■ These iodinated compounds are part of the thyroglobulin molecule (a colloid that serves as a storage depot for thyroid hormone).
         ■ TSH induces proteolysis, leading to the release of iodothyronines into the bloodstream as thyroid hormone (Fig. 20.1).
   ♦ T_4, T_3, and reverse T_3.
      • Removal of one iodine from the phenolic ring of T_4 yields T_3.
      • Removal of iodine from the nonphenolic ring yields reverse T_3, which is biologically inactive.
      • In normal adults, one-third of the T_4 is converted to T_3 in the liver and kidneys.
      • Forty percent of the T_4 is converted to reverse T_3.
      • T_3 is 3 to 5× more active than T_4 (the nuclear receptor affinity is increased tenfold).
      • T_4 is secreted at 20× the rate of T_3, but it serves mainly as a prohormone for T_3.
      • Calories from carbohydrates determine the T_3 levels in adults.
         ■ Low T_3 and increased reverse T_3 are seen in febrile diseases, burns, malabsorption, and anorexia.
         ■ During stress, reverse T_3 increases and T_3 decreases to slow the metabolic rate.
      • Seventy percent of thyroid hormones are bound to thyroid-binding globulin (TBG), and 30% are bound to thyroid-binding prealbumin and albumin; binding proteins have a greater affinity for $T_4 \rightarrow$ allows T_3 entry into cells.
      • TBG is synthesized in the liver.
      • Synthesis is augmented by estrogen.

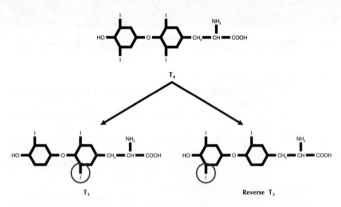

Figure 20.1. Formation of triiodothyronine (T_3) and reverse T_3 from thyroxine (T_4).

- ♦ Thyroid hormone receptor.
  - • A member of the steroid receptor super family.
  - • The nuclear receptor exists in several forms.
    - ■ It is the product of two genes on two different chromosomes as follows:
      1. α Receptor on chromosome 17.
      2. β Receptor on chromosome 3.
    - ■ The T_3 receptor is ubiquitous.
      - ◇ Receptor mutations exist.
      - ◇ They lead to a syndrome of thyroid resistance with elevated thyroid hormones, as well as TSH.
- ♦ Thyroid axis.
  - • Thyrotropin-releasing hormone (TRH) stimulates the axis.
  - • Somatostatin and dopamine inhibit the axis.
  - • Thyroid hormones suppress TRH secretion, probably by decreasing pituitary sensitivity to TRH via short-loop feedback; a decrease in TRH receptors is seen.
  - • TSH receptors are very sensitive to thyroid hormones. A slight change in T_4 will produce a many-fold greater TSH response.
  - • TRH-secreting cells are sensitive to T_4.
    - ■ Sensitivity requires conversion of T_4 to T_3 in the pituitary cells.
    - ■ Brain and pituitary convert T_4 to T_3; however, other tissues depend on serum T_3.
  - • Other influences on TSH response to TRH are as follows:
    - ■ Dopamine agonist and glucocorticoids → INHIBIT.
    - ■ Dopamine antagonists → STIMULATE.
  - • Estrogen increases TRH receptors in the pituitary, so TSH response to TRH is greater in women.

- TRH also stimulates prolactin release, which is not an issue except in hypothyroidism.
- ◆ Functional changes with aging.
  - T_4 metabolism and clearance decrease in older people; T_4 secretion decreases to maintain normal serum levels.
  - Conversion of $T_4 \rightarrow T_3$ decreases with aging.
  - TSH levels increase.
  - TSH response to TRH remains normal.
  - TBG levels decrease, but this decrease is not enough to alter serum levels.

III. Thyroid Function Tests
   - ◆ Free thyroxine (FT_4).
     - Displacement assay using antibody to T_4.
     - Not affected by changes in TBG or thyroid-binding affinity.
     - Normal range: differs between laboratories.
   - ◆ Total T_4.
     - Estimates thyroid concentration in blood by displacement assay.
     - FT_4 preferred to measurements of total T_4 because it is unaffected by factors influencing TBG.
   - ◆ FT_4 index (T_7).
     - Calculated from total T_4 and T_3 resin uptake.
     - Has now been replaced by FT_4 assay.
   - ◆ Total T_3 and reverse T_3.
     - Measured by sensitive immunoassays.
     - Rarely useful in clinical settings as they usually add little information.
   - ◆ TSH.
     - Measured by highly sensitive monoclonal antibody assay.
     - Two antibodies, α and β subunits.
     - Normal levels: vary between laboratories, but levels as low as $0.01 \ \mu U/L$ can be detected.
     - TSH level dependent on pituitary exposure to T_4.
       - Very sensitive as slight changes in T_4 are reflected in a manyfold greater TSH response.
       - Nearly all women with elevated TSH levels have hypothyroidism.
     - Transient changes noted in the following:
       - Psychiatric illnesses.
       - Systemic illnesses.
       - Pharmacologic treatment with dopamine and glucocorticoids.
   - ◆ Radioactive iodine uptake measures and localizes activity within the gland.
   - ◆ Laboratory evaluation (Fig. 20.2).

IV. Hypothyroidism
   - ◆ Clinical consequences of hypothyroidism.
     - Menstrual irregularities; amenorrhea probably secondary to TRH-induced increase in prolactin.
     - Constipation.
     - Cold intolerance.
     - Psychomotor retardation.

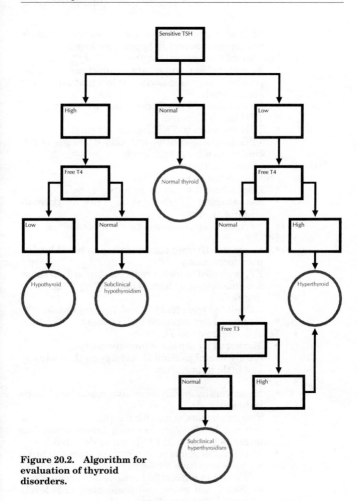

Figure 20.2. Algorithm for evaluation of thyroid disorders.

- Carpal tunnel syndrome.
- Mental slowness.
  - Somnolence.
  - Slow speech.
  - Low-pitched voice.
- Water retention.
- Periorbital edema.
- Hypertension and pericardial effusion.
- Asymmetric septal myocardial hypertrophy.
- Myopathy and neuropathy.
- Ataxia.
- Anemia.
- Elevated cholesterol secondary to impaired low-density lipoprotein (LDL) cholesterol clearance as a result of ↓ LDL receptors.

- Serum enzyme abnormalities.
  - Creatine kinase.
  - Aspartate aminotransferase (AST) and serum glutamic–oxaloacetic transaminase (SGOT).
  - Alanine aminotransferase (ALT) and serum glutamic–pyruvic transaminase (SGPT).
  - Lactate dehydrogenase.
  - Alkaline phosphatase.
- ◆ Other notable clinical implications.
  - In most cases, a specific cause is not apparent.
  - Autoimmune etiology with goiter is known as Hashimoto thyroiditis.
  - Empiric treatment with thyroid hormone is not indicated for euthyroid women with infertility.
  - A questionable association with recurrent pregnancy loss has been noted; evaluation of thyroid function is appropriate.
  - An increased incidence of hypothyroidism occurs with aging; 16.9% of women aged 60 and 17% of women over the age of 75 have elevated TSH levels.
  - Increased antithyroglobulin antibodies are in older women; 7.4% in women over 75.
  - Check TSH every 5 years starting at age the age of 55 and then every 2 years starting at 60 years of age.
  - In patients with amenorrhea and normal or elevated prolactin, check TSH.
- ◆ Diagnosis.
  - Elevated TSH and low T_4 confirm diagnosis.
  - Decreased levels of TSH are seen in pituitary failure.
  - The most common cause of hypothyroidism is autoimmune disease.
- ◆ Subclinical hypothyroidism.
  - Compensated state; increased TSH and normal T_4.
  - Many, but not all, will become clinically hypothyroid.
  - Treat to avoid goiter, but one could observe and recheck in 6 months.
  - Consider the measurement of antithyroid antibodies in asymptomatic patients; 20% per year will become hypothyroid.
- ◆ Treatment.
  - Better to provide T_4 and then to allow peripheral conversion; the desiccated thyroid provides T_3 in excess of normal thyroid secretion.
  - Initial dose of 25 to 50 µg/day × 5 weeks.
    - Start slowly, especially in older women, to avoid an adverse impact or coronary heart disease.
    - Final dose is usually 1.5 µg/lb → 70% of this dose for older patients.
  - Wait 8 weeks between dose changes and checking TSH levels.

V. Hyperthyroidism
   ♦ The two most common etiologies are Graves disease and toxic diffuse goiter.
   ♦ Plummer disease (toxic nodular goiter); usually seen in postmenopausal women with a long history of goiter.
   ♦ Graves disease.
      • Caused by autoantibodies with TSH activity.
      • Hyperthyroidism.
      • Exophthalmos.
      • Pretibial myxedema.

Symptoms	Signs
Menstrual pattern is unpredictable	Proptosis
Nervousness	Lid lag
Heat intolerance	Tachycardia
Weight loss	Tremor
Sweating	Warm, moist skin
Palpitations	Goiter
Diarrhea	

      • Occasional mental status changes.
      • Goiter absent in 40%.
      • Sinus tachycardia in <50%.
      • Atrial fibrillation in 40%; resistant usually to cardioversion and spontaneous reversion.
      • Older women.
         ■ Apathetic or atypical hyperthyroidism in 25%.
         ■ Weight loss, constipation, and loss of appetite in 15%; may suggest a gastrointestinal malignancy.
   ♦ Diagnosis of hyperthyroidism.
      • Requires laboratory testing.
      • Decreased TSH and increased T_4 or T_3; increased T_3 is more common in older women.
      • Most patients should have a radioactive iodine thyroid uptake and scan performed.
         ■ Suppressed uptake indicates the need for drug therapy.
         ■ Diffuse nodule or solitary hot nodule; toxic multinodular goiters seen more frequently in elderly patients.
   ♦ Subclinical hyperthyroidism.
      • Normal T_3 or T_4 concentrations are found, but TSH levels are suppressed.
      • Certain medications can suppress TSH to 0.1 to 5 µU/L.
         ■ Glucocorticoids.
         ■ Dopamine.
         ■ Anticonvulsants.
      • Levels <0.1 µU/L are not secondary to medication.
      • This is less common than subclinical hypothyroidism.
      • Patients may present with atrial fibrillation; consider treatment in older patients to avoid cardiac and bone complications.

- If levels are 0.1 to 5 µU/L, consider close observation with repeat TSH assessment every 6 months.
- ◆ Treatment of hyperthyroidism.
  - Multiple objectives for the treatment of hypothyroidism are as follows:
    - Control of thyroid hormone effects on peripheral tissue.
    - Inhibition of thyroid gland secretion and the release of thyroid hormone.
    - Specific treatment of nonthyroidal systemic illness.
  - Usually one administers antithyroid drugs, followed by definitive therapy with radioactive iodine treatment.
  - Defer pregnancy until several months after treatment.
  - Monitoring of response requires an 8-week interval.
- ◆ Antithyroid drugs.
  - Methimazole.
    - Fewer adverse side effects, so this is the drug of choice.
    - Inhibits organification of iodine.
    - Decreased T_3 and T_4 production.
    - Oral dose is 10 to 20 mg QD.
    - Onset of action: 2 to 4 weeks.
    - Maximum effect at 4 to 8 weeks.
    - Maintenance dose usually 5 to 10 mg QD.
  - Propranolol useful for symptoms; dose of 20 to 40 mg every 12 hours with adjustment to maintain heart rate of 100 beats/minute.
  - Inorganic iodine (Lugol solution).
    - Rarely used.
    - Blocks release of iodine.
    - Dose of two drops per day.
    - Onset at 1 to 2 days, maximum effect in 3 to 7 days.
    - Precludes treatment with radioactive iodine for several months.
  - Radioactive iodine.
    - This is useful once the patient is euthyroid.
    - Consider surgery for multinodular goiter, as hyperthyroidism tends to recur in new nodules.

  All patients treated for hyperthyroidism must be monitored for the development of hypothyroidism.

VI. Osteoporosis and Excessive Thyroxine
  - ◆ Thyroid hormone increases bone mineral resorption.
  - ◆ Increased total and ionized calcium.
    - Increased PO_4^{-3}, increased alkaline phosphatase, and increased bone Gla protein (osteocalcin).
    - Decreased parathyroid hormone.
      - Decreased vitamin D.
      - Decreased calcium absorption while urinary hydroxyproline and calcium increase = **decreased bone density**.

- Take care not to oversuppress and/or overtreat in thyroid disease.
  - Bone density is reduced by 9% in premenopausal women with suppressed TSH for >10 years.
  - This is especially true for postmenopausal women.

VII. Thyroid Nodules
  - The major concern is the potential for cancer.
  - Single nodules are 4× more common in women.
  - Thyroid cancer is 3× more common in women than in men.
    - The incidence rises from the age of 55.
    - The four major types of primary thyroid carcinoma are as follows:
      1. Papillary.
      2. Follicular.
      3. Anaplastic.
      4. Medullary.
    - Cold nodules are malignant in 12% of cases; surgery may have complications, so careful selection of patients is important.
  - Risk factors.
    - Family history.
    - A history of head and/or neck irradiation.
    - In those with thyroid radiation, one-third will have abnormalities; one-third of those with abnormalities will have cancer (10%).
    - The carcinogenic risk is 1% per 100 rad in 20 years.
    - The following increase the chances that the nodule will be cancerous:
      - Rapidly growing nodule.
      - Hard nodule.
      - Palpable nodes.
      - Vocal chord paralysis.
    - *Thyroid nodules in multinodular thyroid glands that have not been previously exposed to thyroid irradiation have no increased risk of cancer.*
    - Follow the nodules closely in a multinodular gland; biopsy or surgery is appropriate if the nodule grows.
  - Diagnostic strategy.
    - Thyroid nodule.
      - Check the thyroid function.
      - If abnormal, the nodule is most likely benign.
    - If risk factors (as above), surgical tissue diagnosis.
    - Fine-needle aspiration (FNA) or radionucleotide scan useful in other cases.
  - Cold nodules require surgical diagnosis, but one could consider suppressive therapy with levothyroxine.
    - If FNA is suspicious, perform a subtotal thyroidectomy.
    - If FNA is benign, begin thyroid replacement therapy and rebiopsy in 1 year; however, biopsy sooner if growth occurs.

- Medullary carcinoma is associated with a poor outcome; serum calcitonin is a good tumor marker (Fig. 20.3).
- ◆ FNA has a sensitivity of 83% and a specificity of 92% in diagnosing malignancy.
  - One-third of indeterminate FNA cases is found to be malignant at thyroidectomy.
  - With a benign biopsy outcome, the biopsy should be repeated in 1 year.
    - Most use suppressive therapy with close observation for 1 year.
    - TSH suppression will inhibit the growth of early carcinoma.

VIII. The Thyroid Gland and Pregnancy
  - ◆ During pregnancy, the thyroid gland increases in size with hyperplasia and increased vascularity.
  - ◆ No change in laboratory values is seen.
  - ◆ The goiter is pathologic in pregnancy and requires evaluation; its prevalence is increased in areas of iodine deficiency.
  - ◆ Increased thyroid activity occurs in pregnancy but is compensated for by the increase in TBG.
    - Chorionic TSH and human chorionic gonadotropin (hCG) are secreted by the placenta.
    - hCG contains 1/4,000 of the thyrotropic activity of TSH.
    - Increased TBG synthesis during pregnancy peaks at 15 weeks with levels twice that of a nonpregnant woman.
      - The increase in T_4 is surpassed by that of T_3.
      - FT_4 and free T_3 (FT_3) levels decrease but are still in the normal range.
    - Decreased clearance is secondary to glycosylation.
  - ◆ TSH levels.
    - TSH levels show an inverse relationship to hCG levels.
    - TSH levels decrease with increasing hCG, which peaks at 10 weeks; placental transfer of TSH, T_4, and T_3 is very limited in both directions.
  - ◆ Fetus and the neonate.
    - By 8 to 10 weeks of gestation, the fetal thyroid is able to concentrate iodine and to make hormone.
      - The development of the pituitary thyroid system is complete by 12 to 14 weeks.
      - This is seen at the same time as pituitary TSH production occurs.
    - An abrupt increase in fetal TSH occurs at 20 weeks; the timing is consistent with the development of the hypothalamic portal system and the maturation of hypothalamus.
    - Fetal TSH is increased and then reaches a plateau at 28 weeks.
    - Fetal T_4 increases to term; at term, it exceeds maternal levels, indicating a state of fetal thyroid hyperactivity.

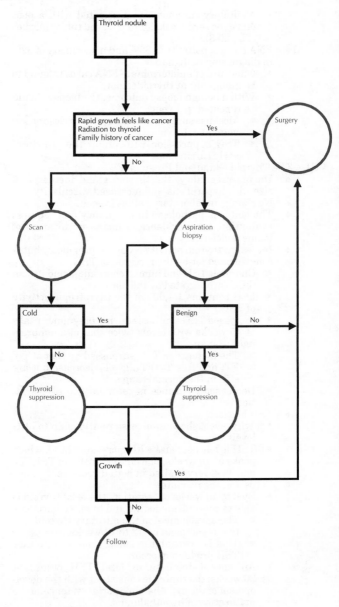

Figure 20.3. Algorithm for evaluation of thyroid nodules.

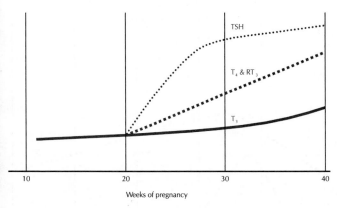

Figure 20.4.   Fetal thyroid hormone levels.

- The major hormone secreted by the fetus is T_4.
- Total T_3 and FT_3 are low.
  - Reverse T_3 is elevated, paralleling the rise in T_4.
  - This allows the fetus to conserve fuel reserves (Figs. 20.4 and 20.5).
♦ Delivery.
  - At delivery, a change from relative T_3 deficiency to T_3 toxicosis occurs.
    - TSH increases to its peak at 30 minutes.
    - It falls to a baseline by 48 to 72 hours.
      ◊ Total T_4 and FT_4 increase to peak values by 24 to 48 hours of age.
      ◊ T_3 levels peak by 24 hours of age.
  - Normal thyroid activity is present by 3 to 4 weeks.
  - Prolactin is also increased; this probably occurs in response to TRH release induced by neonatal cooling.
  - Cutting the cord influences T_4-to-T_3 conversion in the periphery (liver); this is a defense mechanism against entry into the cold world.
  - The high levels of reverse T_3 slowly change.
♦ Summary of fetal and newborn thyroid changes.
  1. TSH and T_4 appear at 10 to 13 weeks and increase abruptly at 20 weeks.
  2. T_4 in the fetus is > T_4 in the mother at term.
  3. T_3 levels rise but remain low.
  4. Reverse T_3 levels exceed normal adult levels.
  5. Low T_3 and high reverse T_3 are similar to situations of malnourishment.
  6. After delivery, TSH peaks at 30 minutes.
     - T_3 peaks at 24 hours → TSH independent.
     - T_4 peaks at 24 to 48 hours.
  7. High reverse T_3 persists for 3 to 5 days and then returns to normal by 2 weeks postpartum.

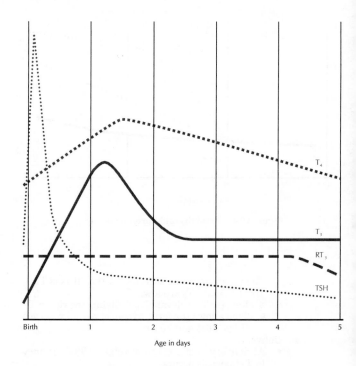

Figure 20.5.   Newborn thyroid hormone levels.

IX.   Newborn Screening
  ♦ Neonatal hypothyroidism is present in 1 of 4,000 deliveries.
  ♦ Congenital hypothyroidism is not evident at birth.
  ♦ Low T_4 and increased TSH must be treated by 3 months of age.
  ♦ An intraamniotic injection of thyroxin can raise fetal levels.
  ♦ Look for fetal goiter.
    • Especially in pregnant women treated with antithyroid drugs.
    • Or in case of polyhydramnios.
  ♦ Fetal cord blood sampling provides an accurate diagnosis.
  ♦ Prenatal treatment provides protection to fetal brain development; these children attain better motor skills.
X.   Hyperthyroidism in Pregnancy
  ♦ Untreated patients have a higher risk of preeclampsia, heart failure, intrauterine growth retardation (IUGR), and stillbirth.
  ♦ Graves disease is the most common; trophoblastic disease can also cause hyperthyroidism.

- ◆ Choice of treatment is between surgery and anti-thyroid drugs.
  - • Control is required prior to surgery.
  - • Propylthiouracil and methimazole are equally effective.
- ◆ Maintain a mild hyperthyroidism to avoid fetal thyroid dysfunction (can occur with a dose of 100 to 200 mg QD).
- ◆ These patients have no problem with breast-feeding; observe neonates closely for a few days until the anti-thyroid drugs have cleared.

XI. Hypothyroidism in Pregnancy
- ◆ Serious hypothyroidism rarely encountered.
- ◆ Questionable increased rate of recurrent pregnancy loss.
- ◆ Increased rate of preeclampsia and IUGR noted in women with significant hypothyroidism.
- ◆ Monitor TSH; keep in normal range during pregnancy. Most women require a dose increase of 20% to 50% during pregnancy.

XII. Postpartum Thyroiditis
- ◆ Affects 5% to 10% of women.
- ◆ Normally manifests 3 to 6 months after delivery.
  - • Transient hyperthyroidism eventually will lead to hypothyroidism.
  - • It is associated with thyroid microsomal autoantibodies.
  - • Family history of autoimmune disease indicates a high risk.
  - • Most women undergo a spontaneous cure.
  - • A risk of recurrence exists.
  - • Treatment with levothyroxine is very helpful; reassess after 1 year for requirements for continued thyroid maintenance.

Family Planning, Sterilization, and Abortion

I. Introduction
   - Fertility decreases as societies become more affluent; rates of contraception and abortion are increased.
   - !Kung women (African hunter–gatherers).
     - Fifteen years of lactational amenorrhea.
     - Four years of pregnancy.
     - Forty-eight menstrual cycles versus 420 menstrual cycles in modern urban women.
   - Teenage pregnancy in the United States is markedly higher than in other Western countries.
     - The difference disappears after age 25 due to surgical sterilization.
     - An estimated 78% of teen pregnancies are unintended; half of these pregnancies are aborted.
     - The abortion rate in U.S. women aged 20 to 35 is higher than in other countries.
     - A major factor in the higher unintended pregnancy rate in the United States is the failure of U.S. women to use contraceptives (of any sort); lower rates of oral contraceptive use in the United States may result from economic and accessibility issues.

II. Efficacy of Contraception
   - Definition and measurement.
     - The Pearl Index.
       - This is defined as the number of failures per 100 woman-years of exposure; the denominator is the total months or cycles of exposure from the onset of a method until study completion, discontinuation, or unintended pregnancy.
       - The quotient is multiplied by 1,200 (if the denominator is months) or 1,300 (if the denominator is cycles).
       - The limitation is that the Pearl Index fails to compare methods accurately at various durations of exposure.
     - Life-table analysis calculates a failure rate for each month of use (Table 21.1).

III. Contraceptive Use in the United States
   - The use of oral contraceptives peaked in 1992; this was the leading method among never-married women.
   - Increased condom use is observed in all race and ethnic groups, reflecting concern about the human immunodeficiency virus (HIV).
   - Sterilization is utilized by 39% of women.
   - Intrauterine device (IUD) use has fallen dramatically (Figs. 21.1–21.3).

**Table 21.1. Failure rates during
the first year of use, United States**

Method	Percentage of Women with Pregnancy	
	Lowest Expected	Typical
No method	85.0%	85.0%
Combination pill	0.1%	3.0%
Progestin only	0.5%	3.0%
IUDs		
Progesterone IUD	1.5%	2.0%
Levonorgestrel IUD	0.6%	0.8%
Copper T 380A	0.1%	0.1%
Norplant	0.05%	0.05%
Female sterilization	0.05%	0.05%
Male sterilization	0.1%	0.15%
Depo-Provera	0.3%	0.3%
Spermicides	6.0%	26.0%
Periodic abstinence		25.0%
Calendar	9.0%	
Ovulation method	3.0%	
Symptothermal	2.0%	
Postovulation	1.0%	
Withdrawal	4.0%	19.0%
Cervical cap		
Parous women	26.0%	40.0%
Nulliparous women	9.0%	20.0%
Sponge		
Parous women	9.0%	28.0%
Nulliparous women	6.0%	18.0%
Diaphragm and spermicides	6.0%	20.0%
Condom		
Male	3.0%	14.0%
Female	5.0%	21.0%

Abbreviation: IUD, intrauterine device.

IV. Impact of Worldwide Use of Contraception
   ♦ The world population is expected to stabilize at 11 to
      12 billion around 2150.
      • Approximately 95% of the growth will be in devel-
         oping countries.
      • Female sterilization and IUDs are most popular
         in developing countries.
         ■ Less than 15% of reproductive-aged women
            worldwide use oral contraceptives.
         ■ More than half live in the United States, Brazil,
            France, and Germany.

(text continues on page 370)

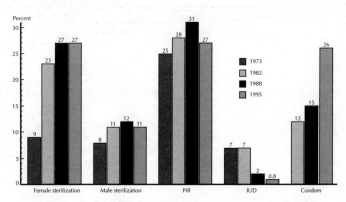

Figure 21.1. Changes in contraceptive use by United States women between the ages of 15 and 44 from 1973 to 1995.

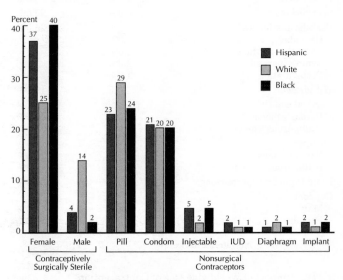

Figure 21.2. Contraceptive methods in women between the ages of 15 and 44 by race in 1995.

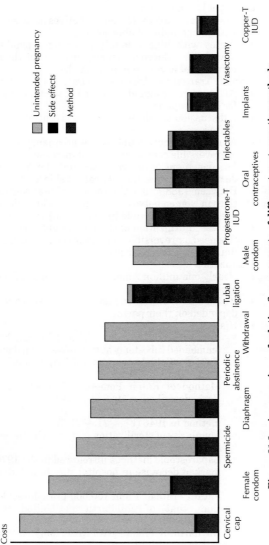

Figure 21.3.   A comparison of relative five-year costs of different contraceptive methods.

♦ Seventy-six percent of the world's population in developing countries accounts for the following:
  • Eighty-five percent of all births.
  • Ninety-five percent of all infant/childhood deaths.
  • Ninety-nine percent of all maternal deaths.

V. Impact of Use and Nonuse
  ♦ Inadequate access to contraceptives is associated with a high induced abortion rate.
  ♦ States with higher family planning expenditures have fewer induced abortions, fewer low birthweight babies, and fewer premature births.

VI. Sexually Transmitted Diseases (STDs) and Contraception
  ♦ STD screening should be offered at the time of a visit for contraception.
  ♦ A discussion of safe sex practices is crucial.

VII. The Future
  ♦ As more and more couples defer pregnancy, the need for reversible contraception will increase.
  ♦ Postponement of marriage accounts for 83% of the decline in the total fertility rate (Table 21.2).
  ♦ Between 1988 and 1995, the use of oral contraceptives in women between the ages of 35 to 39 doubled, and it increased sixfold in women >40 years of age.
  ♦ Increased utilization of the IUD would also address this need for reversible contraception; misconceptions limit appropriate utilization.

VIII. Sterilization
  ♦ Nearly one million Americans undergo sterilization each year.
  ♦ By 1995, 28% of women had tubal occlusion and 11% depended on their partner's vasectomy.
  ♦ History.
    • First suggested by James Blundell in 1823; he recommended tubectomy at time of cesarean delivery.
    • First published report in 1881 by Samuel Lungren of Toledo, Ohio.
    • Method of Ralph Pomeroy of Brooklyn, New York, described in 1929 (4 years after his death).
    • Irving method described in 1924 and Uchida method in 1946 (Figs. 21.4–21.6).
    • Popularity of sterilization increased by the end of the 1960s.
    • Laparoscopic methods introduced in the 1970s; a marked decrease in hospital stay from 6 days to <1 day.
    • Fatality rate of 1.5 in 100,000 procedures; lower than that of childbirth in United States (10/100,000).
    • No harmful effects with vasectomy; mortality rate is essentially zero.

IX. Efficacy of Sterilization (Table 21.3)
  ♦ Fifty percent of the failures are due to technical errors; more complicated methods have higher failure rates.

Table 21.2.   Change in United States female demographics 1985–2000

Age	1985	1990	1995	2000	% Change 1985–2000
15 to 24	19.5 million	17.4 million	16.7 million	17.7 million	–9.2%
25 to 29	10.9 million	10.6 million	9.3 million	8.6 million	–21.1%
30 to 34	10.0 million	11.0 million	10.8 million	9.4 million	–6.0%
35 to 44	16.2 million	19.1 million	21.1 million	21.9 million	+35.2%
Total 15 to 44	56.6 million	58.1 million	57.9 million	57.6 million	+1.8%

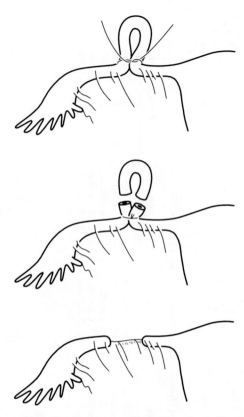

Figure 21.4.   The Pomeroy method of female sterilization.

♦ Age and lactation contribute to failures.
  • Younger women have increased pregnancy rates.
  • Women who are not breast-feeding have higher pregnancy rates.
♦ Pregnancy at the time of the procedure also contributes to the failure rate.
♦ Ectopic pregnancies can occur.
  • More likely after bipolar coagulation.
  • More likely to occur >2 years after the procedure.
  • Majority of pregnancies >2 to 3 years after occlusion will be ectopic; overall risk is still lower than in nonsterilized women because efficacy is high.
♦ Vaginal procedures have higher failure rates; the abscess formation rate is 1%.
♦ Sterilization and ovarian cancer.
  • Associated with a 67% reduced risk of ovarian cancer.
  • A 30% reduction in fatal ovarian cancer.

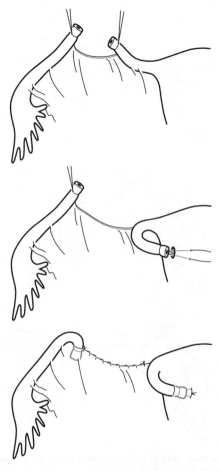

Figure 21.5.   The Irving method of female sterilization.

X. Female Sterilization Techniques
    ♦ Laparoscopy allows direct visualization.
    ♦ Methods of sterilization at laparoscopy include the
       following:
       1. Occlusion and partial resection by unipolar elec-
           trosurgery.
       2. Occlusion and transection by unipolar electro-
           surgery.
       3. Occlusion by bipolar electrocoagulation.
       4. Occlusion by mechanical means (clips or silastic
           rings).

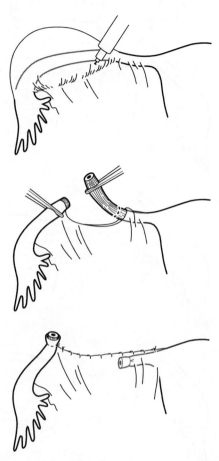

Figure 21.6.   The Uchida method of female sterilization.

- ◆ Failure rates are higher than was previously thought.
  - • Approximately 1.85% experience a failure within 10 years.
  - • Thirty percent are ectopic pregnancies (Table 21.4).
- ◆ Electrosurgical methods.
  - • Unipolar method.
    - ■ Use the lowest possible voltage.
    - ■ The return electrode must be in good contact.
    - ■ Capacitance coupling can result in bowel injuries; use a metal trocar sleeve rather than a nonconductive sleeve.

Table 21.3.   Failure rates during the first year, United States

Method	Percentage of Women with Pregnancy	
	Lowest Expected	Typical
Female sterilization	0.2%	0.4%
Male sterilization	0.1%	0.15%

- - Coagulate the isthmic portion of tube for 2 to 3 cm.
  - Coagulation and transection do not reduce the failure rate.
  - Bipolar method.
    - This method eliminates the return electrode.
    - Inadequate coagulation can result.
    - Desiccated tissue can adhere to the bipolar forceps.
    - It is safer than the unipolar method but has increased failure rates.
- Tubal occlusion with clips and rings.
  - Subject to flaws in materials.
  - The following three are common choices:
    1. Hulka–Clemens clip.
    2. Filshie clip.
    3. Falope (or Yoon) ring.
  - Hulka–Clemens clip.
    - Two plastic jaws with small metal pin.
    - Spring pushed over the jaws to hold them closed.
    - Applied at the proximal isthmus.
    - Destroys 3 mm of tube.
    - One-year pregnancy rate of 2 in 1,000, but 10-year cumulative failure rate is the highest.
    - Good chance for surgical reversal if desired.
  - Filshie clip.
    - Made of titanium.
    - Four millimeters of tube destroyed.
    - One-year failure rate of 1 in 1,000.

Table 21.4.   Female tubal sterilization methods, 10-year cumulative failure rates

Unipolar coagulation	0.75%
Postpartum tubal excision	0.75%
Silastic (Falope or Yoon) ring	1.77%
Interval tubal exclusion	2.01%
Bipolar coagulation	2.48%
Hulka–Clemens clip	3.65%

- Falope (or Yoon) ring.
  - This is a nonreactive silastic rubber band with an elastic memory of 100% if stretched to no more than 6 mm.
  - A 2.5-cm loop of tube is trapped.
  - Ten percent to 15% of patients experience severe postoperative cramping, which is decreased by topical application of a local anesthetic.
  - The ring should be placed at the junction of the proximal and middle third of each tube.
  - The ring has a failure rate of 1% after 2 years; the 10-year cumulative rate is excellent.
  - Bleeding from mesosalpinges can occur.
- ◆ Minilaparotomy.
  - Most frequent method of interval sterilization around the world.
  - Often a simple Pomeroy procedure.

XI. Counseling for Sterilization
- ◆ Patients should be made aware of the nature of the procedure, the alternatives, the efficacy, safety, and complications.
- ◆ Emphasize that sterilization is not intended to be reversible.
- ◆ Sexuality.
  - No detrimental effect on sexuality.
  - In fact, usually positive effects seen.
- ◆ Menstrual function.
  - The range of findings makes counseling couples difficult.
  - Some women experience changes, while others do not.
- ◆ Reversibility.
  - Active participation by both partners is crucial.
  - Two percent of U.S. women experience regret 1 year later (2.7% after 2 years).
  - Tubal reanastomosis is associated with excellent results if only a small portion of the tube is damaged.
    - Pregnancy rates correlate with the length of remaining tube; >4 cm is optimal.
    - The best rates are 70% to 80% with previous clips, rings, or Pomeroy.

XII. Male Sterilization
- ◆ It is safer and less expensive, and it has a lower failure rate.
- ◆ It is performed under local anesthesia.
- ◆ It rarely results in hematoma or infection.
- ◆ Most men develop antisperm antibodies.
- ◆ Whether this causes an increase in prostate cancer is questionable; the data are weak.
- ◆ Reversal is associated with pregnancy rates of 70% to 80%.
  - This decreases to 30% after 10 years.
  - Best results are achieved when the reversal is performed within 3 years.

XIII. Induced Abortion
♦ Induced abortion has been practiced for thousands of years; it did not become illegal until the 19th century.
♦ Vacuum aspiration was introduced in the 1950s.
• The method is much safer.
• It was gradually legalized in the developed countries of the world.
• The U.S. Supreme Court decision in 1973 (*Roe versus Wade*) limited local abortion laws.
• By 1980, legal abortion had become the most common surgical procedure in the United States.
♦ U.S. abortion rate.
• It has been decreasing since a peak in 1990.
• One-third of pregnancies not ending in miscarriage or stillbirth are terminated by abortion.
• More than 50% are obtained by women younger than 25 years of age.
• Twenty percent are performed in women under the age of 20.
   ▪ Rate peaks at 18 to 19 years old.
   ▪ Eighty percent are unmarried.
• American teenagers are especially dependent on abortion.
• The legalization of abortion reduced maternal morbidity and mortality; the number of abortion-related deaths declined from 300 in 1961 to 6 in 1985 and 11 in 1991.
   ▪ Mortality is 0.8 deaths per 100,000 legal abortions.
   ▪ It is related to gestational age and anesthesia.

Major Complications (Hospitalization Required)

Retained tissue	27.7/100,000 induced abortions
Sepsis	21.2
Uterine perforation	9.4
Hemorrhage	7.1
Inability to complete	3.5
Intrauterine plus tubal pregnancy	2.4

Minor Complications
(Managed in the Clinic or Office)

Mild infection	462.0/100,000 induced abortions
Reaspiration— same day	180.8
Reaspiration—later	167.8
Cervical stenosis	16.5
Cervical tear	10.6
Underestimated gestation	6.5
Convulsive seizure	4.0

- No evidence exists for long-term complications, such as infertility, increased rate of ectopics, or adverse pregnancy outcome.
- Psychological sequelae have been studied and debated.
- No increased risk of breast cancer has been observed.

♦ Preoperative care of the abortion patient.
  - Ninety percent of abortions are performed during the first trimester; morbidity and mortality are one-tenth of the rates in later trimester procedures.
  - One needs to diagnose the presence of an intrauterine pregnancy and the gestational age; these are the most common sources of complications and litigation.
  - Most women are candidates for an outpatient procedure; exceptions include the following:
    - Severe cardiorespiratory disease.
    - Severe anemias or coagulopathies.
    - Mental disorders.
    - Severe concern about operative pain.
    - Known uterine anomalies or leiomyomata.

♦ Counseling abortion patients.
  - Counseling has played a critical role in the development of efficient and acceptable abortion services.
  - It should include help with decision-making, technical concerns, and emotional support, as well as referral for patients deciding against abortion.
  - Informed consent includes a discussion of complications.

♦ Methods of first trimester abortions.
  - Ninety-nine percent with vacuum curettage.
  - Local anesthesia.
  - Cervical dilation with Pratt dilators.
    - Some surgeons use cervical tents.
    - Mifepristone (RU486) may also be used for cervical dilation.
  - Nonsurgical methods in clinical testing; recent U.S. Food and Drug Administration approval of mifepristone.
  - Mifepristone.
    - Forms hormone receptor complex.
    - Prevents full gene activation; some agonist activity.
    - Dimethyl side chain at carbon 11—principal factor in antiprogesterone action.
    - Single 600-mg oral dose; followed a day later by prostaglandin (PG) analog.
      ◊ An 800-mg dose of misoprostol administered vaginally = best studied.
      ◊ A 400-mg oral dose also used; a 1% failure rate under 7 weeks of gestation.

- A lower dose of mifepristone (200 mg) also effective.
- Mechanism of action.
  - It creates a blockade of progesterone receptors in the endometrium.
    - ◇ Leads to disruption of the embryo.
    - ◇ Corpus luteum support withdrawn.
  - Other conditions that can potentially be treated with mifepristone include the following:
    - ◇ Cushing disease.
    - ◇ Endometriosis.
    - ◇ Induction of labor.
    - ◇ Contraception.
    - ◇ Cancer.
- Methotrexate.
  - Used in combination with a PG.
  - Efficacy decreased beyond 7 weeks.
  - Prolonged time to abortion.
  - No direct studies comparing it with mifepristone.
- Other medical methods.
  - Tamoxifen and misoprostol.
  - PG alone—infants born to pregnant women exposed to misoprostol have an increased risk of abnormal vascular development.
- ◆ Complications of abortions.
  - Bleeding.
    - This is most commonly caused by retained products of conception.
    - Rates vary from 0.2% to 0.6%.
    - Prompt aspiration is the best therapy.
  - Infection.
    - Fever and uterine tenderness are the most common signs or symptoms.
    - Prophylactic antibiotics may reduce the risk; metaanalysis concluded that their routine use should be standard.
      - ◇ Doxycycline.
      - ◇ Tetracycline.
    - Peritoneal signs and fever >38°C (101°F) require hospitalization and intravenous antibiotics; provide outpatient therapy for patients with signs or symptoms that are localized to uterus.
  - Dysfunctional bleeding.
    - Treat hormonally.
    - Curettage is not required.
  - Ectopic pregnancy.
    - Examine aspirate carefully for villi.
    - Measure serum β-human chorionic gonadotropin (hCG) and perform a vaginal sonogram.
  - Cervical stenosis.
    - Very rare (0.02%).

- More frequent in early first trimester abortions with minimal cervical dilation.
- Easily treated with paracervical block and gentle dilation.
- Other late complications.
  - Asherman syndrome.
    - ◇ Very rare; usually follows endometrial infection.
    - ◇ Best treated with hysteroscopy.
  - Rh sensitization.
    - ◇ Can be prevented by administration of 50 mg Rh immunoglobulin (RhoGAM) to all Rh-negative, Du-negative women.
    - ◇ Standard dose of RhoGAM is given in the second trimester.

XIV. Abortion in the Second Trimester
- Only 4% of abortions are performed at 16 to 20 weeks of gestation, and 1% at >21 weeks; 94% of second-trimester abortions are accomplished by dilation and evacuation (D&E).
- Safety of D&E is dependent upon training, experience, and skills of the surgeon.
  - Complication rates are higher with advancing gestational age.
  - Preoperative cervical dilation is essential.
- Medical methods are favored in the United Kingdom.
  - Mifepristone and misoprostol.
  - Intramuscular PG.
  - Intraamniotic PG, hydroxyurea, or hypertonic saline.

Oral Contraception

I. History
- ♦ 1931—Ludwig Haberlandt proposed administration of hormones for birth control and produced an extract called Infecundin.
- ♦ 1939—Russell Marker devised a method to convert sapogenin into progestin (Marker degradation).
  - At this time, 2,500 pregnant pig ovaries were needed to make 1 mg progesterone.
  - He began looking for sources of diosgenin.
    - He expanded his search to Mexico in the 1940s.
    - Mexican yam roots were distilled into a syrup.
    - One 5-gallon can yielded 3 kg progesterone.
  - 1943—Without pharmaceutical industry support, he collected 10 tons of *Dioscorea mexicana* roots.
    - Found a chemical company in the Mexico City phone book to work with him on this project.
    - Eventually founded a joint company called Syntex.
  - Within 2 months, Marker made several pounds of progesterone (worth $300,000); by 1944, he made over 30 kg progesterone.
  - Marker was cheated by his partners and founded a new company: Botanic-Mex.
    - Price of progesterone fell to $5 per gram (it had been $200/g).
    - Sold this company to Organon in 1946.
  - Marker returned to the United States in 1949 and made replicas of antique works in silver.
    - He endowed chairs at Penn State and University of Maryland.
    - He was granted an honorary Ph.D. in 1987 from the University of Maryland; he died in 1995.
- ♦ 1949—Carl Djerassi worked on the synthesis of cortisone with diosgenin as starting point.
  - A better method of microbiologic fermentation was discovered at Upjohn; this method used progesterone as a starting point.
    - Upjohn needed 10 tons of progesterone each year.
    - The price was $0.48/g.
  - Djerassi began work on new steroids.
    - Ethisterone had been available for a dozen years.
    - Removal of C-19 increased the progestational activity—norethindrone.
    - This became the first patent for a drug listed in the National Inventor's Hall of Fame in Akron, Ohio.

♦ 1934—Gregory Pincus achieved *in vitro* fertilization of rabbit eggs.
  • Was recruited to Clark University after failing to receive tenure at Harvard by his friend Hudson Hoagland.
  • 1944—Worcester Foundation established; Hoagland, Pincus, and Min-Chueh Chang were three of the principals.
♦ 1951—Min-Chueh Chang demonstrated that progesterone inhibits ovulation in rabbits.
♦ 1952—Pincus met Katherine McCormick.
  • Margaret Sanger and Katherine McCormick provided research grant funding.
  • McCormick eventually contributed over $3 million to this work.
♦ 1940s—John Rock, chief of obstetrics and gynecology at Harvard, became involved in reproductive physiology; 1944—Rock first demonstrated *in vitro* fertilization of human oocytes from oophorectomy specimens.
♦ 1954—Synthetic progestin prevented ovulation in 50 of Rock's patients; 7 of 50 subsequently conceived after stopping the medication.
♦ 1955—This study was reported at the International Planned Parenthood meeting.
♦ 1956—The first human trial was performed in Puerto Rico.
  • Initial progestin products were contaminated with mestranol (50 to 500 μg).
  • Purification efforts yielded breakthrough bleeding.
  • Combination oral contraceptive pills (OCPs) contained both components to decrease the incidence of breakthrough bleeding.
♦ 1957—Mestranol/norethynodrel (Enovid) was approved for treatment of miscarriage and menstrual disorders (150 μg mestranol/9.85 mg norethynodrel).
♦ 1960—Mestranol/norethynodrel was approved for contraception.
♦ 1962—Syntex and Ortho combined forces to release norethindrone/mestranol (Ortho-Novum).
♦ 1968—Wyeth introduced norgestrel.
II. Pharmacology
  ♦ Estrogen component.
    • 1938—Addition of ethinyl group at position 17 made estradiol active orally.
    • Mestranol is the 3-methyl ether of ethinyl estradiol.
    • Both are different from natural estradiol; metabolism of ethinyl estradiol varies from individual to individual.
    • Thrombosis risk is related to the estrogen component (Fig. 22.1).
  ♦ Progestin component.
    • Late 1930s—Ethisterone was discovered to be an orally active ethinyl derivative of testosterone.

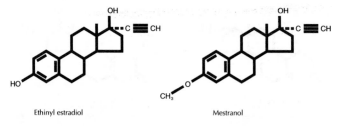

Ethinyl estradiol   Mestranol

Figure 22.1.   Structure of the estrogen component of oral contraceptives.

- 1951—Removal of C-19 from ethisterone yielded norethindrone; this changed the major hormonal impact from androgen to progestin.
  - Minimal anabolic and androgenic potential remains.
  - Slight estrogen activity is due to weak binding to estrogen receptor.
- Norethindrone family of compounds.
  - Norethindrone.
  - Norethindrone acetate.
  - Norethynodrel.
  - Ethynodiol diacetate.
  - Lynestrenol.
  - Norgestrel.
  - Norgestimate.
  - Desogestrel.
  - Gestodene.
- Norgestrel is a racemic mixture; levonorgestrel is the active form.
- Desogestrel undergoes conversion to 3-keto-desogestrel; this differs from levonorgestrel by the methylene group at CH.
- Gestodene is converted into many derivatives but is NOT converted to levonorgestrel.
- Norgestimate is converted into several metabolites.
  - 17-Deacetylated norgestimate.
  - 3-Keto-norgestimate.
  - Levonorgestrel probably the active metabolite (Figs. 22.2 and 22.3).
- ◆ Definitions.
  - Low-dose contraceptives: <50 µg ethinyl estradiol.
  - First-generation: >50 µg ethinyl estradiol.
  - Second-generation: 30 to 35 µg ethinyl estradiol and levonorgestrel, norgestimate, or another norethindrone family progestin.
  - Third-generation: 20 to 30 µg ethinyl estradiol and gestodene or desogestrel.
- ◆ Medroxyprogesterone acetate.
  - It is formed from the acetylation of the 17-hydroxy group of 17-hydroxyprogesterone.

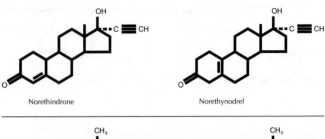

Norethindrone   Norethynodrel

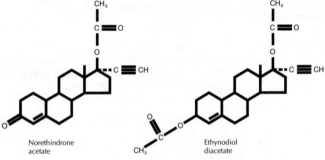

Norethindrone   Ethynodiol
acetate   diacetate

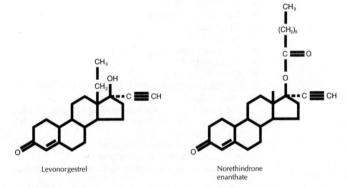

Levonorgestrel   Norethindrone
                         enanthate

Figure 22.2.   Structures of the various progestins found in first and second generation oral contraceptives.

- • Methylation at position 6 is needed to provide sufficient progestational strength.
- • It inhibits metabolism.
- ♦ Potency.
  - • An accurate assessment of potency is difficult to achieve; progestins act on numerous target organs.
  - • Progestin potency is no longer a consideration.
  - • Clinical advice based on potency has not withstood the test of time.
- ♦ New progestins.

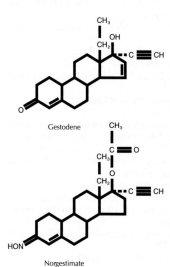

Desogestrel

Gestodene

Norgestimate

Figure 22.3.   Additional newer progestins used in oral contraceptives.

- Desogestrel, gestodene, norgestimate.
- Comparable with previous products in regard to breakthrough bleeding and amenorrhea.
- Negligible impact on carbohydrate metabolism.
- Increased sex hormone–binding globulin (SHBG) and thus decreased free testosterone; may be of clinical value in acne and hirsutism, but no clinical studies exist.
- May promote favorable lipid changes, but clinical significance is uncertain.
- ♦ New formulations.
  - Multiphasic preparations are meant to reduce breakthrough bleeding and amenorrhea.
  - The metabolic effects are minimal.
- ♦ Mechanism of action.
  - They inhibit gonadotropin secretion via an effect on both the pituitary and hypothalamic centers.
    - Progestin suppresses luteinizing hormone (LH).

- Estrogen suppresses follicle-stimulating hormone (FSH).
  - ◇ Also stabilizes the endometrium.
  - ◇ Potentiates progestin action and increases progesterone receptors (PR).
- Progestin also produces a decidualized endometrium.
- It thickens the cervical mucus and possibly alters tubal motility.
- ♦ Efficacy.
  - Failures usually occur because of a delay in initiation of the next cycle.
    - Other prevalent problems include vomiting and/or diarrhea.
    - Use a backup method for 7 days after an episode of gastroenteritis.
  - Failure rate of 0.1% to 3.0% during the first year of use (Table 22.1).

III. Metabolic Effects of Oral Contraception
  - ♦ Cardiovascular disease.
    - 1995—The UK Committee on Safety of Medicines sent a letter to all UK physicians and pharmacists that suggested that gestodene and desogestrel were associated with an increased risk of venous thromboembolism (VTE).
    - This led to an immediate decrease in use of all OCPs and to an increased rate of abortion.
    - Thromboembolism can be divided into the following two categories:
      1. Venous—pulmonary embolism and deep vein thrombosis (DVT).
      2. Arterial—myocardial infarction (MI) and stroke.
  - ♦ The coagulation system.
    - The goal of the clotting mechanism is to produce thrombin, which converts fibrinogen to a fibrin clot.
    - Deficiencies of antithrombin III, protein C, and protein S are inherited as autosomal dominant.
      - Account for 10% to 15% of familial thrombosis.
      - Resistance to actuated protein C (factor V Leiden mutations) found in 30% of individuals with VTE.
        - ◇ Factor V is resistant to degradation.
        - ◇ Heterozygotes have an 8× increased risk.
        - ◇ This is rare in those who are not of European descent.
    - OCPs increase the production of clotting factors secondary to estrogen, but changes from low-dose pills are of uncertain significance.
  - ♦ VTE—conventional wisdom.
    - VTE is an estrogen-related risk.
      - Limited to current users.
      - Effect is gone after 3 months.

**Table 22.1.   Failure rates during
the first year of use, United States**

Method	Percentage of Women with Pregnancy	
	Lowest Expected	Typical
No method	85.0%	85.0%
Combination pill	0.1%	3.0%
Progestin only	0.5%	3.0%
IUDs		
Progesterone IUD	1.5%	2.0%
Levonorgestrel IUD	0.6%	0.8%
Copper T 380A	0.1%	0.1%
Norplant	0.05%	0.05%
Female sterilization	0.05%	0.05%
Male sterilization	0.1%	0.15%
Depo-Provera	0.3%	0.3%
Spermicides	6.0%	26.0%
Periodic abstinence		25.0%
Calendar	9.0%	
Ovulation method	3.0%	
Symptothermal	2.0%	
Postovulation	1.0%	
Withdrawal	4.0%	19.0%
Cervical cap		
Parous women	26.0%	40.0%
Nulliparous women	9.0%	20.0%
Sponge		
Parous women	9.0%	28.0%
Nulliparous women	6.0%	18.0%
Diaphragm and spermicides	6.0%	20.0%
Condom		
Male	3.0%	14.0%
Female	5.0%	21.0%

Abbreviation: IUD, intrauterine device.

- Lower-dose preparations and screening of high-risk patients have lowered the risk; the risk is reduced to twofold but is still present.
- ◆ Epidemiology primer.
  - Clinical reports.
    - Case reports.
    - Case series.
  - Observational studies (nonexperimental).
    - Cross-sectional studies—description at one point in time.

- ◇ Advantages:
  - ○ Reliable method to estimate prevalence.
  - ○ Quick and inexpensive.
- ◇ Disadvantages:
  - ○ Cannot assess changes over time.
  - ○ Susceptible to sampling error.
- ■ Case-control studies—a retrospective comparison of those with a condition that is compared with a control group.
  - ◇ Advantages:
    - ○ Relatively quick.
    - ○ Relatively inexpensive.
  - ◇ Disadvantages:
    - ○ Subject to biases and errors.
    - ○ Small sample size.
- ■ Cohort studies—prospective follow-up and exposure information is compared with those who develop a disease.
  - ◇ Advantages:
    - ○ Relatively accurate estimate because of large numbers.
    - ○ Can evaluate changes over time.
    - ○ Avoid recall bias.
  - ◇ Disadvantages:
    - ○ Expensive.
    - ○ Lengthy amount of time.
    - ○ Subject to surveillance bias.
- ■ Randomized controlled trials—a true clinical experiment.
  - ◇ Advantage: provide scientific, epidemiologic proof.
  - ◇ Disadvantages:
    - ○ Expensive.
    - ○ Time-consuming.
    - ○ Can evaluate only a limited number of hypotheses.
- ◆ Possible confounders and biases.
  - • Confounders—factors associated with the disease and the exposure.
    - ■ Age.
    - ■ Weight.
    - ■ Smoking.
    - ■ Family history.
    - ■ Duration of use.
    - ■ Healthy user effect.
  - • Biases—errors due to study design.
    - ■ Detection and/or surveillance bias.
    - ■ Publication bias.
    - ■ Reporting or recall bias.
    - ■ Selection bias.
      - ◇ Also includes the "healthy user" effect.
      - ◇ Choice of controls.
    - ■ Information and/or observer bias; patients lost to follow-up.

- Commonly used terms:
  - Relative risk (RR)—the ratio of risk among those exposed to the risk of those who are unexposed.
  - Odds ratio (OR)—the measure of association in case-control studies when the prevalence of disease events is low.
  - Confidence interval (CI)—the range of RR that would include 95% of the subjects being studied.
    - ◇ A tighter range corresponds to a more precise conclusion.
    - ◇ RR that includes 1 in the 95% CI, is not statistically significant.
  - Attributable risk—the difference in incidence between exposed and unexposed groups; when events are rare, a modest increase in RR will produce only a small number of cases.
- ◆ VTE—the controversial studies.
  - World Health Organization (WHO) collaborative study.
    - Hospital-based case-control study.
    - Twenty-one centers in 17 countries.
    - Risk of idiopathic VTE examined.
    - Compared levonorgestrel OCP with desogestrel or gestodene OCP.
    - Levonorgestrel: OR 3.5 versus nonusers.
    - Desogestrel: OR 9.1 versus nonusers.
    - Gestodene: OR 9.1 versus nonusers.
  - Transnational study of OCPs.
    - Analyzed 471 cases of DVT and/or VTE from the United Kingdom and Germany.
    - Second-generation: OR 3.2 versus nonusers.
    - Third-generation: OR 1.5-fold greater than second generation.
  - General practice research database.
    - Fifteen unexpected idiopathic cardiovascular deaths were noted (a nonsignificant change).
    - The risk of VTE with desogestrel and gestodene was 2× greater than for levonorgestrel.
- ◆ VTE—subsequent studies.
  - Denmark study.
    - Hospital-based case-control study.
    - Increased risk found in new users; new progestins frequent in new users.
  - Randomized transnational case-control study; adjustment for duration of use found no difference between second-generation and third-generation products.
- ◆ Evaluation of the studies—how can one explain the inherent biologic implausibility?
  - Former users are often switched to "safer" products—"preferential prescribing."
  - "Attrition of susceptibles" leads to disparate cohorts of individuals.

- Because desogestrel and gestodene products were marketed as less androgenic and "better," clinicians prescribed these to high-risk and older patients.
- Also, new studies preferentially prescribed third-generation products.
- The apparent differences were due to these factors.

♦ VTE and factor V Leiden mutation.
- Risk of VTE increases by 3 to 4× over the normal, general incidence.
- Factor V Leiden mutation may account for a significant portion of these patients (Table 22.2).
- Should we screen all perspective users for this mutation (Table 22.3)?
- Of the 10,000,000 women using OCPs, about 450,000 are likely to carry the mutation.
  - However, the incidence rate is very low: 4 to 5 per 100,000 young women per year.
  - Of women with the mutation, the event rate is 1 per 1,000 women per year.
- Screening is appropriate in women with a previous episode or a family history of VTE.
- The role of the choice of OCPs in activated protein C resistance had been suggested in a report from the Netherlands.
  - This suggested a difference in second-generation versus third-generation OCPs.
  - On further analysis, considerable overlap was found among all of the groups tested; these results could not be replicated by another laboratory.

♦ Arterial thrombosis.
- The incidence of cerebral thrombotic attacks is higher than VTE or MI; the risk is even greater in women >40 years of age.

Table 22.2.   Relative risk and actual incidence of venous thromboembolism

Population	Relative Risk	Incidence per 100,000 per year
Young women—general population	1	4 to 5
Pregnant women	12	48 to 60
High-dose oral contraceptives	6 to 10	24 to 50
Low-dose oral contraceptives	3 to 4	12 to 20
Leiden mutation carrier	6 to 8	24 to 40
Leiden carrier and oral contraceptives	30	120 to 150
Leiden mutation—homozygous	80	320 to 400

**Table 22.3. Carrier frequency for the
Leiden mutation in the United States**

White Americans	5.27%
Hispanic Americans	2.21%
Native Americans	1.25%
Black Americans	1.23%
Asian Americans	0.45%

- • The dose response relationship is difficult to establish.
- ◆ MI—the risk is important in older patients who smoke (Table 22.4).
- ◆ Stroke.
  - • Risk is clearly influenced by the presence of hypertension.
  - • Increased risk is observed in smokers or in users of high-dose products (Table 22.5).
- ◆ Current assessment.
  - • New studies fail to find any substantial risk of ischemic or hemorrhagic stroke with low-dose OCPs in young healthy women.
  - • The benefit of screening patients is evident from the increased arterial thrombotic risk in developing countries.
  - • Smoking.
    - ■ Twenty-four percent of 35-year-old to 45-year-old OCP users are smokers; 85% of these are heavy smokers.

**Table 22.4. Incidence of myocardial
infarction in women of reproductive age**

Overall incidence	5 per 100,000 per yr
Women less than age 35	
Nonsmokers	4 per 100,000 per yr
Nonsmokers and OCPs	4 per 100,000 per yr
Smokers	8 per 100,000 per yr
Smokers and OCPs	43 per 100,000 per yr
Women aged 35 and older	
Nonsmokers	10 per 100,000 per yr
Nonsmokers and OCPs	40 per 100,000 per yr
Smokers	88 per 100,000 per yr
Smokers and OCPs	485 per 100,000 per yr

Note: The above incidences are estimates based on oral contraceptive pill (OCP) use paired with cardiovascular risk factors prevalent in the general population. Effective screening would produce smaller numbers. The increased risks in the smokers and OCP groups reflect the impact of undetected cardiovascular risk factors, especially hypertension.
OCP, oral contraceptive pill.

Table 22.5. Incidence of stroke in women of reproductive age

Incidence of ischemic stroke	5 per 100,000 per yr
	1 to 3 per 100,000 per yr in women under age 35
	10 per 100,000 per yr in women over age 35
Incidence of hemorrhagic stroke	6 per 100,000 per yr
Excess cases per year due to OCPs, including smokers and hypertensives	2 per 100,000 per yr in low-dose OCP users
	1 per 100,000 per yr in low-dose OCP users under age 35
	8 per 100,000 per yr in high-dose OCP users

Abbreviation: OCP, oral contraceptive pill.

- A former smoker must have quit at least 12 months previously to be regarded as a non-smoker; women using nicotine patches or gum are considered smokers.
  - Lipoproteins.
    - Levonorgestrel triphasic has no effect.
    - Levonorgestrel higher-dose monophasic produces the following effects:
      ◇ Increases low-density lipoprotein (LDL) and apoprotein B.
      ◇ Decreases high-density lipoprotein (HDL) and apoprotein A.
    - Desogestrel pills have a favorable impact.
    - Triphasic norgestimate and gestodene produce beneficial changes.
    - Monophasic norethindrone has no effect.
    - Estrogen offers protection in spite of any lipid changes.
  - Hypertension.
    - OCP-induced hypertension is observed in 5% of the users of high-dose pills.
    - Annual assessment is still appropriate.
    - The mechanism involves the renin–angiotensin system.
      ◇ Marked increase in angiotensinogen.
      ◇ Excessive vasoconstriction prevented by compensatory decrease in plasma renin.
    - Patients with well-controlled hypertension may choose OCPs; they need an evaluation every 3 months.
  IV. Cardiovascular Disease—Summary
    1. Pharmacologic estrogen increases the production of clotting factors.

2. Progestins have no significant impact on clotting factors.
3. Past users have no increased risk of cardiovascular disease.
4. All low-dose OCPs increase the risk of VTE.
5. Smoking has no effect on VTE.
6. Smoking and estrogen have an additive effect on the risk of arterial thrombosis.
7. Hypertension is an important additive risk factor for studies in OCP women.
8. Low-dose OCPs do not increase the risk of MI or stroke in healthy nonsmokers, regardless of age.
9. Almost all MIs and cerebrovascular accidents occur in OCP users of high-dose products or in users with risk factors and > age 35.
10. Arterial thrombosis has a dose response relationship with estrogen.
   ◆ Insufficient data to assess the risk difference of 20-µg, 30-µg, or 35-µg products.
   ◆ Evaluation of idiopathic thromboembolism or family history.
      • Screening tests are listed below.
      • Consider a hematologist evaluation.

Hypercoaguable Conditions	Thrombophilia Screening
Antithrombin III deficiency	Antithrombin III
Protein C deficiency	Protein C
Protein S deficiency	Protein S
Factor V Leiden mutation	Activated protein C resistance ratio
Prothrombin gene mutation	Activated partial thromboplastin time (PTT)
Antiphospholipid syndrome	Hexagonal activated PTT
	Anticardiolipin antibodies
	Lupus anticoagulant
	Fibrinogen
	Prothrombin G mutation (DNA test)
	Thrombin time
	Homocysteine level
	Complete blood cell count

V. Carbohydrate Metabolism
   ◆ In newer low-dose pills, the insulin and glucose changes are of no clinical significance.
   ◆ Progestin does alter insulin sensitivity.
      • Is the resulting slight hyperinsulinemia a risk factor for later cardiovascular disease?
      • Current studies are reassuring.
   ◆ No increase in diabetes mellitus is observed; no increase is seen even in women with previous gestational diabetes.

◆ Patients with diabetes.
  • No effect on their insulin requirement has been noted.
  • In women <35 years old, no significant increase in VTE is seen.
  • OCPs have no effect on retinopathy and nephropathy.

VI. The Liver
  ◆ Estrogen influences the synthesis of hepatic DNA and RNA, hepatic cell enzymes, serum enzymes formed in the liver, and the plasma proteins.
  ◆ No increase in serious liver disease has been observed.
  ◆ Impairment of active transport biliary components is occasionally found in higher-dose OCPs; this rarely occurs with low-dose OCPs.
  ◆ Absolute contraindication for OCPs is acute or chronic cholestatic disease.
  ◆ The link to gallstones is inconsistent; however, OCPs may accelerate existing disease.

VII. Other Metabolic Effects
  ◆ Nausea, breast discomfort, weight gain; all are less frequent with low-dose OCPs.
  ◆ Weight gain—an anabolic response to sex steroids in some patients; nonresponsive to dieting.
  ◆ No association with peptic ulcer disease or inflammatory bowel disease.
  ◆ Not recommended for those with malabsorption.
  ◆ Chloasma now a rare problem.
  ◆ Slight changes in vitamin metabolism; routine supplementation is increasing.
  ◆ Androgenic side effects no longer an issue with low-dose pills.

VIII. The Risk of Cancer
  ◆ Endometrial cancer.
    • OCPs protect against endometrial cancer.
    • Use for 12 months reduces the risk by 50%.
    • Protection persists for 20 years after discontinuation.
    • They are protective against all three adenocarcinoma subtypes.
  ◆ Ovarian cancer.
    • Protection against ovarian cancer is one of the most important benefits of OCPs.
    • The risk is reduced by 40% in users.
      ■ Increases with the duration of use.
      ■ Continues for 10 to 15 years.
    • Some protection is seen in as little as 3 to 6 months of use.
    • An 80% reduction in risk occurs with >10 years of use.
    • This is especially true in women with high-risk family history; it is also true for women with *BRCA1* or *BRCA2* mutation.
  ◆ Cancer of the cervix.

- An increased risk has been observed, but this may be the result of confounding factors, including the following:
    - Age at first coitus.
    - Number of sex partners.
    - Failure to use barrier methods (protective).
    - Detection and/or surveillance bias.
- Increased risk of adenocarcinoma of the cervix has been observed in several studies.
- Consider Pap tests every 6 months in patients on OCPs who have other risk factors.

♦ Liver adenomas.
- Produced by steroids of the estrogen and androgen family.
- Several different lesions: peliosis, focal nodular hyperplasia, and adenomas.
- May regress with discontinuation of OCPs.
- Risk related to duration of use and dose in the pill.
- Exceedingly rare in low-dose pills.

♦ Liver cancer.
- WHO study demonstrated no association.
- No change in death rates from liver cancer has occurred since the pill was introduced.

♦ Breast cancer.
- The issue is not totally resolved.
- OCPs have a protective effect on benign breast disease.
- Several large cohorts showed no significant difference in breast cancer rates, but these women were often using OCPs after a previous full-term pregnancy.
- The use of OCPs early in life, prior to the first pregnancy, is still under evaluation.
- A reanalysis of the world's data has been done (Table 22.6).
- Young women who begin use before the age of 20 have a higher risk of breast cancer during use and for 5 years after stopping; this possibly results from the acceleration of a preexisting malignancy.
- In older women, previous use may have a protective effect.

♦ Conclusions.
1. Current and recent use may be associated with a 20% increased risk of early premenopausal breast cancer.

Table 22.6. Oral contraceptives and the risk of breast cancer: reanalysis of the world's data

Current users	RR = 1.24 (95% Cl, 1.15–1.33)
1 to 4 yr after stopping	RR = 1.16 (95% Cl, 1.08–1.23)
5 to 9 yr after stopping	RR = 1.07 (95% Cl, 1.02–1.13)

Abbreviations: CI, confidence interval; RR, relative risk.

- Limited essentially to localized disease.
- May represent detection bias.
2. Previous OCP use may be associated with a reduced risk of later breast cancer.
3. OCP use does not increase the risk of breast cancer in women with a positive family history.
4. Breast-feeding and the control of alcohol intake protect against breast cancer in premenopausal women.

IX. Endocrine Effects
- ◆ Adrenal gland.
  - Estrogen increases cortisol-binding globulin.
  - Free and active cortisol levels are both increased.
  - The effects of elevated levels are unknown.
  - A normal response to adrenocorticotropic hormone (ACTH) occurs in women on OCPs.
- ◆ Thyroid.
  - Estrogen increases synthesis and circulatory levels of thyroxine-binding globulin.
  - Free thyroxine level is unchanged.

X. Oral Contraception and Reproduction
- ◆ Inadvertent use during cycle of conception and early pregnancy.
  - Initial reports suggesting a link to congenital malformation have not been substantiated; these could be the result of a recall bias.
  - Virilization is also not an issue—this would require 20 to 40 mg norethindrone per day.
  - A metaanalysis of 26 studies demonstrated no increased risk; this level of reassurance can also be extended to patients exposed to medroxyprogesterone or 17-hydroxyprogesterone caproate.
- ◆ Reproduction after discontinuing OCPs.
  - Fertility—no effect on overall fertility has been seen, but a delay in the return of full fertility has been noted.
    - Interval of >13 months from discontinuation of contraception to conception in the following:
      - ◇ An estimated 24.8% of OCP users.
      - ◇ Approximately 12.4% of intrauterine device (IUD) users.
      - ◇ An estimated 8.5% of diaphragm users.
      - ◇ Approximately 11.9% of users of other methods.
    - Within 24 months, 90% of OCP users become pregnant.
  - Spontaneous miscarriage.
    - No increase.
    - Possible protective benefit in women who become pregnant after age 30.
  - Pregnancy outcome.
    - No increased rate of abnormal children.
    - Dizygous twinning is increased (1.6% versus 1.0%) in women who conceive soon after the cessation of OCPs.

- ◆ Breast-feeding.
  - Diminished quantity and quality of breast milk, but no demonstrable impairment of growth.
  - Contraceptive effectiveness of lactation depends upon the following:
    1. Length of intervals between births.
    2. The level of nutrition in mother.
    3. The intensity of suckling.
    4. The level of supplemental feeding.
  - Total protection for exclusively breast-feeding women is present for only 10 weeks.
    - Fifty percent of women who are not fully breast-feeding ovulate prior to the sixth week postpartum.
    - Consider a postpartum visit during the third week.
- ◆ Initiation of OCPs in the postpartum period
  - Mean time from delivery to menses = 45 ± 10 days.
  - No woman will ovulate <25 days after delivery.
  - ***The Rule of Threes:***
    In the presence of FULL breast-feeding, a contraceptive method should be used beginning in the *third postpartum month*.
    With PARTIAL breast-feeding or NO breast-feeding, a contraceptive method should begin during the *third postpartum week*.
  - Start OCPs immediately after termination of a pregnancy of <12 weeks; they can probably be started immediately in cases of midtrimester or preterm delivery as well.
  - Consider use of the progestin-only minipill, following a 3-day postpartum delay.
  - Consider especially in patients with history of gestational diabetes.
- XI. Other Considerations
  - ◆ Prolactin-secreting adenomas.
    - No relationship between OCPs and prolactin-secreting adenomas.
    - No reported cases of tumor growth in the author's history.
  - ◆ Postpill amenorrhea.
    - Incidence of 0.7% to 0.8% for spontaneous secondary amenorrhea.
    - No evidence of cause and effect.
    - Should evaluate for other causes as with any patient.
  - ◆ Pubertal use of OCPs.
    - The need for contraception takes precedence.
    - No evidence of impairment of growth and development of the reproductive system is seen in pubertal, sexually active girls.
- XII. Infections and Oral Contraception
  - ◆ Viral sexually transmitted diseases (STDs).
    - Dual approach of the barrier method with OCPs offers the best protection.

- No association has been found between viral STDs and OCP use.
- ◆ Bacterial STDs.
  - 1995—7.6% of reproductive age U.S. women were treated for pelvic inflammatory disease (PID).
  - Pelvic infection is the greatest risk for infertility.
  - Twelve months of OCP use decreased the incidence of PID by 50% to 60%.
    - ■ Protection is limited to current users.
    - ■ The mechanism of protection may be cervical mucus changes.
  - The protection of OCP against upper-tract PID may not apply to chlamydial cervicitis.
    - ■ Possible role of cervical ectopia.
    - ■ Additional risk factor—multiple partners.
- ◆ Other infections.
  - Relationship with urinary tract infections and viral diseases is unclear, especially with the appearance of low-dose preparations.
  - OCPs protect against bacterial vaginosis and *Trichomonas*.

XIII. Patient Management
  - ◆ Absolute contraindications.
    1. Thrombophlebitis, thromboembolic disorders (including a close family history [parent or sibling], which is suggestive of an inherited susceptibility for venous thrombosis), cerebrovascular disease, coronary occlusion, or a history of these conditions or conditions predisposing to these problems.
    2. Markedly impaired liver function. Steroid hormones are contraindicated in patients with hepatitis until liver function tests return to normal.
    3. Known or suspected breast cancer.
    4. Undiagnosed abnormal vaginal bleeding.
    5. Known or suspected pregnancy.
    6. Smokers over the age of 35.
  - ◆ Relative contraindications.
    1. Migraine headaches—avoid in women with complex migraines, prolonged aura, other stroke factors (older age, smoking, hypertension).
    2. Hypertension—OCPs are okay in women <35, who are otherwise healthy and whose blood pressure is under control with medications.
    3. Fibroids.
       - Not a contraindication.
       - OCPs do not stimulate growth of fibroids; bleeding decreases.
    4. Gestational diabetes—use of OCPs is allowed, but monitor fasting glucose; consider use of the progestin-only minipill.
    5. Elective surgery.
       - Consider discontinuing 4 weeks prior to major surgery if a period of immobilization is anticipated; the data are based on high-dose pills.

- Continue low-dose pills up to the time of laparoscopic tubal sterilization.
6. Epilepsy—OCPs do not exacerbate epilepsy, but antiepileptic drugs may decrease effectiveness of OCPs.
7. Obstructive jaundice—not all patients will develop jaundice on OCPs, especially with the low-dose formulation.
8. Sickle cell disease or sickle C disease.
   - Patients with the sickle trait can use OCPs.
   - The risk of thrombosis in sickle cell or sickle C disease is theoretic (and medicolegal); protection against pregnancy warrants the use of OCPs.
9. Diabetes mellitus—small risk exists of complicating vascular disease in women <35 years of age who are otherwise healthy.
10. Gallbladder disease—OCPs do not cause gallstones, but they may accelerate the symptoms in patients with gallstones.
XIV. Clinical Decisions
   - ◆ Surveillance.
     - Because of the safety of low-dose OCPs, see patients every 12 months; see women with risk factors every 6 months.
     - Reassess new users within 1 to 2 months.
     - Monitor glucose, lipids, and lipoproteins.
       - ■ Young women—at least once.
       - ■ Women >35 years.
       - ■ Women with a strong family history of heart disease, diabetes, or hypertension.
       - ■ Women with gestational diabetes.
       - ■ Women with xanthomatosis.
       - ■ Obese women.
       - ■ Diabetic women.
   - ◆ Choice of pill.
     - Choose a pill with <50 µg estrogen.
     - Little difference is seen between low-dose monophasics and multiphasics.
     - Progestin potency has been accounted for by dose adjustments; the biologic effects are similar.
   - ◆ Pill taking.
     - The contraceptive benefit is present during the first cycle as long as the pills are started on day 5 or earlier and no pills are missed.
     - No rationale exists for advocacy of a "pill-free rest period."
     - Precise pill-taking minimizes breakthrough bleeding and helps to promote the formation of habits (Fig. 22.4).
     - When pills are missed, what should the patient do?
       - ■ Only 33% of women miss no pills in cycle 1; by cycle 3, one-third of women missed three or more pills.
       - ■ See "Current Recommendations" in Fig. 22.4.

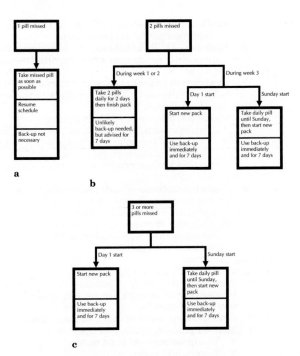

Figure 22.4. Algorithm for correcting oral contraceptive use for a patient who has missed taking the pill for one or more days.

- In gastroenteritis patients → use a backup method for 7 days.

XV. Clinical Problems
- ◆ Breakthrough bleeding.
  - • The onset of bleeding, although annoying, does not indicate a decrease in efficacy.
  - • This occurs most frequently in the first few months of use.
    - ■ Ten percent to 30% in first month.
    - ■ Ten percent in the third month.
  - • It is more common in smokers and in patients on 20-µg pills.
  - • The bleeding is best managed by encouragement and reassurance.
    - ■ Also review the need to take the pills consistently.
    - ■ Exclude cervical infections.
  - • Other options include restarting a new pill pack after 7 days or considering a short course of exogenous estrogen.
  - • No evidence that different formulations differ in the rates of breakthrough bleeding.

- ♦ Amenorrhea.
  - • Estrogen content may not be sufficient for stimulating endometrial growth; therefore, the progestational effect dominates.
  - • Permanent atrophy does not occur.
  - • The only harm for patients who remain amenorrheic on OCPs is the anxiety that it induces.
  - • Incidence is <2% in first year and 5% after several years.
  - • Remind patients that a basal body temperature <36.6% (98°F) at the end of the pill-free week is not consistent with pregnancy.
  - • Options include the addition of exogenous estrogen for 1 month but do not change to the 50-μg pill.
- ♦ Weight gain—studies do not support an association between OCP use and weight gain.
- ♦ Acne.
  - • All low-dose products improve acne.
  - • Low protection doses are insufficient to generate an androgenic response.
- ♦ Ovarian cysts—the risk of cysts is not eliminated, but they may offer some protection.
- ♦ Drugs that affect efficacy.
  - • No evidence demonstrates that antibiotics reduce efficacy.
  - • Drugs that stimulate the liver enzyme actually can alter efficacy; consider alternative contraceptive methods for patients on the following:
    - ■ Rifampin.
    - ■ Phenobarbital.
    - ■ Phenytoin (Dilantin).
    - ■ Primidone (Mysoline).
    - ■ Carbamazepine (Tegretol).
    - ■ Possibly also ethosuximide, griseofulvin, and troglitazone.
- ♦ Other drug interactions.
  - • OCPs may potentiate the action of some drugs, including the following:
    - ■ Diazepam (Valium).
    - ■ Chlordiazepoxide (Librium).
    - ■ Tricyclic antidepressants.
    - ■ Theophylline.
  - • The OCP user may require higher doses of acetaminophen and aspirin.
- ♦ Migraine headaches.
  - • The risk of stroke in migraineurs on OCPs is uncertain.
  - • The onset of visual symptoms or severe headaches requires a response; this can include switching pills or decreasing the dose.
  - • True vascular migraines are an indication to stop OCP use.
    - ■ OCPs should also be avoided in women with complex migraine or prolonged aura or if additional stroke risk factors (older age, smoking, hypertension) are present.

- ■ **Clues to severe vascular headaches:**
  Headaches that last a long time
  Dizziness, nausea, or vomiting with headaches
  Scotomata or blurred vision
  Episodes of blindness
  Unilateral, unremitting headaches
  Headaches that continue despite medication
- Menstrual migraines may improve with continuous OCP use.

XVI. Summary—Oral Contraceptive Use and Medical Problems
  - ♦ Gestational diabetes.
    - No contraindications.
    - Concern about breast-feeding women using the progestin-only minipill.
  - ♦ Diabetes mellitus.
    - Can be used by well-controlled diabetics who are <35 years old.
    - No evidence of accelerated vascular disease in OCP users with insulin-dependent diabetes mellitus.
  - ♦ Hypertension.
    - Can be used in well-controlled patients <35 years of age.
    - Choose lowest-dose preparations.
  - ♦ Pregnancy-induced hypertension—safe as long as the blood pressure has returned to normal.
  - ♦ Hemorrhagic disorders—can be used by women taking anticoagulants.
    - Avoids corpus luteum hemorrhage.
    - Decreases menstrual blood loss.
  - ♦ Gallbladder disease.
    - Use very cautiously or not at all.
    - May precipitate a symptomatic attack.
  - ♦ Obesity—obese but otherwise healthy women can use low-dose OCPs.
  - ♦ Liver disease.
    - May be used when liver function tests return to normal.
    - Recheck in 2 to 3 months.
  - ♦ Seizure disorders.
    - No impact of OCPs on pattern or frequency of seizures.
    - Possible increased risk of contraceptive failure resulting from anticonvulsant-induced hepatic enzyme activity.
  - ♦ Mitral valve prolapse.
    - Limit their use to nonsmoking asymptomatic patients; a small subset of patients is at increased thromboembolic risk.
    - Use progestin-only contraception or an IUD in patients with atrial fibrillation, migraine headaches, or clotting factor abnormalities.
  - ♦ Systemic lupus erythematosus.
    - OCPs can exacerbate systemic lupus.
    - Vascular disease and lupus are a contraindication to use; progestin-only methods are a good choice.

- Lupus patients with stable and/or inactive disease, no renal involvement, and an absence of high antiphospholipid antibodies can use OCPs.
- Migraine headaches.
  - Low-dose (lowest estrogen formulation) OCPs can be used in the common migraine with careful surveillance.
  - Avoidance is best in patients with classic migraine that is associated with neurologic symptoms.
- Sickle cell disease.
  - Depot medroxyprogesterone inhibits sickling, but OCPs can be considered as well.
  - The risk of thrombosis is theoretic.
- Benign breast disease.
  - Not a contraindication.
  - May actually improve with OCP use.
- Congenital heart disease and/or valvular heart disease—use is contraindicated in cases of marginal cardiac reserve or with predisposition to thrombosis.
- Hyperlipidemia.
  - OCPs have a negligible impact, so this is not an absolute contraindication.
    - High triglycerides are an exception.
    - Avoid in cases of vascular disease or smoking.
  - Monitor lipid profiles every few months.
  - Desogestrel, norgestimate, or gestodene can increase HDL levels.
- Depression—minimal impact on mood and/or depression.
- Smoking.
  - This is an absolute contraindication in women >35 years old.
  - Heavy smoking (>15 cigarettes/day) in women <35 years of age is a relative contraindication; the actual incidence of adverse events is low, but the risk is real.
  - Consider someone who is an exsmoker × 1 year as a nonsmoker.
  - Consider the 20-µg estrogen formulation regardless of age.
- Pituitary prolactin-secreting adenomas—low-dose contraception is safe.
- Infectious mononucleosis—OCPs are safe as long as liver function tests are normal.
- Ulcerative colitis—no association has been found between OCPs and ulcerative colitis.
- Alternative route of administration.
  - Certain circumstances preclude oral administration (e.g., nausea and/or vomiting with chemotherapy).
  - The pills can be administered vaginally.
- Athletes and OCPs.
  - Provide contraception and protection against bone loss.
    - Measurement of bone minimal density may be worthwhile.

- ■ Motivate the amenorrheic athlete to take hormone-replacement therapy (HRT).
  - No adverse effect on oxygen uptake or respiratory rate.
    - ■ A possible decrease in soreness has been reported.
    - ■ They have no effect on prevalence and/or severity of low back pain.
- ◆ Noncontraceptive benefits of OCPs.
  Effective contraception.
  Less need for induced abortion.
  Less need for surgical sterilization.
  Less endometrial cancer.
  Less ovarian cancer.
  Fewer ectopic pregnancies.
  More regular menses.
  Less flow.
  Less dysmenorrhea.
  Less anemia.
  Less salpingitis.
  Probably less endometriosis.
  Possibly less benign breast disease.
  Possibly less rheumatoid arthritis.
  Possibly protection against atherosclerosis.
  Possibly increased bone density.
  Possibly fewer fibroids.
  Possibly fewer ovarian cysts.
- ◆ Cancer prevention.
  - Forty percent reduction in ovarian cancer.
  - Fifty percent reduction in endometrial cancer.
- ◆ Neoplasms and OCPs—low-dose preparations.
  - No impact on fibroids.
  - Fail to prevent functional cysts.
- ◆ Bone density—possibly improved, but today's low-dose products may have little impact on bone density.
- ◆ Rheumatoid arthritis—probably beneficial.
- ◆ Other clinical entities that may benefit from use of OCPs.
  Definitely beneficial:
  Dysfunctional uterine bleeding.
  Dysmenorrhea.
  Mittelschmerz.
  Endometriosis prophylaxis.
  Acne and hirsutism.
  HRT for hypothalamic amenorrhea.
  Prevention of menstrual porphyria.
  Control of bleeding (dyscrasias, anovulation).
  Possibly beneficial:
  Functional ovarian cysts.
  Premenstrual syndrome.
- ◆ Acne and hirsutism.
  - The low-dose preparations are effective (including low-dose preparations with levonorgestrel).
  - SHBG increases, and free testosterone decreases.
  - Theoretic benefit of desogestrel, gestodene, and norgestimate is as follows:

- Associated with greater $\uparrow$ in SHBG and $\downarrow$ in free testosterone.
- No clinical evidence supporting this claim.

XVII. Continuation: Failure or Success?
- Worldwide, millions of pregnancies occur in women on OCPs because of poor compliance; these are more likely in unmarried, poor, and/or minority women (10% to 20% failure rate).
- Three major factors affecting compliance are as follows:
  1. Side effects.
     - Breakthrough bleeding.
     - Amenorrhea.
     - Headaches, nausea, and breast tenderness.
     - Weight gain.
  2. Fears and concerns about safety.
     - Cancer.
     - Cardiovascular disease.
     - Future fertility.
  3. Nonmedical issues.
     - Inadequate instructions.
     - Pill packaging.
     - Package insert.
- Overcoming these issues to improve compliance
  1. Explain how OCPs work.
  2. Review the risks and benefits, putting the risks in proper perspective; emphasize the noncontraceptive benefits.
  3. Show the patient the package of pills she will use and demonstrate its use to her.
  4. Explain how to take the pills.
     - When to start.
     - Daily routine.
     - What to do if she misses pills.
  5. Review the possible side effects.
  6. Discuss the warning signs of potential problems.
  7. Ask the patient to call if she has other medications prescribed.
  8. Ensure understanding by having the patient repeat this information.
  9. Schedule a follow-up visit in 1 to 2 months; 3 months is too late.
  10. Keep the lines of communication open.

XVIII. The Progestin-Only Minipill
- Minipills available worldwide.

1. Micronor, Nor-QD, Noriday, Norod	0.350 mg norethindrone
2. Microval, Norgeston, Microlut	0.030 mg norgestrel
3. Ovrette, Neogest	0.075 mg levonorgestrel
4. Exluton	0.500 mg lynestrenol
5. Femulen	0.500 mg ethynodiol diacetate
6. CerazetteR	0.075 mg desogestrel

- Mechanism of action.
  - Contraceptive benefit is dependent upon endometrial and cervical effects.

- Forty percent of patients will ovulate normally.
- Tubal motility may be affected.
- **These pills must be taken at same time each day.**
- The risk of ectopic pregnancy in cases of contraceptive failure is higher; a previous ectopic pregnancy is not a contraindication.
- No significant metabolic effects have been found.
- An immediate return to fecundability is experienced.
- A threefold increase in diabetes exists in women with gestational diabetes who breast-feed; this could result from the unimpeded progestin effect on insulin resistance.

♦ Efficacy.
- Failure rates of 1.1 to 9.6 per 100 women in the first year; higher in younger women (3.1 per 100 woman-years).
- Failure rate equal to that of combination OCPs in motivated women.

♦ Taking the pill.
- Start on day 1 of menses.
- Use a backup method for first 7 days.
- Some women ovulate as early as 7 to 9 days after the onset of menses.
- Missed pills.
  - Resume as soon as possible.
  - Use a backup method for at least 2 days.
  - If >2 pills are missed and no menstrual bleeding occurs in 4 to 6 weeks, then check with a pregnancy test.
  - If pill is taken >3 hours late, then use a backup method for 48 hours.

♦ Problems.
- Irregular bleeding is common.
- Forty percent of women have normal cycles.
- Forty percent have short, irregular cycles.
- Twenty percent have problems ranging from irregular bleeding to spotting to amenorrhea.
- Functional cysts are more common; consider combination OCPs or medroxyprogesterone acetate (Depo-Provera) in patients with a history of recurrent cysts.
- Acne may occur on the levonorgestrel minipill; SHBG is decreased by levonorgestrel.

♦ Clinical decisions.
- Near total effectiveness in the following two clinical situations:
  - Lactating women.
  - Women over 40 years of age.
- Lactation and the minipill.
  - No adverse effect on milk volume or infant growth and development.

- Positive impact seen as women on the minipill breast-feed longer.
- Can start 3 days postpartum.
- Minipill use in situations where estrogen is contraindicated:
  - Diabetes with vascular disease.
  - Severe lupus.
  - Cardiovascular disease.
  - No impact on the coagulation system.
- Other issues.
  - Can be beneficial in women with decreased libido on the combination pill.
  - Should be avoided in women on medications that increase liver metabolism, such as the following:
    ◇ Rifampin.
    ◇ Phenobarbital.
    ◇ Phenytoin (Dilantin).
    ◇ Primidone (Mysoline).
    ◇ Carbamazepine (Tegretol).
    ◇ *Possibly* ethosuximide, griseofulvin, and troglitazone.
  - Protective benefits possibly similar to the combination pill, but data are lacking.

XIX. Emergency Postcoital Contraception
- ♦ The following regimens have been documented to be effective:

  Norgestrel/ethinyl estradiol (Ovral): two tablets followed by two more tablets 12 hours later

  Levonorgestrel/ethinyl estradiol (Alesse): five tablets followed by five additional tablets 12 hours later

  Estrogen/progestin (Lo/Ovral), levonorgestrel/ethinyl estradiol (Nordette, Levlen, Triphasil, Tri-Levlen): four tablets followed by four more tablets 12 hours later

- ♦ Levonorgestrel, 0.75 mg given twice 12 hours apart, is more successful and is better tolerated than the combination method.
- ♦ Uses of emergency contraception:
  - Condom breakage.
  - Sexual assault.
  - Dislodgement of cervical cap or diaphragm.
  - Failure to use contraceptives.
- ♦ Emergency contraception could prevent 1.7 million unwanted pregnancies annually; abortions would decrease by 40%.
  - Patients can be directed to the office of Population Research at Princeton University for additional information (http://ec.princeton.edu/).
  - Consider providing "kits" to patients in advance.
- ♦ Mechanism and efficacy.
  - Not known with certainty, but probably represents interference with ovulation or implantation.

- Failure rates of 0.1% to 3%.
- In general, risk of pregnancy reduced by 75%; 98% effective.
- ◆ Treatment method.
  - Initiate as soon as possible, but no later than 72 hours.
  - Exclude existing pregnancy prior to therapy.
  - Helpful to add an antiemetic like meclizine; if the patient vomits within 1 hour, then redose as soon as possible.
  - Theoretic risk of increasing clotting factors.
    - Avoid in high-risk patients.
    - Consider the levonorgestrel method.
  - Schedule 3-week follow-up visit.
  - Mifepristone also very effective.
    - Six hundred milligrams in a single dose.
    - Less nausea and/or vomiting; equally effective.
  - IUD insertion (copper IUD) effective; not useful for rape victims or patients with multiple sex partners.
- XX. Oral Contraception for Older Women
  - ◆ Aging of the baby boom generation has three specific reproductive impacts as follows:
    1. Need for effective contraception.
    2. Problems of achieving pregnancy later in life.
    3. Problems of being pregnant later in life.
  - ◆ Between the ages of the 20 to 44, American women have the highest proportion of pregnancies aborted.
    - Half of all U.S. pregnancies are unplanned.
    - More than half of these are aborted.
  - ◆ OCPs for the transition years.
    - These are considered as the years from the age of 35 to menopause.
    - Preventive health issues are important.
      - Need for contraception.
      - Management of anovulation.
      - Menopausal and postmenopausal HRT.
    - The frequency of ovulation decreases in women over 40 years of age; inadequate luteal function is more common.
    - Smoking is a contraindication to use in women over 35 years of age.
      - A former smoker must have stopped at least 12 months previously.
      - Current use of gum or patches qualifies as a smoker.
    - Consider the use of the 20-µg pill as many women may not be honest about tobacco use; 20 µg has no impact on clotting factors.
    - The progestin-only minipill is also a very good choice.
    - The incidence of dysfunctional uterine bleeding increases during this period.
      - Consider serum progestin levels to document ovulation.

- ■ Avoid endometrial hyperplasia.
- • Anovulatory woman with proliferative or hyperplastic endometrium.
  - ■ Ten milligrams medroxyprogesterone acetate for 10 days/month; document the regression of hyperplasia.
  - ■ Consider the use of combination OCPs.
- • Use of postmenopausal regimens is not appropriate.
  - ■ These will not prevent ovulation.
  - ■ The addition of estrogen without concomitant progestin is inappropriate in the absence of menopausal symptoms.
- ◆ When to change from OCPs to HRT.
  - • Even a 20-μg estrogen dose is four times greater than the standard HRT doses.
  - • Measure FSH level annually after the age of 50.
    - ■ Obtain sample on day 6 to 7 of the pill-free week.
    - ■ Change to HRT when FSH is >20 IU/L.

XXI. Concluding Thoughts
- ◆ Use of OCPs yields an overall improvement in individual health.
- ◆ They are a component of good preventive care.
- ◆ The clinician's attitude toward the use of OCPs is very important.

Long-Acting Methods of Contraception

I. Introduction
   - Long-acting methods simplify compliance.
   - The following two methods are available:
     1. Progesterone implant (Norplant).
     2. Medroxyprogesterone acetate injection (Depo-Provera).
   - These are as effective as sterilization and intrauterine devices and are more effective than barrier or oral contraceptives (OCPs); they require little user effort.
II. Norplant
   - Six capsules, 34-mm length, 2.4-mm outer diameter.
   - Thirty-six milligrams of crystalline levonorgestrel are in each capsule.
   - The capsules are made of medical-grade silastic tubing and are sealed with silastic medical adhesive.
   - The hormone is stable for 9 years.
     - Shelf life of 5 years.
     - Five to 7 years of effective life once inserted.
     - Store in cool dry area.
   - Mechanism of action.
     - Levonorgestrel diffuses through the wall of the tubing.
     - Plasma concentrations reach 0.4 ng to 0.5 ng/mL within 24 hours; the patient should use a backup method for 3 days.
     - Eighty-five micrograms of levonorgestrel are released every 24 hours during the first 12 months; this declines to 50 µg every 24 hours by 9 months and to 30 µg per 24 hours for the remainder. The dose is equivalent to the progestin-only minipill and is 25% to 50% of the dose in low-dose combined OCPs.
     - A mean concentration <0.20 ng/mL is associated with increased pregnancy rates.
     - Body weight affects circulating levels; the greatest decrease is found in women >70 kg (154 lbs).
     - Sex hormone–binding globulin (SHBG) levels also affect levonorgestrel levels; SHBG levels drop in the first week and then increase to one-half of the preinsertion levels by 1 year of use.
   - Three possible mechanisms are as follows:
     1. Suppresses luteinizing hormone (LH) surge at the level of the hypothalamus and pituitary.
        - Ten percent of women ovulate in the first 2 years, 50% by 5 years.
        - A high incidence of luteal insufficiency is seen.
     2. Thickens the cervical mucus.
     3. Suppresses estradiol-induced endometrial maturation → atrophy; could prevent implantation, but

no evidence of fertilization is seen in Norplant users.

- ◆ Advantages.
  - • Safe and highly effective (close to theoretic effectiveness).
  - • Requires little user effort.
  - • Progestin-only method.
  - • Constant hormone levels.
  - • Excellent postpartum choice, breast-feeding is okay.
  - • No adverse lipid effects.
  - • Prompt return of fertility.
- ◆ Disadvantages.
  - • Eighty percent of patients experience abnormal bleeding patterns.
  - • It must be inserted and/or removed by a surgical procedure; a 5% complication rate of removal is found.
  - • Implants can be visible under the skin.
  - • It provides no protection against STDs.
  - • It has a high initial cost.
- ◆ Indications—consider in women who are characterized by the following:
  1. Desire spacing of future pregnancies.
  2. Desire a highly effective long-term method.
  3. Experience estrogen-related side effects with OCPs.
  4. Have difficulty remembering to take a daily pill.
  5. Have completed childbearing but do not desire sterilization.
  6. Have a history of anemia and heavy bleeding.
  7. Have chronic illnesses and wish to avoid pregnancy.
- ◆ Absolute contraindications are as follows:
  1. **ACTIVE** thrombophlebitis or thromboembolic disease.
  2. Undiagnosed genital bleeding.
  3. **ACUTE** liver disease.
  4. Benign or malignant liver tumors.
  5. Known or suspected breast cancer.
- ◆ Relative contraindications include the following:
  1. Heavy tobacco use in women >35 years of age.
  2. History of ectopic pregnancy.
  3. Diabetes.
  4. Hypercholesterolemia.
  5. Hypertension.
  6. History of cardiovascular disease.
     - • Myocardial infarction (MI), cerebrovascular accident, angina, or a previous thromboembolic event.
     - • Artificial heart valve.
  7. Gallbladder disease.
  8. Chronic disease.
- ◆ Other methods preferable to Norplant may be considered in patients with the following:
  1. Severe acne.

2. Severe vascular or migraine headaches.
3. Severe depression.
4. Concomitant use of medications that induce microsomal liver enzymes (because of a significant reduction in efficacy). These include phenytoin, carbamazepine, and rifampin.

♦ Efficacy.
  • Norplant is highly effective: 0.2 pregnancies per 100 woman-years; most pregnancies occur at the time of insertion.
  • The failure rate is higher in U.S. trials.
    ▪ Denser capsules.
    ▪ Heavier patients; but pregnancy rates are still lower than for OCPs.
  • Thirty percent of the failures are ectopic pregnancies (Table 23.1).

♦ Menstrual effects.
  • Eighty percent report irregular menses in the first year; this decreases to 33% by the fifth year.
  • Enlarged venous sinusoids are responsible for abnormal bleeding; it can also result from reduced expression of a protein factor involved in the initiation of hemostasis.
  • Overall menstrual blood loss decreases.
  • Prolonged bleeding may respond to conjugated estrogens or prostaglandin (PG) inhibitors.
  • Evaluate for pregnancy if the patient becomes amenorrheic.

♦ Metabolic effects.
  • No significant effects on metabolism; lipoprotein profile is unchanged.
  • No decrease in adolescent bone density.

♦ Future fertility.
  • Circulating levels are undetectable within 48 hours of removal.
  • No long-term effect on fertility has been observed; Depo-Provera can result in 18-month delay of fertility.

♦ Side effects.
  • Serious side effects are rare.
  • The most common side effect is headache; 20% of women who discontinue use do so because of headache.
  • An increase in appetite can occur; a 5-year follow-up reveals no increase in body mass index (BMI).
  • Mastalgia usually improves over time; effective treatments include the following:
    ▪ Danazol, 200 mg/day.
    ▪ Vitamin E, 600 U/day.
    ▪ Bromocriptine, 2.5 mg/day.
    ▪ Tamoxifen, 20 mg/day.
  • Galactorrhea can be common in postpartum insertions.
  • Acne is a common complaint; it is caused by a decrease in the SHBG levels.

**Table 23.1.   Failure rates during
the first year of use, United States**

Method	Percentage of Women with Pregnancy	
	Lowest Expected	Typical
No method	85.0%	85.0%
Combination pill	0.1%	3.0%
Progestin only	0.5%	3.0%
IUDs		
Progesterone IUD	1.5%	2.0%
Levonorgestrel IUD	0.6%	0.8%
Copper T 380A	0.1%	0.1%
Norplant	0.05%	0.05%
Female sterilization	0.05%	0.05%
Male sterilization	0.1%	0.15%
Depo-Provera	0.3%	0.3%
Spermicides	6.0%	26.0%
Periodic abstinence		25.0%
Calendar	9.0%	
Ovulation method	3.0%	
Symptothermal	2.0%	
Postovulation	1.0%	
Withdrawal	4.0%	19.0%
Cervical cap		
Parous women	26.0%	40.0%
Nulliparous women	9.0%	20.0%
Sponge		
Parous women	9.0%	28.0%
Nulliparous women	6.0%	18.0%
Diaphragm and spermicides	6.0%	20.0%
Condom		
Male	3.0%	14.0%
Female	5.0%	21.0%

Abbreviation: IUD, intrauterine device.

- Ovarian cysts can form since follicle-stimulating hormone (FSH) is not suppressed; adrenal masses are 8× more frequent in comparison with normally cycling women.
- It is possibly linked to an increase in herpes simplex virus outbreaks.
- Cancer risk is as follows:
  - Epidemiologic data is needed, but the risk of endometrial cancer should be reduced.
  - The risk of ovarian cancer may also be lowered.
- Patient evaluation.
  - Risks and benefits need to be reviewed.

- Insertion can occur at any time in the menstrual cycle.
  - Insert in the third postpartum week in non–breast-feeding women.
  - Insert in the third postpartum month in breast-feeding women.
- Upper inner arm placement is usually preferred.
◆ Reasons for termination.
  - Only 30% of women continue for the full 5 years.
  - Menstrual changes account for discontinuing therapy in most women.
  - Other common reasons are as follows:
    - Headache.
    - Weight change.
    - Mood changes.
    - Ovarian cyst formation.
    - Lower abdominal pain.
    - Skin conditions.
◆ User acceptance.
  - Highly acceptable ease of use.
  - Implants noticed by friends and family of 20% of U.S. patients; only 25% of the patients are bothered by this attention.
◆ Counseling women.
  - Frank and open discussion is needed to address the concerns of women.
  - Many women may not be aware of the advantages and disadvantages.

III. Levonorgestrel Rod
  ◆ A new system of two implants to replace the discontinued Norplant-2 is under clinical-trial evaluation.
  ◆ Removal is faster and easier.

IV. New Developments in Implant Contraception
  ◆ 3-Keto-desogestrel (Implanon).
    - Single implant of 60 mg of 3-keto-desogestrel; hormone is released at a rate of 60 µg/day.
    - Provides contraception for 2 to 3 years.
    - Efficacy and side effects similar to Norplant.
  ◆ Nomegestrol acetate (Uniplant).
    - Thirty-eight milligrams of nomegestrol acetate; releases 100 µg/day.
    - Provides contraception for 1 year.
  ◆ Levonorgestrel (Capronor).
    - Single capsule, biodegradable.
    - Levonorgestrel-releasing.
    - Provides 1 year of contraceptives.
    - Circulating levels of 0.2 to 0.3 ng/mL.
    - Capsule disappears after 12 months.
  ◆ Norethindrone (Anuelle).
    - Biodegradable norethindrone pellet.
    - Could provide contraception for up to 3 years.

V. Depo-Provera
  ◆ Most thoroughly studied progestin-only contraceptive.
  ◆ Approved in United States in 1992; studied for decades in other countries.

- ◆ Microcrystals suspended in an aqueous solution; 150 mg intramuscularly (IM) every 3 months.
- ◆ Contraceptive level maintained for at least 14 weeks.
- ◆ Mechanism of action.
  - Thickens the cervical mucus.
  - Effectively blocks the LH surge; some follicular growth is maintained.
  - Treatment initiated during the first week of menses.
- ◆ Efficacy.
  - Equal to sterilization; better than all of the temporary methods.
  - Not influenced by weight or by medications that stimulate hepatic enzymes; good for epileptics because high progestin levels raise the seizure threshold.
- ◆ Indications.
  1. One year of spacing between births is desired.
  2. Highly effective and long-acting.
  3. Estrogen-free.
  4. Breast-feeding.
  5. Sickle cell disease.
  6. Seizure disorder.
- ◆ Absolute contraindications.
  1. Pregnancy.
  2. Unexplained genital bleeding.
  3. Severe coagulation disorders.
  4. Previous sex steroid–induced liver adenoma.
- ◆ Relative contraindications.
  1. Liver disease.
  2. Severe cardiovascular disease.
  3. Rapid return to fertility desired.
  4. Difficulty with injections.
  5. Severe depression.
- ◆ Advantages.
  - No compliance issues.
  - Useful in those who have difficulty remembering contraceptive requirements.
  - No estrogen-related side effects; in fact, it may have a beneficial impact on those with sickle cell anemia.
  - Increases milk quantity in nursing mothers.
  - Decreases the risk of endometrial cancer.
- ◆ Major problems.
  - Irregular bleeding (70% in the first year).
  - Breast tenderness.
  - Weight gain.
  - Depression.
  - Discontinuation.
    - ■ Thirty-three percent by the first year.
    - ■ Fifty percent by 2 years.
    - ■ Eighty percent by 3 years.
  - No evident increase in depression.
  - Slow return of menses; 25% take a year to resume normal cycles.

♦ Breast cancer.
  • Causes breast tumors in beagle dogs.
  • Reassuring evidence in women.
    ■ Very slight increase in the first 4 years of use; possibly reflects an enhancement of growth of existing tumors.
    ■ No increased risk with increased duration of use.
♦ Metabolic effects.
  • Uncertain impact on lipoprotein profile; suggest annual surveillance.
  • Bone loss unlikely to be sufficient to raise the risk of osteoporosis.
♦ Effect on future fertility.
  • Delay in return of fertility is unique to injectable contraception.
  • Ninety percent are pregnant by 18 months after the last dose.
  • The delay does not increase with increasing duration of use.

VI. Short-Term Injectable Contraceptives
  ♦ Cyclo-Provera and Cyclofem.
    • Twenty-five milligrams Depo-Provera and 5 mg estradiol cypionate.
    • Monthly administration.
    • Rapidly reversible.
    • Will inhibit lactation.
  ♦ Norethindrone ethanthate (Mesigyna).
    • Two hundred milligrams IM every 2 months.
    • Combination of 50 mg norethindrone ethanthate with 5 mg estradiol valerate—can be given monthly.
    • Fewer bleeding problems than Cyclofem.
  ♦ Dihydroxyprogesterone acetophenide with estradiol enanthate.
    • Most widely used in Latin America.
    • Regular monthly bleeding; often even reduced.

VIII. New Developments
  ♦ Microspheres and microcapsules are under evaluation.
  ♦ These can provide constant circulating levels.
  ♦ Menstrual changes are frequent.

The Intrauterine Device (IUD)

I. Historic Perspective
   - Forerunners of modern IUDs were small stem pessaries that were used in the 1800s.
   - 1902—Hollweg developed a pessary that extended into the uterus.
     - Great risk of infection.
     - Required self-insertion.
   - 1909—Richter reported success with a silkworm catgut ring that had nickel and bronze wire protruding through the cervix.
   - 1920s—Gräfenberg removed the tail and pessary but fell victim to the Nazi political philosophy opposing contraception.
   - 1934—Ota made improvements to the Gräfenberg ring to limit expulsion (Fig. 24.1).
   - IUDs were rediscovered in the decades following World War II.
   - IUD use thrived in the 1960s and 1970s.
     - 1962—First International Conference on IUDs.
     - Lippes Loop introduced; had a monofilament tail.
     - 1970—Dalkon Shield was introduced.
       - High incidence of pelvic infection.
       - Multifilament tail.
       - Sales of the Dalkon Shield stopped in 1975.
         - ◇ The call for removal was not issued until the 1980s.
         - ◇ The Dalkon Shield problem has tainted all IUDs since.

II. Sexually Transmitted Diseases (STDs) and the IUD
   - The use of control groups that used oral contraceptives or barrier contraception tainted the initial epidemiologic studies; they also failed to control for the following risk factors:
     - Multiple partners.
     - Early age at first coitus.
     - Increased frequency of coitus.
   - Concern about infection and legal actions against manufacturers led to the removal of IUDs from the U.S. market.
     - Did not return until 1988.
     - Use has decreased:
       - 1982—7.1%.
       - 1988—2%.
       - 1995—0.8%.
   - IUDs are the most widely used method of reversible contraception in the rest of world → 100 million users (Fig. 24.2 and Table 24.1).

III. The Modern IUD
   - The addition of copper was suggested by Jaime Zipper of Chile; copper IUDs could be made smaller

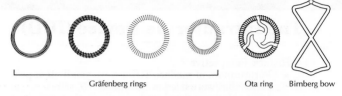

Figure 24.1. Various early intrauterine devices, including the Gräfenberg rings, the Ota ring, and the Birnberg bow.

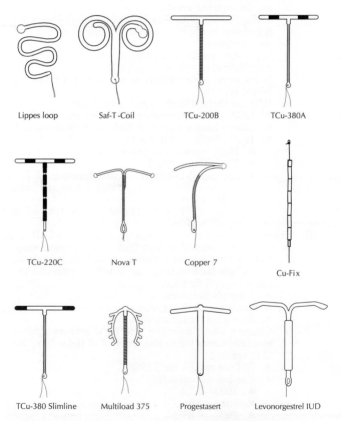

Figure 24.2. Additional intrauterine devices, to the present time.

**Table 24.1.   Use of the IUD
in the United States and the world**

Year	United States	China	Total World
1981	2.2 million women	42 million	60 million
1988	0.7 million women	59 million	83 million
1995	0.3 million women	75 million	106 million

Abbreviation: IUD, intrauterine device.

       since copper may be spermicidal or it may diminish fertilizing ability or motility.
- ♦ Copper IUDs Cu-7 and Tatum-T were removed from the U.S. market in 1986.
- ♦ The Population Council developed TCu-380A.
  - 380 mm^2 of exposed copper surface, including the sleeve on each arm.
  - Used in 30 countries since 1982; marketed in the United States in 1988 as ParaGard.
- ♦ The progesterone-releasing IUD (Progestasert) was developed by Alza Corporation.
  - T-shaped device releases progesterone, 65 μg/day, for 1 year.
  - It decreases blood loss and cramping.
IV. Types of IUDs
  - ♦ Unmedicated IUDs.
    - The Lippes Loop is still used throughout the world, except in the United States.
    - Flexible stainless steel rings are used in China.
  - ♦ Copper IUDs.
    - Initially wound with 200 to 250 mm^2 of wire; TCu-200 and Multiload 250 are still used outside the United States.
    - Modern copper IUDs have more copper.
      - TCu-380A.
      - TCu-220C.
      - Nova-T.
      - Multiload-375.
      - Sof-T (Swiss).
      - Several copper IUD variants are used in China.
    - TCu-380A.
      - Has 380 mm^2 of exposed copper.
      - Has a 0.36-mm stem.
      - Monofilament tail.
      - Barium for x-ray detection in the frame.
      - Variations on this model:
        - ◊ TCu-380 Ag (silver core).
        - ◊ TCu-380 Slimline.
  - ♦ Hormone-releasing IUDs.
    - Progestasert.
      - The T-shaped IUD is made of ethylene/vinyl acetate copolymer; it contains titanium dioxide.

- ■ The vertical stem contains 38 mg progesterone.
- ■ The horizontal arms are solid.
- ■ It releases progesterone, 65 µg/day.
- • LNG-20.
  - ■ T-shaped IUD with a collar containing 52 mg levonorgestrel; releases 15 µg/day.
  - ■ Lasts up to 10 years.
  - ■ Reduces menstrual blood loss and pelvic inflammatory disease (PID) infection rates.
- ◆ Future IUDs: modifications of copper IUDs are being studied.
  - • Ombrelle-250 and Ombrelle-380 are more flexible.
  - • FlexiGard, Cu-Fix, and GyneFix.
    - ■ Frameless IUD with six copper sleeves.
    - ■ Low rate of removal but more difficult insertion.

V. Mechanism of Action
- ◆ The contraceptive action is limited to the uterine cavity.
  - • Ovulation not affected.
  - • Not an abortifacient.
- ◆ A sterile inflammatory response is created.
  - • Very few (if any) sperm reach the ovum.
  - • The inflammatory response would also prevent implantation.
- ◆ The copper IUD releases free copper and copper salts.
  - • Biochemical and morphologic effect on the endometrium.
  - • Produces alterations in the cervical mucus.
  - • No measurable increase in serum copper levels.
  - • Enhanced inflammatory response.
- ◆ Progestin-releasing IUDs.
  - • The endometrium is decidualized, and implantation is inhibited.
  - • Sperm capacitation and survival are reduced.
  - • Levonorgestrel IUD users have serum levels of progestin equal to half those of Norplant users.
  - • The cervical mucus is thicker.
  - • Decreased menstrual blood loss occurs; hemoglobin and iron levels rise within 1 year.
- ◆ No delay in return to normal fertility; no evidence of infection leading to infertility.

VI. Efficacy of IUDs
- ◆ Intrauterine pregnancy.
  - • The actual failure rate for all IUDs is 3%.
    - ■ Ten percent expulsion rate.
    - ■ Fifteen percent removal rate (Table 24.2).
  - • The TCu-380A has an even better record; failure rate is less than with the use of oral contraceptives (Table 24.3).
- ◆ Ectopic pregnancy.
  - • Previous IUD use does not increase the risk of a subsequent ectopic pregnancy.
  - • The current use of a non–progestin-releasing IUD offers protection against ectopic pregnancy.

**Table 24.2.   First-year clinical
trial experience in parous women**

Device	Pregnancy Rate	Expulsion Rate	Removal Rate
Lippes Loop	3%	12% to 20%	12% to 15%
Cu–7	2% to 3%	6%	11%
TCu–200	3%	8%	11%
TCu–380A	0.5% to 0.8%	5%	14%
Progesterone IUD	1.3% to 1.6%	2.7%	9.3%
Levonorgestrel IUD	0.2%	6%	17%

Abbreviation: IUD, intrauterine device.

- IUD users are 50% less likely to have an ectopic pregnancy than are those using no contraception; however, when an IUD user becomes pregnant, the pregnancy is more likely to be ectopic.
- TCu-380A users are 90% less likely to have an ectopic pregnancy when compared with non–contraceptive users.
- In 8,000 woman-years of experience with TCu-380A, only 1 ectopic pregnancy has been reported; a 7-year study with the levonorgestrel IUD had NO ectopics.
- **The protection against ectopic pregnancy provided by the TCu-380A and the levonorgestrel IUD makes these IUDs acceptable choices for contraception in women with previous ectopic pregnancies (Table 24.4).**

VII. Side Effects
- No associated risk of infertility is observed even if IUDs are removed for problems.
- The most common complaints (5% to 15% of women) are as follows:
  - Increased uterine bleeding.
  - Increased menstrual pain.
- Treatment with nonsteroidal antiinflammatory drugs (NSAIDs) or a progesterone IUD may aid in reducing these problems.
- Menstrual blood loss with the copper IUD increases by 55%, and menstrual bleeding is prolonged × 1 to 2 days.
- Amenorrhea can develop with progestin-containing IUDs; these can also result in androgenic side effects.
- The copper IUD is safe for magnetic resonance imaging (MRI) examination.
- The copper IUD may also reduce endometrial and cervical cancer rates.

VIII. Infections
- IUD-related bacterial infections are linked to insertion; infections occurring after 3 to 4 months are believed to be acquired STDs.

Table 24.3.   Ten-year experience with Paragard, TCu-380A: rate per 100 users per year

	Year									
	1	2	3	4	5	6	7	8	9	10
Pregnancy	0.7	0.3	0.6	0.2	0.3	0.2	0.0	0.4	0.0	0.0
Expulsion	5.7	2.5	1.6	1.2	0.3	0.0	0.6	1.7	0.2	0.4
Bleeding/pain removal	11.9	9.8	7.0	3.5	3.7	2.7	3.0	2.5	2.2	3.7
Medical removals	2.5	2.1	1.6	1.7	0.1	0.3	1.0	0.4	0.7	0.3
Continuation	76.8	78.3	81.2	86.2	89.0	91.9	87.9	88.1	92.0	91.8
Number starting each year	4,932	3,149	2,018	1,121	872	621	563	483	423	325

Data from Population Council (n = 3,536) and World Health Organization (n = 1,396) trials.

Table 24.4. Ectopic pregnancy rates per 1,000 woman-years

Non–contraceptive users, all ages	3.00 to 4.50
Progesterone IUD (based on small numbers; thus, probably the same as non–contraceptive users)	6.80
Levonorgestrel IUD	0.20
TCu–380A IUD	0.20

Abbreviation: IUD, intrauterine device.

- ◆ The risk of infection is very low (81 per 23,000 insertions); prophylactic antibiotics are of little benefit in low-risk patients.
- ◆ IUDs offer little protection against STDs.
  - • Copper may inhibit chlamydia.
  - • Levonorgestrel IUD may have an STD-protective benefit.
- ◆ IUDs can be used in patients at risk of bacterial endocarditis; prophylaxis should be provided 1 hour prior to insertion.
- ◆ The treatment of STDs is unchanged, and the IUD can be left in place as long as no symptoms of upper tract infection are observed.
- ◆ PID treatment.
  - • *Appropriate outpatient management of less severe infections is as follows:*
    Cefoxitin (2 g intramuscularly [IM]) plus probenecid (1 g orally), **or**
    Ceftriaxone (250 mg IM) plus doxycycline (200 mg BID orally) for 14 days.
  - • *Severe infections require hospitalization and treatment with the following:*
    Cefoxitin (2 g intravenously [IV] every 6 hours) **or**
    Cefotetan (2 g IV every 12 hours)
    Plus doxycycline (100 mg BID orally or IV)
    Followed by 14 days of an oral regimen of antibiotics.
  - • *The following is an alternative regimen:*
    Clindamycin (900 mg IV every 8 hours) plus Gentamicin (2 mg/kg IV or IM followed by 1.5 mg/kg every 8 hours).
  - • Use of an IUD is acceptable in human immunodeficiency virus (HIV)-positive women; no association has been found between IUD use and the acquisition of HIV.
- ◆ *Actinomyces.*
  - • The significance of actinomycosis infection in IUD users is unclear.
    - ▪ Thirty percent of plastic IUD users have this organism on Pap test.
    - ▪ This declines to only 1% or less with copper devices.

- Infection is usually asymptomatic; if it is, leave the IUD in place—no evidence of a need to treat this finding exists.
- Treat symptomatic patients with oral penicillin G 500 mg QID × 1 month; remove the IUD after the initiation of treatment.

IX. Pregnancy with an IUD *In Situ*
   ♦ Spontaneous miscarriage.
      - More frequent in IUD users with an IUD in place (40% to 50%).
      - Remove IUD if pregnancy is diagnosed and IUD string is visible; rate of loss is 35% after removal, but with easy removal or spontaneous expulsion of the IUD in the first trimester, the loss rate is not increased.
   ♦ Septic abortion.
      - No increased risk of septic abortion is observed except with the Dalkon Shield.
      - Removal of an IUD from an infected uterus requires the initiation of antibiotic therapy prior to removal; prepare for the possibility of septic shock.
   ♦ Other complications.
      - No increased risk of congenital anomalies.
      - Fourfold increase in preterm labor and delivery.

X. IUD Insertion
   ♦ Patient selection.
      - Selection requires careful attention to menstrual history and risk for STDs.
      - Contraindications include current, recent, or recurrent PID.
      - Nulliparous and nulligravid women can use the IUD.
      - Women with a distorted uterine cavity are not good candidates.
      - Women with Wilson disease should not use the copper IUD; the risk is theoretic.
      - Immunosuppressed patients should not use an IUD.
      - Diabetics can use an IUD; in fact, an IUD may be an ideal choice.
   ♦ Patient insertion.
      - A careful speculum and bimanual examination is essential.
      - The uterine position must be documented; perforation is more common with a severely retroverted uterus.
      - The depth of the uterus should be between 6 and 9 cm.
      - The absence of infection should be established.
   ♦ Key points in patient counseling—prospective IUD users should be aware of the following important possibilities:
      1. Protection against unwanted pregnancy begins immediately after insertion.

2. Menses can be longer and heavier (except with hormonal IUDs); tampons can be used.
3. A slightly increased risk of pelvic infection exists in the first few months after insertion.
4. Protection against infections transmitted through the vaginal mucosa requires the use of condoms.
5. Ectopic pregnancies can still occur.
6. The IUD can be spontaneously expelled; monthly palpation of the IUD strings is important to avoid unwanted pregnancies. If the strings are not felt or if something hard is palpable (suggestive of the IUD frame), a clinician should be notified as soon as possible. Backup contraception should be provided until the patient can be examined.

♦ Timing of insertion.
  • It can be inserted at any time after pregnancy, but insertion is usually done 4 to 8 weeks postpartum.
  • Insertion may be easier during or shortly after menses.
    ■ The expulsion rate may be lower if done after day 11.
    ■ The infection rate may be lower if done after day 17.
♦ Insertion technique for TCu-380A and Progestasert.
  • Clean the cervix with chlorhexidine or povidone–iodine.
  • Leave an antiseptic-soaked, cotton-tipped applicator in the cervical canal.
  • Place a paracervical block; it may include 0.4 mg atropine to decrease vaginal response.
  • Wait 2 to 3 minutes before proceeding.
  • Sound the uterus.
  • Load the IUD.
  • Insert to the level of the fundus and then withdraw a few millimeters and release the IUD.
  • Trim the string to 4 cm from the external os.
  • Check after each menses for the presence of string; follow up after 3 months.
♦ Prophylactic antibiotics—no clear benefit of doxycycline or azithromycin usage.

XI. Summary: IUD Use and Medical Conditions
1. A woman with a previous ectopic pregnancy can use a copper IUD or the levonorgestrel IUD.
2. Women with heavy menses and dysmenorrhea, including women who have a bleeding disorder or are anticoagulated, should consider a progestin-releasing IUD.
3. Women at risk of bacterial endocarditis should receive prophylactic antibiotics at the times of insertion and removal.
4. Current, recent, or recurrent PID is a contraindication for IUD use.
5. Women with diabetes mellitus, whether insulin-dependent or non–insulin-dependent, can use IUDs.

6. IUD insertion is relatively easier in breast-feeding women, and the rates of expulsion and uterine perforation are not increased.

XII. IUD Removal
- ♦ Grasp the string with ring forceps and exert firm traction; use a cytobrush or cotton-tipped applicator to probe for strings.
- ♦ Sonographic or hysteroscopic guidance may be helpful for embedded IUDs.
- ♦ Fertility returns promptly after removal.
- ♦ Use antibiotics if placement of a new IUD is desired.
- ♦ Displaced IUDs.
  - • A sonogram is very helpful.
  - • Abdominal x-rays may be needed.
  - • Perforated IUDs require laparoscopy for removal; this most often occurs at insertion.

XIII. IUD Myths
1. **IUDs are *NOT* abortifacients.**
2. **An increased risk of infection with the modern IUD is related *ONLY* to the insertion.**
3. **The modern IUD *HAS NOT* exposed clinicians to litigation.**
4. **IUDs *DO NOT* increase the risk of ectopic pregnancy.**

XIV. IUDs for Older Women
- ♦ A good reversible choice for older women.
- ♦ Removal may be necessary because of changes in bleeding patterns.

Barrier Methods of Contraception

I. Historic Perspective
   - Widespread and ancient means of contraception.
   - Described in Egyptian papyri from 1850 B.C.
   - Soranus of Ephesus (A.D. 98–138).
     - Explicit instructions on contraceptive technology.
     - Described 40 different combinations.
   - Description of condoms indicates initial attempts to protect against infection.
     - A linen condom was described in 1564 by Fallopius; the origin of the term "condom" remains mysterious.
     - 1850—Rubber condoms were available in the United States.
   - The diaphragm was first described in papers published in the 1880s.
     - C. Haase described its use under the pseudonym of Wilhelm P.J. Mensinga.
     - It was predated by the cervical cap (1860), which was very popular in Europe by the 1930s.
   - Spermicidal products were marketed by the 1950s.
   - 1961—C. Lee Buxton (Chair at Yale) and Estelle Griswold (Executive Director of Connecticut Planned Parenthood) were arrested and fined for opening Planned Parenthood clinics.
     - 1965—The Supreme Court overturned the Connecticut law on contraceptives.
     - Until 1975, some states still had laws preventing contraceptive distribution (Table 25.1).
II. Risks and Benefits Common to All Barrier Methods
   - Fifty percent reduction of sexually transmitted diseases (STDs) and pelvic inflammatory disease (PID); only condoms have been shown to prevent human immunodeficiency virus (HIV).
   - Reduction in the risk of cervical cancer.
   - Should avoid use of the diaphragm or cervical cap in women with a history of toxic shock syndrome.
   - No protection against preeclampsia.
III. The Diaphragm
   - Distribution of diaphragms led to Margaret Sanger's arrest in New York City in 1918.
   - By 1940, it was used by one-third of U.S. women employing contraceptives; this decreased to 10% with introduction of oral contraceptive pills (OCPs) and fell to 1.9% in 1995.
   - Failure rates of 2% to 23% are seen; however, no studies have examined the use of spermicide with the diaphragm.

**Table 25.1.   Failure rates during
the first year of use, United States**

Method	Percentage of Women with Pregnancy	
	Lowest Expected	Typical
No method	85.0%	85.0%
Combination pill	0.1%	3.0%
Progestin only	0.5%	3.0%
IUDs		
Progesterone IUD	1.5%	2.0%
Levonorgestrel IUD	0.6%	0.8%
Copper T 380A	0.1%	0.1%
Norplant	0.05%	0.05%
Female sterilization	0.05%	0.05%
Male sterilization	0.1%	0.15%
Depo-Provera	0.3%	0.3%
Spermicides	6.0%	26.0%
Periodic abstinence		25.0%
Calendar	9.0%	
Ovulation method	3.0%	
Symptothermal	2.0%	
Postovulation	1.0%	
Withdrawal	4.0%	19.0%
Cervical cap		
Parous women	26.0%	40.0%
Nulliparous women	9.0%	20.0%
Sponge		
Parous women	9.0%	28.0%
Nulliparous women	6.0%	18.0%
Diaphragm and spermicides	6.0%	20.0%
Condom		
Male	3.0%	14.0%
Female	5.0%	21.0%

Abbreviation: IUD, intrauterine device.

- ♦ Side effects.
  - • Vaginal irritation.
  - • Urinary tract infections (UTIs) possibly increased 2 to 3×.
    - ■ Consider prophylactic antibiotics in patients who are at risk.
    - ■ Single postcoital dose of one of the following:
      - ◇ Trimethoprim/sulfamethoxazole, one tablet.
      - ◇ Nitrofurantoin, 50 to 100 mg.
      - ◇ Cephalexin, 250 mg.

- No link with toxic shock syndrome but best to remove after 24 hours.
- Reduces PID and STDs (except HIV—no data).
- The three types of diaphragms (sizes from 50 to 105 mm; most women, 65 to 80 mm) are as follows:
  1. Flat metal or coil spring.
  2. Arching diaphragm (All-Flex).
  3. Hinged—may be easier to insert.
- Fitting—successful use depends on a proper fitting, which needs to be rechecked every year.
- Timing.
  - Insert no longer than 6 hours prior to coitus; place spermicide in dome and along the rim.
  - Leave in place for 6 to 24 hours after coitus.
- Care of the diaphragm—wash with soap and water after each use and store in a cool, dark place.

IV. The Cervical Cap
- Only the Prentif cavity-rim cervical cap has been approved for U.S. use.
- It is as effective as the diaphragm, but it is harder to fit; it is less effective in parous women.
- It can be left in place for 48 hours.
- Spermicide is beneficial.
- Fitting is critical; four sizes are available.
- Remove 8 to 48 hours after coitus.
- No evidence exists of the cap causing toxic shock or dysplasia.

V. The Contraceptive Sponge
- Polyurethane disc impregnated with nonoxynol-9.
- Currently not available in the United States.
- Efficacy is lower than with the diaphragm or condom.
- Provides protection for 24 hours.
- Possible concern about increased HIV transmission due to vaginal mucosal damage.

VI. Spermicides
- Modern spermicides were introduced in the 1950s.
  - Certain surface active agents damage sperm cell membranes.
  - They also provide STD protection.
- Their efficacy ranges from 1% to 25% rate of failure in the first year of use.
- They require application from 10 to 30 minutes prior to coitus; tablets and suppositories are effective for less than 1 hour.
- Douches are ineffective.
- Spermicides are inexpensive and widely available; they should not be used without condoms if the primary objective is STD prevention.
- Side effects are rare.

Representative Products

Vaginal contraceptive film	VCF (70 mg nonoxynol-9)
Foams	Delfen (nonoxynol-9, 12.5%)
	Emko (nonoxynol-9, 8%)
	Koromex (nonoxynol-9, 12.5%)

Jellies and Creams	Conceptrol (nonoxynol-9, 4%)
	Delfen (nonoxynol-9, 12.5%)
	Ortho Gynol (nonoxynol-9, 3%)
	Ramses (nonoxynol-9, 5%)
	Koromex Jelly (nonoxynol-9, 3%)
Suppositories	Encare (nonoxynol-9, 2.27%)
	Koromex Inserts (nonoxynol-9, 125 mg)
	Semicid (nonoxynol-9, 100 mg)

VII. Condoms
   - The male condom is the only contraceptive proven to prevent HIV.
   - Goals are correct use, consistent use, and affordable, easy availability.
   - Latex condoms are 0.3 to 0.8 mm thick.
   - Organisms can penetrate "natural skin" condoms made from lamb intestines.
   - The use of spermicide is helpful; it may increase the incidence of *Escherichia coli* bacteriuria and UTIs.
   - The polyurethane condom may have higher rate of breakage.
   - Proper usage is important.
   - **Summary—Key steps for maximal condom efficacy**
     1. Use condoms for every act of coitus.
     2. Place the condom before vaginal contact.
     3. Withdraw while the penis is still erect.
     4. Hold the base of the condom during withdrawal.
     5. Use a spermicide or a condom lubricated with a spermicide.
   - Inconsistent use explains most failures.
     - Breakage rates of 1 to 8 per 100 episodes of vaginal intercourse.
     - The major risks are pregnancy and STD transmission.
   - Provide emergency OCP therapy in cases of breakage.
   - The female condom.
     - Made of polyurethane.
     - High cost and low acceptability (Table 25.2).

Table 25.2. Comparison of methods of female barrier contraceptive devices

	Diaphragm	Cap	Sponge	Female Condom
Insertion before coitus, no longer than	6 h	6 h	24 h	8 h
After coitus, should be left in place for	6 h	8 h	6 h	6 h
Maximal wear time	24 h	48 h	30 h	8 h

Female Infertility

I. Introduction
   - Infertility is defined as 1 year of unprotected coitus without conception.
   - It affects between 10% and 15% of couples of reproductive age.
   - Fecundability—the probability of achieving pregnancy within one menstrual cycle (about 25%).
   - Fecundity—the ability to achieve a live birth with one menstrual cycle.
   - Three major changes in infertility practice include the following:
     1. Introduction of *in vitro* fertilization (IVF) and other assisted-reproductive technology (ART) procedures.
     2. Increased public awareness.
     3. Increased proportion of women over the age of 35; one-fifth of U.S. women are having their first child after 35 years of age.

II. Epidemiology
   - The decline in U.S. fertility is accounted for by several social changes.
     - Sixteen percent is accounted for by the increased age at marriage.
     - Eighty-three percent is the result of change in marital fertility rates.
   - The proportion of births accounted for by the older population has increased; the aging baby boom generation is seeking to accomplish pregnancy in the shortest time possible.
   - Concern with infertility.
     - A marked increase in the demand for fertility services.
       - Total of 600,000 visits in 1968.
       - Approximately 1,000,000 visits per year in the 1970s.
       - More than 2,000,000 visits every year in the 1980s.
     - The data on fertility services in 1995 show that 15% of women of reproductive age used some infertility service.
       - ART—1%.
       - Ovulation drugs—3%.
     - The overall percentage of infertile women increased from 8.4% in 1984 and 1988 to 10.2% in 1995.
       - Aging of the baby boomers.
       - Increase in sexually transmitted diseases (STDs).
       - Increased awareness about infertility.
     - Fifty-six percent of women with impaired fecundity do not seek care.

III. Aging and Fertility
- ♦ The following two factors affect fertility:
    1. Aging of the reproductive system.
        - • One-third of women in their mid to late 30s will have infertility.
        - • It affects half of women >40.
    2. Increase in spontaneous pregnancy loss.
        - • Women >30 years of age: 10%.
        - • Late 30s: 18%.
        - • Early 40s: 34%.
            - ■ Rate of preclinical and clinical pregnancy loss in women >40: 75%.
            - ■ Possibly the result of impaired meiotic spindle formation in older eggs.
- ♦ The Hutterites are an example of ideal fertility.
- • Infertility rate: 2.4%.
- • Average age at last pregnancy: 40.9.
    - ■ Women who are infertile after the age of 34: 11%.
    - ■ Infertile by 40: 33%.
    - ■ Infertile by 45: 87%.
- ♦ French donor insemination data provide 1-year pregnancy rates:
    - • Women <31 → 74%.
    - • Women 31 to 35 → 62%.
    - • Women >35 → 54%.
- ♦ Netherlands donor insemination data demonstrated the following:
    - • The probability of live birth decreases by 3.5% per year after the age of 30.
    - • A woman who is 35 years of age has half the chance of live birth that a woman who is 25 years old does.
- ♦ The following changes occur in the male reproductive system with aging.
    - • Paternal age >40 is associated with a 20% increase in birth defects.
    - • The decline in testosterone and the increase in gonadotropin are associated with decreased sperm production.
- ♦ Endocrine changes with aging.
    - • Accelerated follicular loss occurs in the last 10 to 15 years before menopause.
        - ■ Begins when the total number of follicles is approximately 25,000 (age 37 to 38).
        - ■ Decreased inhibin and increased follicle-stimulating hormone (FSH); reduced quality and/or capability of aging follicles.
    - • Subtle changes in menstrual cycles; shorter follicular phases.
        - ■ Increased FSH, normal luteinizing hormone (LH), and normal luteal phase.
        - ■ Cycles are shortest in the late 30s; lengthen again prior to menopause.
    - • Incipient ovarian failure.
        - ■ Elevated FSH, decreased inhibin, and normal estradiol.

◊ Inhibin B is the specific inhibin involved in the early follicular phase.
◊ Inhibin A is decreased in the luteal–follicular transition.
- Controversy exists as to whether the rise in FSH represents development of less competent follicles versus a reduced follicular pool. Inhibin A and inhibin B levels are similar in follicular fluid from both old and young patients, so this change in FSH may represent a decrease in the pool of follicles.
- Ovarian volume decreased; <3 cm^3 predicts a poor response to ovulation induction.
♦ Testing the ovarian reserve.
  • FSH levels on cycle day 3 are predictive of response to gonadotropins.
    - Less than 10 IU/L = normal.
    - More than 10 IU/L = abnormal.
    - More than 25 IU/L (or age >44) is independently associated with a near zero chance of pregnancy.
  • Women with a single ovary have higher 3-day FSH levels and reduced IVF success.
  • Elevated estradiol (>80 pg/mL) is also associated with poorer outcome and premature or accelerated follicular recruitment.
♦ Clomiphene citrate challenge test (CCCT).
  • A bioassay of FSH response.
  • Dosage of 100 mg/day on cycle days 5 to 9.
    - Check FSH on days 3 and 10.
    - Sum of FSH levels >26 IU/L = poor prognosis.
  • High incidence of abnormal response in women >35 (26% in women >39); 85% of women with increased FSH respond poorly to stimulation.
♦ Screening recommendations.
  • Cycle day 3 FSH, estradiol, and CCCT.
    - All infertile women >30.
    - Women of any age with unexplained infertility.
    - Women with histories of poor response to ovulation induction.
  • Utility unclear in women >40 years of age.
    - A normal test is not reassuring.
    - An abnormal test may bolster the recommendation for ovum donation.
IV. Assisted Reproduction in Older Couples
  ♦ Uterine factors are not associated with declining fecundity.
    • Older women could probably benefit from an increased progesterone dose (100 mg).
    • A decline in hormone receptors has been suggested.
  ♦ Spontaneous abortion rate is related to the age of the ova donor, which supports the above contention.
V. The Role of the Physician
  ♦ Spontaneous cure pregnancy rate.

- Fifty percent of couples with 1 year of infertility will spontaneously conceive during the next year.
- Only 20% of couples with 2 years of infertility never conceive.
- Infertile couples with a normal evaluation will have a pregnancy rate of 74% over 2 years.
- Forty percent of couples conceive after discontinuing treatment.

♦ The four goals of the physician are as follows:
  1. Seek and correct the causes of infertility.
  2. Provide accurate information.
  3. Provide emotional support.
  4. Advise when to stop.

VI. The Female Infertility Investigation
  ♦ Evolution of practice.
    - Decreased emphasis on diagnosis.
    - Increased movement toward empiric therapy—superovulation with intrauterine insemination (IUI).
  ♦ Etiologies. See Fig. 26.1 and Table 26.1.

VII. The Postcoital Test
  ♦ Perform at the time of the expected LH surge and 2 to 8 hours after coitus.
  ♦ Spinnbarkeit, or the stretchability, should be 8 to 10 cm.
  ♦ Treatment of poor mucus.
    - Consider 0.625 mg conjugated estrogens daily on cycle days 5 to 13; evidence of value for this treatment is lacking.
    - The preferred treatment is IUI; a cumulative pregnancy rate of 40% to 50% over three to four cycles is observed.
  ♦ Limitations of the postcoital test.
    - Not a substitute for semen analysis.
    - Can be repeatedly abnormal in normal couples.
    - An academic exercise to assess sperm–cervical mucus interaction if superovulation or IUI is already planned.

VIII. Hysterosalpingography (HSG)
  ♦ Tubal disease is clearly associated with infertility.
    - Westrom's studies with laparoscopically confirmed pelvic inflammatory disease (PID) and subsequent tubal infertility provide the following data:
      ■ A 12% incidence after one episode.
      ■ A 23% incidence after two episodes.
      ■ A 54% incidence after three episodes.
    - The risk of ectopic pregnancy increases sixfold.
    - Half of the patients with tubal disease have no history of antecedent disease.
  ♦ HSG details.
    - Perform 2 to 5 days after the cessation of menstrual flow.
    - Check the serum sedimentation rate if patient has a history of PID; treat an elevated sedimentation rate with antibiotics and repeat prior to HSG.

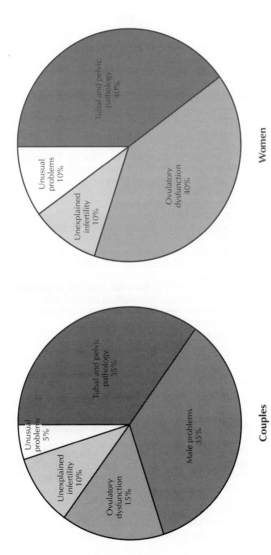

Figure 26.1. Causes of infertility in couples (left) and in women (right).

Couples

- Tubal and pelvic pathology 35%
- Male problems 35%
- Ovulatory dysfunction 15%
- Unexplained infertility 10%
- Unusual problems 5%

Women

- Tubal and pelvic pathology 40%
- Ovulatory dysfunction 40%
- Unexplained infertility 10%
- Unusual problems 10%

Table 26.1. Time required for conception in couples who will attain pregnancy

Time of Exposure	% Pregnant
3 mo	57%
6 mo	72%
1 yr	85%
2 yr	93%

- Defer HSG in cases of documented PID and perform a laparoscopy instead.
- The overall risk of infection is <1% (3% in high-risk patients); it is as high as 11% in patients with dilated tubes.
- Consider prophylactic antibiotics, 100 mg BID for 5 days; start 2 days before the HSG.
- The following three films are usually required:
  1. Preliminary.
  2. A film showing spill.
  3. A delayed film demonstrating spread.
- Inject slowly—usually only 3 mL to 6 mL of dye is required.
- A unilateral spill is usually associated with a normal contralateral tube in spite of the absence of filling.
- A normal study does not rule out pathology.
- The therapeutic benefit is likely limited to use of oil-based dye; this has been confirmed in some studies and refuted by others.
  ◆ Benefits of oil dye.
  1. Mechanical lavage.
  2. Straightens tubes.
  3. Stimulates cilia.
  4. Improves cervical mucus.
  5. Bacteriostatic effect of iodine.
  6. Decreases macrophage release of cytokines.
  ◆ Sonohysterography—better than HSG for the identification of uterine polyps on the myomata.
IX. Hysteroscopy
  ◆ Complements HSG and sonohysterography.
  ◆ More effective than HSG for the pursuit of abnormalities, especially if operative intervention is planned.
X. Falloposcopy
  ◆ Requires considerable expertise.
  ◆ Utility unclear.
XI. Outpatient Tubal Canalization
  ◆ Can be done with a fluoroscopic or hysteroscopic technique.
  ◆ Most clinical experience is with fluoroscopic tubal canalization.
    - It is 80% to 90% successful.
    - An estimated 30% of patients will become pregnant within 3 to 6 months.

XII. Disorders of Ovulation
- These account for 20% of all infertility problems.
- Prompt treatment with clomiphene is very successful; most will conceive within 3 months (see Chapter 30).
- Basal body temperature (BBT).
  - Women with regular monthly menstrual periods are almost always ovulating; a 5% rate of anovulation is seen.
  - The BBT provides indirect evidence of correlation.
  - It may be helpful as a preliminary indicator of ovulation; several months of charts is sufficient.
  - The increase in temperature coincides with the rise of peripheral progesterone to >4 ng/mL; the temperature is usually sustained for 11 to 16 days.
- Coital timing.
  - Should occur every 36 to 48 hours during the interval lasting from the 3 to 4 days prior to and the 2 days after expected ovulation.
  - Most pregnancies occur during coitus 3 days prior to ovulation.
- Endometrial biopsy.
  - Perform 2 to 3 days prior to expected menses.
  - Read the histology using the Noyes criteria.
  - The danger of interrupting a pregnancy is not great.
- Progesterone measurements.
  - Levels <3 ng/mL are consistent with the follicular phase.
  - Midluteal levels should be at least 6.5 ng/mL and preferably are >10 ng/mL.
  - A single midluteal measurement is insufficient for determining the adequacy of the luteal phase.
- Luteal Phase Defect (LPD).
  - LPD is historically defined as a lag of 2 days; it can be found in up to 30% of isolated cycles in normal women.
  - Three percent to 4% of infertile women are diagnosed with LPD, as are 5% of patients with recurrent pregnancy loss.
  - Underlying causes.
    - Decreased follicular phase FSH.
    - Decreased LH surge.
    - Decreased endometrial response to progesterone.
    - Elevated prolactin and hypothyroidism.
  - Does this entity exist?
    - Diagnosis is difficult as histologic dating is variable.
    - Incidence in the fertile population may be similar to that of the infertile population.
    - Out-of-phase biopsies are seen in conception cycles; no difference in term delivery rate has been noted.
  - Treatment—the use of both clomiphene and progesterone has been advocated.

- Clomiphene, 50 mg for 5 days (start day 3, 4, or 5).
- Progesterone.
  ◇ Twenty-five–milligram suppository BID starting 2 to 3 days postovulation.
  ◇ If pregnant, consider switching to 250 mg intramuscular 17-hydroxyprogesterone caproate per week.
- Oral micronized progesterone, 100 mg TID.
- Crinone 8% (90 mg) gel QD.

XIII. Luteinized Unruptured Follicle
   - The diagnosis is made on the basis of ultrasound monitoring.
   - Diagnosis is difficult.
   - This is unlikely to be a significant cause of infertility.
   - Patients are recommended to avoid nonsteroidal antiinflammatory drugs (NSAIDs) around ovulation.

XIV. Mycoplasma
   - A pleuropneumonia-like organism.
   - Higher prevalence in infertile couples (cervical mucus).
     • Other studies do not support this finding.
     • A culture may be unrewarding.
   - Empiric treatment of infertile couples not warranted.

XV. Endoscopy
   - Endoscopy is usually performed 6 months after HSG; exceptions are those who are at high risk for tubal disease or those who are older.
   - The findings agree with HSG two-thirds of the time.
   - Fifty percent of women with infertility will have some pathology.
   - Treatment success of tubal disease depends on the severity (Table 26.2).

XVI. Unexplained Infertility
   - Infertility is unexplained in 10% to 15% of patients without laparoscopy and in <10% of patients undergoing laparoscopy.
   - The monthly pregnancy rate is 1.5% to 3%.
   - After 3 years of infertility, the prospect of pregnancy decreases by 24% per year.
   - Sixty percent of couples with unexplained infertility conceive within 3 years; consider waiting 3 years in women <30 years of age.
   - These couples may benefit from sperm penetration assays.
   - Superovulation and IUI.

Table 26.2.   Laparoscopic treatment of distal tubal pathology

Lysis of adhesions	50% pregnancy rate
Distal tubal obstruction	
Mild disease	80% pregnancy rate
Moderate disease	30% pregnancy rate
Severe disease	15% pregnancy rate

Table 26.3.   Pregnancy rate per cycle

No treatment	1.3% to 4.1%
IUI	3.8%
Clomiphene	5.6%
Clomiphene and IUI	8.3%
Gonadotropins	7.7%
Gonadotropins and IUI	17.1%
IVF	20.7%

Abbreviations: IUI, intrauterine insemination; IVF, *in vitro* fertilization.

- Success rates and cost are less than IVF.
- Patients with unexplained infertility may have subtle hormonal abnormalities ($\uparrow$ FSH, $\downarrow$ progesterone), which becomes the rational basis for providing ovarian stimulation.
- A cumulative pregnancy rate of 40% is seen after six cycles of superovulation.
- For monthly pregnancy rates in unexplained infertility, see Table 26.3.
- Few pregnancies occur after four cycles.
- The success of treatment is dependent on number of sperm inseminated; success rare if <1 to 3 million sperm.
- Treatment of women >40 may be unwarranted because of extremely low pregnancy rates.

XVII.   Adoption
- ◆ A range of options is available.
- ◆ The incidence of a birth mother reclaiming an infant is about 5%.

XVIII.   Myths
- ◆ Anxiety has little influence on infertility.
- ◆ Empiric treatment with levothyroxine is worthless.
- ◆ Dilation and curettage is not part of the routine fertility evaluation.
- ◆ A retroverted uterus is not a cause of infertility, but it may be associated with adhesions and/or endometriosis.

Recurrent Early Pregnancy Losses

I. Introduction
- Early pregnancy loss is defined as the termination of pregnancy prior to 20 weeks of gestation or below a fetal weight of 500 g.
  - Fifteen percent of all pregnancies between 4 and 20 weeks of gestation will undergo clinically recognized loss.
  - True early loss is close to 50% because of the high rate of unrecognized losses in the 2 to 4 weeks following conception.
- "Habitual" abortion is classically defined as three or more spontaneous miscarriages.
  - Early risk assessments were theoretic.
  - Clinical studies demonstrate the actual loss rate to be lower (Table 27.1).

II. Normal Statistics
- Reproduction is inefficient.
- Fifty percent of fertilized ova do not progress to viable pregnancy; 30% of pregnancies are lost between implantation and the sixth week.
- Both euploid and aneuploid losses increase with maternal age.
- Eighty percent of losses occur in the first 12 weeks; 70% of these are due to chromosomal anomalies.
- The miscarriage rate is only 12% in women <20 years of age; it increases to 26% in women >40; the overall loss rate (preclinical and clinical) is 75% in women >40.
- Demonstration of fetal cardiac activity is associated with a 3% to 5% loss rate in normal women; the loss rate increases by 4 to 5× in women with a history of recurrent pregnancy loss (RPL).
  - Estimated at 22.7% in those patients with more than two losses.
  - Roughly 29% in women >40 undergoing *in vitro* fertilization (IVF).

III. Genetic Factors
- The spontaneous success rate is 55% to 70%, but checking karyotypes is still worthwhile; 3% to 8% of couples will have an abnormality.
  - Usually balanced translocation.
  - Other findings.
    - Sex chromosome mosaicism.
    - Chromosome inversions.
    - Ring chromosomes.
- Single gene defects will not be found by karyotype analysis.

**Table 27.1. The risk of recurrent
early pregnancy loss in young women**

	Number of Prior Miscarriages	% Risk of Miscarriage in Next Pregnancy
Women who have had at least one liveborn infant	0	12%
	1	24%
	2	26%
	3	32%
	4	26%
	6	53%
Women who have not had at least one liveborn infant	2 or more	40% to 45%

- ◆ Evidence of meiotic disorders will also not be found in blood cells.
- ◆ If abnormalities are found, then chance of success depends on the specific abnormality.
  - • Can be as high as 50% or as low as 32%.
  - • Options for treatment.
    - ■ Donor gametes.
      - ◇ Donor sperm.
      - ◇ Donor egg.
    - ■ IVF with preimplantation genetic diagnosis.
- ◆ Fetal chromosomal abnormalities.
  - • Account for 70% of early spontaneous losses.
  - • Account for 30% of second trimester losses.
  - • Seen in 3% of stillbirths.
  - • Specific anomalies.
    - ■ Autosomal trisomy (50%); usually 13, 16, 18, 21, or 22.
    - ■ Monosomy X (25%).
    - ■ Polyploidies.
  - • Indications for karyotype analysis.
    - ■ Three consecutive early losses.
    - ■ A family history of miscarriage or a malformed or mentally retarded child.
- IV. Environmental Factors
  - ◆ Definitely associated.
    - • Smoking.
    - • Accutane.
  - ◆ Possibly associated.
    - • Anesthetic gases and tetrachloroethylene.
    - • Caffeine (controversial).
    - • Alcohol.
  - ◆ Not associated.
    - • Exercise.
    - • Video display terminals.
    - • Electric blankets.
    - • Heated water beds.

V. Endocrine Factors
- Mild or subclinical endocrine diseases are not causes of RPL; the assessment of thyroid states or carbohydrate metabolism is not likely to be helpful.
- No association is found between endometriosis and RPL.
- Elevated levels of luteinizing hormone (LH) are associated with RPL in patients with polycystic ovary syndrome (PCOS).
  - No evidence suggesting that LH is a factor for recurrent pregnancy loss in ovulatory women currently exists.
  - Treatment of women with PCOS with gonadotropin-releasing hormone (GnRH) agonist does not alter their rate of loss.
- Inadequate luteal phase.
  - This may cause RPL.
  - Attempts to implicate low progesterone levels or to treat with progesterone have been fruitless.
  - Approximately 20% to 30% of women with RPL may have an inadequate luteal phase; however, treatment has not been shown to alter the outcome.
  - Diagnosis is usually based on repeated endometrial biopsies showing a lag in histology or basal body temperature rise.
  - Treatment.
    - Clomiphene or progesterone.
    - Dopamine agonist in cases of galactorrhea or ↑ prolactin.
  - Empiric treatment may be appropriate because of diagnostic limitations.
VI. Anatomic Causes
- An estimated 12% to 15% of women with RPL have a uterine developmental abnormality or a distorted cavity.
  - Diagnosis is usually by ultrasound (with saline infusion) or magnetic resonance imaging (MRI).
  - Hysterosalpingography is relatively inaccurate.
- Surgical correction by hysteroscopy yields delivery rates of 70% to 80%.
  - A septate uterus is most common.
  - Repeat procedures may be necessary.
- Cerclage may be indicated in patients with late losses and müllerian anomalies (Fig. 27.1).
- Asherman syndrome is an uncommon cause.
VII. Infectious Causes
- Currently, no hard evidence exists to show that bacteria or viruses cause RPL.
- Treatment with antibiotics may be beneficial in the case of infection with *Ureaplasma urealyticum*.
- Empiric treatment of both partners with antibiotics may be both more cost-effective and time-effective.
  - Doxycycline, 100 mg BID × 14 days.
  - Erythromycin, 250 mg QID × 14 days.

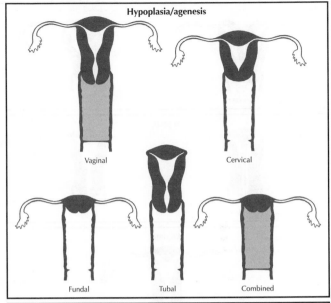

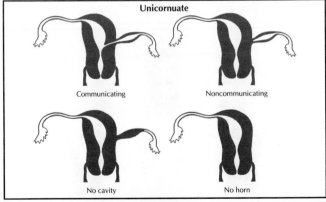

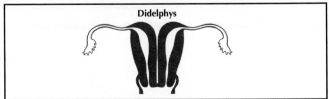

Figure 27.1.   Classification of müllerian anomalies.

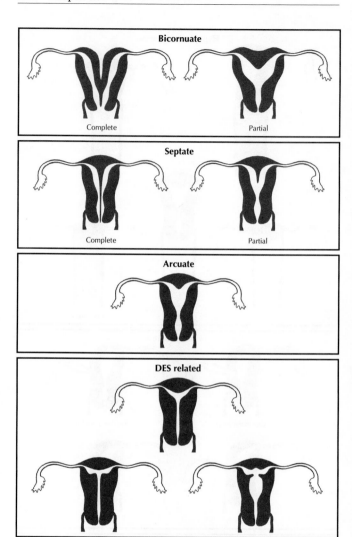

Figure 27.1. Classification of müllerian anomalies (continued).

VIII. Thrombophilia
- ♦ The major cause of thrombosis in pregnancy is an inherited clotting disorder.
  - • Antithrombin III deficiency.
  - • Factor V Leiden mutation → activated protein C deficiency.
  - • Protein C and protein S deficiencies.
- ♦ Factor V Leiden mutation.
  - • Found in 30% of patients with venous thromboembolism.
    - ■ The mutation makes factor V resistant to degradation by protein C.
    - ■ The entire clotting cascade is resistant to the actions of protein C.
  - • Degree of risk of venous thromboembolism.
    - ■ Eightfold ↑ in heterozygotes.
    - ■ Eightyfold ↑ in homozygotes.
  - • Highest prevalence in Europeans (3% to 4%); rare in Africans and Asians.
  - • Risk of loss possibly not increased in early pregnancy.
- ♦ Screening for thrombophilia is not clear cut, but potential screening would include the following:

Hypercoagulable Conditions	Thrombophilia Screening
Antithrombin III deficiency	Antithrombin III
Protein C deficiency	Protein C
Protein S deficiency	Protein S
Factor V Leiden mutation	Activated protein C resistance ratio
Prothrombin gene mutation	Activated partial thromboplastin time (PTT)
Antiphospholipid syndrome	Hexagonal activated PTT
	Anticardiolipin antibodies
	Lupus anticoagulant
	Fibrinogen
	Prothrombin G mutation (DNA test)
	Thrombin time
	Homocysteine level
	Complete blood cell count

IX. Immunologic Problems
- ♦ Autoimmunity (self-antigens)—a humoral or cellular response directed against a specific host component.
- ♦ Antiphospholipid antibodies.
  - • Directed against platelets and the vascular endothelium, causing thrombosis and pregnancy loss.
  - • Blockage of prostaglandin (PG) formation, resulting in unbalanced thromboxane activity.
  - • May be found in 10% to 16% of patients with RPL.

- The mechanism is probably decidual and placental insufficiency.
- It may result from reduced levels of annexin V on trophoblasts.
- Antiphospholipid antibodies may prolong the prothrombin time and PTT; the kaolin clotting time is also sensitive.
- The association of other antiphospholipid antibodies besides anticardiolipin and lupus anticoagulant is still questionable.
- Treatment.
  - Low-dose aspirin (80 mg) and low-dose heparin at the time of diagnosis of pregnancy; low-dose aspirin alone is not helpful.
  - Treatment with glucocorticoids is not necessarily effective.
  - Roughly 75% of these patients will deliver a viable infant.

Table 27.2. Summary of laboratory evaluation and management for repeated early pregnancy losses

Category	Evaluation	Treatment
Normal statistics	Numbers review, no laboratory tests	Education and support
Genetic factors	Karyotypes of both parents	Counseling, donor gametes where appropriate
Environmental factors	No laboratory tests	Counseling
Endocrine factors	TSH, prolactin, luteal phase assessment	Empiric clomiphene
Anatomic causes	Vaginal ultrasound with saline instillation, confirmed by MRI	Surgery
Infectious causes	Cultures if clinically indicated	Empiric doxycycline or erythromycin
Thrombophilia	Screen for inherited predisposition for thrombosis	Low-molecular-weight heparin anticoagulation
Immunologic	Activated partial thromboplastin time, kaolin clotting time, anticardiolipin antibody, lupus anticoagulant	Low-dose aspirin and heparin

Abbreviations: MRI, magnetic resonance imaging; TSH, thyroid-stimulating hormone.

- Treatment carries risks, so it should not be used indiscriminately.
♦ Alloimmunity (foreign antigens).
    - This term refers to all causes of losses related to an abnormal maternal immune response.
    - Immunotherapy has been advocated in these causes, but no specific immunologic test or clinical method can predict the need for treatment.
    - Treatment remains experimental; it may be helpful in patients with more than five losses.
    - Summary of immunologic causes.
        1. Many previous spontaneous miscarriages.
        2. No recent full-term pregnancies.
        3. Less than 35 years of age.
        4. Aborted conceptus with a normal karyotype.
        5. Usually at least one loss after the first trimester (Table 27.2).

X. Conclusion
    ♦ The patient is usually anxious and frustrated and is on the edge of depression; frequent communication is essential.
    ♦ Continued attempts are successful in 70% to 75% of patients.
    ♦ Fifty percent of patients have no identifiable abnormalities.
    ♦ Close monitoring is indicated because of the increased rate of ectopic pregnancy.
    ♦ Treatment with IVF is uncertain; some studies reveal a benefit.
    ♦ Treatment with oocyte donation has been helpful.

Endometriosis

I. Etiology
- Endometriosis was described in the medical literature in the 1800s.
- John Sampson suggested that peritoneal endometriosis arises from seedings from ovarian endometriosis.
  - Established retrograde menstruation as the probable cause.
  - Conclusions validated by the following observations:
    1. Laparoscopic demonstration of blood flowing from the fimbriated end of the tube is observed in almost all menstruating women.
    2. Endometriosis is most commonly found in dependent portions of the pelvis.
    3. Endometrial fragments from menstrual flow can grow in cultures.
    4. Endometriosis developed in primate studies using cervical transposition or retroperitoneal injection.
    5. Increased incidence is seen in women with outflow tract obstruction.
    6. The risk of endometriosis is higher in women with shorter cycles and larger flows.
    7. Retrograde menstruation occurs more frequently in baboons with spontaneous endometriosis.
- Other developmental pathways exist.
  - Vascular.
  - Lymphatic.
  - Coelomic metaplasia.
- Supporting evidence for the theory of coelomic metaplasia is as follows:
  1. Endometriosis occurs in adolescent girls before any cycle is experienced.
  2. Endometriosis has been reported in a prepubertal girl.
  3. Endometriosis has been encountered in women who never menstruated.
  4. Endometriosis in unusual sites—the thumb, thigh, knee—may be explained by the proximity of mesenchymal limb buds adjacent to the coelomic epithelium.
  5. Endometriosis can occur in men and is usually associated with high-dose estrogen.
- Genetic and immunologic factors are also at work.
  - Sixfold increased incidence in first degree relatives with the disease (6%).
  - Monozygotic twins are concordant.
  - Increased incidence of humoral antibodies.

II. Prevalence
- A rough estimate is that endometriosis occurs in 3% to 10% of women of reproductive age; it is seen in 25% to 35% of infertile women.
- It occurs at a rate of 4 per 1,000 women between the ages of 15 and 64 who are hospitalized each year.
- Endometriosis is not confined to nulliparous women, white women, or women over the age of 30.

III. Diagnosis
- Symptoms and signs.
  - Many women are asymptomatic, but the onset of dysmenorrhea and dyspareunia after years of relatively pain-free menses and coitus is suggestive; a lack of correlation between pain and visible endometriosis exists.
    - Deeply infiltrating lesions may be difficult to diagnose.
    - Pain can be diffuse or localized (low back pain).
  - No clear evidence of menstrual dysfunction or galactorrhea is associated with endometriosis.
- Ca-125 assay.
  - A useful marker for epithelial ovarian cancer.
  - Often elevated in endometriosis; its sensitivity is too low for screening, but it may be a marker of response to treatment.
  - Other causes of elevated Ca-125 include the following:
    - Pregnancy.
    - Leiomyomata.
    - Pelvic inflammatory disease.
    - Menstruation.
- Physical examination.
  - Consider performing a pelvic examination at the time of menses.
  - The uterus may be retroverted.
  - Cul-de-sac or uterosacral nodularity is found in 35% of patients.
  - Endometriosis can be detected by ultrasound or magnetic resonance imaging (MRI); hemorrhagic cysts account for a false-positive rate.
  - The appearance at laparoscopy is varied; the lesions can be red, black, blue, white, or clear.

IV. Classification
- The system of the American Society for Reproductive Medicine has weaknesses.
- High interobserver and intraobserver variability is seen with any system.

V. Endometriosis and Infertility
- Clearly impairs fertility when associated with tubal and/or ovarian adhesions.
- Role of minimal or mild endometriosis unclear with regard to infertility.
  - Dyspareunia.
  - Questionable role in peritoneal fluids and prostaglandins (PGs).

- Peritoneal macrophages.
  - Phagocytosis of sperm.
  - Secretion of interleukin (IL)-1.
  - Elevation of IL-6.
  - Secretion of vascular endothelial growth factor.
- Abnormal follicular dynamics.
- ◆ Should mild or minimal endometriosis be treated?
  - Five-year expectant pregnancy rate of 90%.
  - Canadian randomized trial.
    - Forty-eight percent pregnancy rate in the treated group (blue/black lesions).
    - Thirty-five percent pregnancy rate in the non-treated group.
- ◆ Moderate or severe endometriosis should be treated surgically; if the patient does not become pregnant after surgery, move to gonadotropin, superovulation with intrauterine insemination, or *in vitro* fertilization (IVF).

VI. Surgical Treatment
- ◆ Surgery is best for adhesions or endometriomas >2 cm.
- ◆ Restore the normal anatomy.
- ◆ Consider a presacral neurectomy for midline pain.
- ◆ Success correlates with the extent of the disease.
  - Moderate—60%.
  - Severe—35%.
- ◆ Postoperative medical therapy is helpful in pain cases.
- ◆ Pregnancy usually occurs within the first 2 years following surgery; the recurrence rate is 20% within 5 years.
- ◆ Radical surgery includes hysterectomy and oophorectomy; patients with ovarian conservation have a 6× increased risk of recurrent symptoms.

VII. Medical Treatment
- ◆ Medical treatment is of no proven value in infertility.
- ◆ Medical therapy is valuable for dysmenorrhea, dyspareunia, and pelvic pain.
- ◆ Options.
  1. Continuous oral contraceptives.
     - Can convert implants into decidualized cells with inactive glands.
     - Pregnancy rates of 40% to 50% after stopping.
     - A suppressive, not curative, therapy.
  2. Danazol.
     - Isoxazole derivative of 17α-ethinyltestosterone.
     - Does not alter gonadotropin levels; eliminates the midcycle surge.
     - Sixty metabolic products.
     - Creates high androgen–low estrogen environment; leads to amenorrhea.
     - Side effects for at least 80% of users; bothersome to 10% of patients.
       - Decreased breast size.
       - Increased acne.
       - Increased hirsutism.
       - Atrophic vaginitis.
       - Hot flushes.

- Voice changes.
- Contraindicated in liver disease.
- Dangerous in heart disease.
  ◇ Fluid retention.
  ◇ Lipid changes.
- Efficiency—90% of patients report pain relief.
- Dosage.
  ◇ Four hundred milligrams orally BID or 200 mg orally QID.
  ◇ Recurrence within 1 year in one-third of patients.
  ◇ Doses lower than 800 mg possibly less effective.
3. Progestins.
   • Oral and intramuscular medroxyprogesterone acetate both effective; oral dose of 30 mg/day is as effective as danazol.
   • Luteinizing hormone (LH) secretion suppressed → hypoestrogenic.
   • Side effects.
     ■ Reversible bone loss.
     ■ Weight gain.
     ■ Fluid retention.
     ■ Breakthrough bleeding.
     ■ Depression.
   • Effective for pain but not for fertility.
4. Gonadotropin-releasing hormone (GnRH) agonists.
   • Native GnRH has a short half-life.
     ■ Rapid cleavage occurs between amino acids 5–6, 6–7, and 9–10.
     ■ Substitutions at 6 or the glycine amide inhibit degradation.
   • The best therapeutic effect is associated with estradiol in the 20 to 40 pg/mL range (Table 28.1 and Fig. 28.1).
   • It is equally effective when compared with danazol or progestin (monkey studies); no adverse lipid changes are seen.
   • GnRH agonist therapy is suppressive, not curative.
   • A 6% to 8% decrease in trabecular bone density is seen at 6 months of treatment.
     ■ This is usually, but not always, reversed within 1 year.
     ■ The use of 19-nortestosterone progestin helps to prevent bone loss.
     ■ Bisphosphonates can also be used.
   • This treatment has no benefit for fertility.
VIII. Recurrence
   ♦ The recurrence rate is 5% to 20% per year with medical therapy.
     • Forty percent after 5 years; GnRH agonist data show 5-year recurrence rates of 37% and 74% for minimal and severe disease, respectively.
     • Fifty-six percent after 7 years.

Table 28.1. GnRH agonists in clinical use

Position	1	2	3	4	5	6	7	8	9	10
Native GnRH	pGlu	His	Trp	Ser	Tyr	Gly	Leu	Arg	Pro	Gly-NH$_2$
Leuprolide						D-Leu				NH-Ethylamide
Buserelin						D-Ser (tertiary butanol)				NH-Ethylamide
Nafarelin						D-Naphthylalanine (2)				
Histrelin						D-His (tertiary benzyl)				NH-Ethylamide
Goserelin						D-Ser (tertiary butanol)				Aza-Gly
Deslorelin						D-Trp				NH-Ethylamide
Tryptorelin						D-Trp				

Abbreviation: GnRH, gonadotropin-releasing hormone.

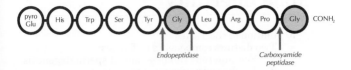

Gonadotropin releasing hormone

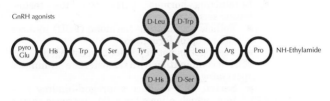

GnRH agonists

Figure 28.1. Structures of gonadotropin-releasing hormone (GnRH) and GnRH agonists.

- ◆ Recurrence rates are 10% within 1 year and 20% within 5 years after laparoscopy.

IX. Hormone Treatment After Surgery
- ◆ Begin hormone-replacement therapy after total abdominal hysterectomy with bilateral salpingo-oophorectomy.
- ◆ Risk of inciting growth of residual disease is negligible.
- ◆ Always add progestin because of reported cases of adenocarcinoma development in areas of endometriosis.

X. Prevention of Infertility
- ◆ Treat an incidental finding of endometriosis surgically; consider postoperative medical therapy.
  - Mild disease—oral contraceptive pills (OCPs).
  - Moderate or severe disease—GnRH agonist, medroxyprogesterone acetate (Provera), or danazol.
- ◆ Consider prophylactic use of OCPs in women with a strong family history of endometriosis.
- ◆ No increased rate of spontaneous abortion is seen.
- ◆ An increased incidence of ovulatory dysfunction or luteal phase defect has not been observed.
- ◆ Superovulation increases fecundity but not the cumulative pregnancy rates.
- ◆ Patients with mild and moderate disease do well with IVF; success with severe disease is more disappointing.

Male Infertility

I. Regulation of the Testes
- Two distinct components as follows:
  1. Seminiferous tubules—site of spermatogenesis.
  2. Leydig cells—source of testosterone.
- The control of both components is gonadotropin-dependent.
  - Luteinizing hormone (LH) stimulates testosterone secretion.
    - Follicle-stimulating hormone (FSH) induces LH-receptor formation.
    - Feedback is not dependent on estrogens.
  - FSH in combination with testosterone stimulates spermatogenesis.
    - Sertoli cells produce androgen-binding protein, which allows for a 50× increase in the local concentration of testosterone and dihydrotestosterone (DHT) (Fig. 29.1).
    - Fertility can occur even in the face of FSH-receptor mutation.
- FSH secretion is not suppressed by steroids at the physiologic level.
  - It depends on inhibin B.
  - Inhibin A is absent in male circulation.
- The role of prolactin is unclear; hypersecretion leads to reduced testosterone.
- Sertoli cells and sperm production.
  - Tight junctions between the Sertoli cells seal the tubules.
    - "Blood–testis barrier."
    - Seminiferous tubes are avascular; regulatory substances must enter by diffusion.
  - X chromosome activity.
    - In female somatic cells → one X is inactive.
    - In female gametes (oocytes) → both Xs are active.
    - In male somatic cells → X is active.
    - In male gametogenesis → X is inactive.
- The testis.
  - Composed mainly of the seminiferous tubule; 70 cm long if uncoiled.
  - Total of 74 days required to produce spermatozoa.
  - Fifty days spent in the tubule.
  - Twelve to 21 days to travel the epididymis (5 to 6 m long).
  - Vas deferens, length of 35 cm (Fig. 29.2).
II. Semen Analysis
- The patient should practice abstinence for 2 to 3 days prior to semen collection.
- Collect the semen into a clean container.
  - It can be collected at home.

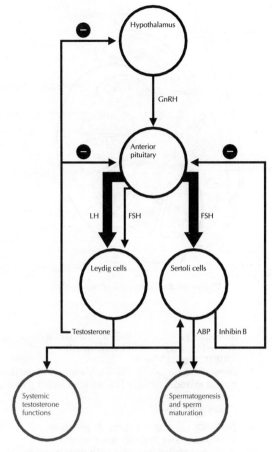

Figure 29.1. The hypothalamic–pituitary–testicular axis.

- Coitus interruptus may result in the loss of specimen.
♦ Liquefaction occurs within 20 to 30 minutes; if the specimen is too viscid, consider repeated passage through a 19-gauge needle, collecting as split ejaculate, or treat with proteolytic enzyme (rare).

Normal values (World Health Organization [WHO] guidelines)

Volume	2.0 mL
Concentration	>20 million/mL
Motility	50% with forward progression or 25% with rapid progression within 60 minutes

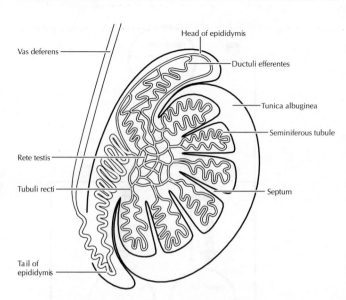

Figure 29.2.   Structure of the testis.

Morphology	30% normal forms
White blood cell (WBC) count	<1 million/mL
Immunobead	<20% with adherent particles
Sperm mixed agglutination reaction (MAR)	<10% with adherent particles

- ♦ Defining normal is a difficult proposition.
  - • Counts and motility are variable.
  - • Pregnancies do occur with poor counts.
- ♦ Consider sequential repeat semen analysis.
- ♦ The coefficient of variation may be >35%; errors can still occur with the use of computer-assisted semen analysis.
- ♦ The use of total motile sperm (TMS) may be helpful; pregnancy rates increase with an increase in TMS.
- ♦ Sperm morphology.
  - • Some improvement in variation is seen with the use of overlay in association with video microscopy.
  - • Kruger morphology is much stricter.
    - ■ More than 14% normal = normal rates of fertilization in *in vitro* fertilization (IVF) cycles.
    - ■ Less than 4% normal = IVF fertilization rate of 7% to 8%.
- ♦ Other parameters.
  - • Volume of <1 mL or >7 mL may inhibit contact of the sperm with the cervix.

- Round cells may be white blood cells (WBC) or immature sperm forms; consider the use of prostatic massage to obtain a culture.

III. Test of Sperm Function
- No test has emerged as a reliable measure of fertilizing ability.
- Sperm penetration assay (SPA).
    - Incubate zona free hamster eggs for 2 to 3 hours with human sperm; compare the resulting specimen with a known fertile control.
    - Although this concept is attractive, the test is difficult to standardize.
    - Its prognostic value is uncertain.
        - A SPA of 0% can be associated with a pregnancy rate of 16%.
        - If SPA = 0% in the optimized test, then consider the use of intracytoplasmic sperm injection (ICSI) or donor sperm.
- Human zona binding assay.
    - Requires a source of human zona.
    - Split zona between the subject and the control.
- Sperm mucus penetration tests.
    - Little practical benefit.
    - Usually treat with intrauterine insemination (IUI) anyway.
- Hypoosmotic swelling test—clinical utility uncertain except in cases of nonmotile sperm.
- Measurement of adenosine triphosphate is not helpful.
- Acrosome reaction.
    - A low percentage of sperm will become reactive while in media or following treatment with calcium ionophore.
    - This is not clinically important.

IV. Sperm Antibodies
- Immunization with sperm can induce infertility.
    - Semen is very antigenic.
    - It is normally isolated by the blood–testis barrier, but antibodies can occur after the following:
        - Vasectomy.
        - Torsion.
        - Infection.
        - Trauma.
- Agglutination is nonspecific; serum antisperm antibodies have no influence on fertility.
- Laboratory testing.
    - Immunobead test.
        - The beads are labeled with anti-IgG, anti-IgA, or anti-IgM.
        - The site of sperm adherence can be noted.
            - ◇ Anti-IgA is usually tail.
            - ◇ Anti-IgG is usually head.
        - Positive test: 40% of motile sperm with beads.
    - Sperm MAR.

- This test uses antibody to IgG to bridge antibody-coated sperm and latex particles conjugated with human IgG.
- The end point in the test is clumping.
- The location of the reactions cannot be determined.
- The test can be performed on unprepared semen.
- Positive test: 10% to 40% motive sperm attached to particles signifies probable immunologic infertility.
- Treatment.
  - The use of condoms has been abandoned.
  - The use of corticosteroids is associated with a high rate of complications.
  - Treatment with IUI is appropriate.
  - The highest pregnancy rates are achieved with superovulation plus IUI, IVF, or IVF plus ICSI (best success).

V. Investigation and Treatment of Male Infertility
  - ◆ Evaluation for environmental and/or social factors:
    1. History of testicular injury, surgery, or mumps.
    2. Exposure to excessive heat.
    3. Severe allergic reactions.
    4. Exposure to radiation and/or environmental toxins.
    5. Heavy marijuana, alcohol, or drug use. Prescription drugs that can depress sperm quantity and quality include the following:
       - Cimetidine.
       - Spironolactone.
       - Nitrofurans.
       - Sulfasalazine.
       - Erythromycin.
       - Tetracycline.
       - Anabolic steroids.
       - Chemotherapy.
       - α-Blockers.
       - Phentolamine.
       - Methyldopa.
       - Guanethidine.
       - Reserpine.
    6. Coital frequency.
       - Too frequent.
       - Too infrequent (every 10 to 14 days).
    7. Questionable effect of diethylstilbestrol exposure.

VI. Urologic Evaluation
  - ◆ Refer to a urologist to evaluate for anatomic abnormality, infection, endocrine or genetic disorder, or varicocele; 1 of 100 patients will have serious medical pathology (tumor).
  - ◆ Anatomic abnormalities.
    - Hypospadias.
    - Retrograde ejaculation.
    - Obstruction of the vas.

- Testicular biopsy helpful at times.
♦ Genetic causes.
  - Oligospermic men have a high prevalence of Y chromosome submicroscopic deletions.
  - The following three regions on Yq are labeled as azoospermic factors: AZFa, AZFb, and AZFc (DAZ); 7% to 10% have AZFb or AZFc deletions.
    - Consider genetic screening prior to ICSI.
    - Cystic fibrosis mutations are associated with conjugated absence of the vas.
    - Other abnormalities are found in azoospermic or oligospermic men.
      ◊ Klinefelter syndrome (1 of 500 males).
      ◊ Mutations in the LH-β subunit.
      ◊ An inactivating mutation of the FSH receptor.
♦ Endocrine disorder.
  - An uncommon cause of infertility.
  - Nonspecific therapies not beneficial.
    - Fertility is not impaired.
    - Most studies lack a control group.
♦ Varicocele.
  - A varicocele is found in 20% to 40% of infertile males.
    - It is usually left-sided.
    - The spermatic vein is inserted into the renal vein.
  - Treatment success is difficult to assess.
  - Sperm parameters may worsen over time.
  - Ligation is associated with a 30% to 35% pregnancy rate.
  - Large varicoceles exert a greater effect than small ones.
♦ Reactive oxygen species.
  - Increased levels can cause damage to the sperm membrane.
  - Consider treatment with vitamin E and glutathione in the face of elevated leucocyte counts.
VII. Intrauterine Insemination of Washed Sperm
  ♦ Untreated sperm has a limited role in infertility.
  ♦ A variety of separation methods exist, including the following:
    - Washing.
    - Swim-up.
    - Density gradients.
    - Glass wool filtering.
  ♦ All methods provide increased motility and more uniform morphology, but the improvement may not translate into better pregnancy rates.
  ♦ Inseminate with at least 1 million motile sperm; highest pregnancy rates are usually found in insemination of >10 million motile sperm.
  ♦ Superovulation and IUI.
    - Increases the number of oocytes.
    - Raises hormone levels.

- Increases the number of sperm reaching the uterine cavity.
- IUI without superovulation may not be beneficial in male infertility; in severely compromised cases, proceed to IVF and ICSI.
- The timing of insemination is usually the day after the LH surge or 36 hours after injection of human chorionic gonadotropin (hCG); uncertain benefit to use of multiple inseminations.
- Gonadotropin-releasing hormone (GnRH)-α treatment does not enhance pregnancy rates.
- Infection is rare (1 of 500).
- The multiple pregnancy rate is 20%.
- Estrogen monitoring may not be necessary.
- Risk of ovarian hyperstimulation syndrome is increased in cases with the following:
  - Excessive number of small follicles (10 to 13 mm).
  - High estrogen level (>2,000 pg/mL).

VIII. Therapeutic Donor Insemination
- The procedure raises emotional, ethical, and legal issues.
- Three points are worth emphasizing as follows:
  1. Donor inseminations do not guarantee pregnancy.
     - The fresh insemination pregnancy rate is 70% over five to six cycles.
     - Frozen semen pregnancy rates are lower.
       - Twenty-one percent after 3 months.
       - Forty percent after 6 months.
       - Sixty-two percent after 12 months.
  2. IUI rates are better than intracervical insemination pregnancy rates; consider two IUIs per cycle if no success is seen after 2 months.
  3. Children from donor IUI have outcomes comparable to the general population.
- Fifty percent of couples do not tell their children.
- Divorce rates in families with children from donor inseminations are lower than the general rate.

30

Induction of Ovulation

I. Introduction
   ♦ In many clinical circumstances, treatment can result in pregnancy rates equivalent to those in the normal population.
   ♦ The disparity between ovulation and pregnancy rates reminds us of the imprecision of the diagnosis.
   ♦ An appropriate medical evaluation must be done to ensure that no contraindication to therapy exists.
   ♦ The World Health Organization (WHO) classification of ovulatory deficiencies.
      • Group I: **Hypothalamic–pituitary failure** (hypothalamic amenorrhea).
         ▪ Stress-induced.
         ▪ Anorexia nervosa.
         ▪ Kallmann syndrome.
         ▪ Isolated gonadotropic deficiency.
      • Group II: **Hypothalamic–pituitary dysfunction**.
         ▪ Normogonadotropic, normoestrogenic, anovulatory, and oligoamenorrheic women.
         ▪ Includes classic polycystic ovary syndrome (PCOS).
      • Group III: **Ovarian failure** (hypergonadotropic hypogonadal).
II. Induction of Ovulation with Clomiphene Citrate
   ♦ Clomiphene.
      • First synthesized in 1956; clinical trials in 1960.
      • Approved for clinical use in 1967.
      • Racemic mixture of two stereochemical isomers; active isomer—zuclomiphene (38%).
      • Weak estrogenic effect.
      • Binds the estrogen receptor.
         ▪ Prolonged occupancy (weeks rather than hours).
         ▪ Concentration of estrogen receptors reduced by inhibition of replenishment.
      • Mechanism of action.
         ▪ The true estrogen signal is falsely lowered.
         ▪ Gonadotropin-releasing hormone (GnRH) secretion is activated.
            ◊ Normally cycling women: ↑ follicle-stimulating hormone (FSH) and luteinizing hormone (LH) pulse frequency.
            ◊ Anovulatory women: ↑ pulse amplitude.
         ▪ FSH and LH rise.
            ◊ This indirectly occurs through GnRH.
            ◊ Animal models also suggest direct action on the pituitary.
         ▪ Clomiphene functions as an antiestrogen in the uterus, cervix, and vagina.

- ■ The adverse impact on the cervical mucus or endometrium is unlikely to alter its clinical efficiency.
- • Slow clearance; plasma concentrations are significant for up to 1 month.
- • Could interfere in the luteal phase with the induction of LH receptors.
- • No evidence of teratogenicity.
- ♦ Selection of patients.
  - • Those with absent or infrequent ovulation are candidates for use.
  - • Patients should not have evidence of liver disease.
  - • Consider endometrial biopsy in patients with a long history of anovulation.
  - • Check a semen analysis to rule out azoospermia.
  - • Evaluate further if the patient fails to conceive after 3 months of ovulation on clomiphene.
  - • Use progesterone withdrawal bleed and gonadotropin level to assess for ovarian failure.
  - • Treatment can be helpful in patients with an inadequate luteal phase; it is as effective as progesterone supplementation.
  - • Hypoestrogenic women rarely respond to treatment with clomiphene.
  - • Clomiphene can be used in Orthodox Jewish patients to delay ovulation in the face of a short follicular phase.
- ♦ Use of clomiphene.
  - • Begin on the fifth day of cycle following spontaneous or induced bleeding with a dosage of 50 mg × 5 days.
    - ■ Approximately 50% of patients conceive with 50 mg.
    - ■ An estimated 20% of patients conceive with 100 mg.
    - ■ Occasionally, patients conceive with 25 mg.
  - • Earlier administration is associated with multiple follicular development.
  - • Increase the dose if ovulation is not achieved; a 15% pregnancy rate is achieved with a 150-mg to 200-mg dose.
  - • The required dose correlates with body weight.
  - • The ovulatory surge usually occurs at day 16 or 17.
  - • Coitus should take place every other day for 1 week starting 5 days after the last dose.
  - • Assess for residual ovarian enlargement after the first cycle; cysts of 3 to 5 cm do not require a rest cycle.
  - • Consider basal body temperature charting to document the luteal phase; if <11 days, consider an empiric increase in dose or supplemental progesterone.
  - • Consider endometrial biopsy to document the adequacy of the luteal phase.

- Ultrasound monitoring may aid in the evaluation of treatment failures; sonogram, LH testing, and human chorionic gonadotropin (hCG) administration are unlikely to impact the pregnancy rate significantly.
- ◆ Results with clomiphene.
  - Eighty percent are expected to ovulate.
  - Forty percent conceive.
    - Twenty percent to 25% per ovulatory cycle.
    - Ten percent are multiples—usually twins.
    - No increase in miscarriage rates is seen.
  - Failure to conceive indicates the following:
    - The presence of other fertility factors.
    - A lack of persistence; the 6-month conception rate is 60% to 75%.
- ◆ Complications.
  - Not dose-related.
  - Vasomotor flushes—10%.
  - Abdominal distention, bloating, pain, and soreness—5.5%.
  - Breast discomfort—2%.
  - Nausea/vomiting—2.2%.
  - Visual symptoms—1.5% → further treatment not recommended.
    - Blurring vision, scotoma, and abnormal perception are from an unknown cause.
    - These symptoms disappear after the discontinuation of medicine—may take 1 to 2 weeks.
  - Headache—1.3%.
  - Dryness or hair loss—6.3%.

III. What to Do with Clomiphene Failures
  - ◆ Most likely, failures are in those with excess hyperandrogenemia and obesity.
  - ◆ Etiology of failure.
    - Excess LH in the follicular phase.
    - Dysfunctional effects of an untimely LH surge.
    - Excess local androgens.
    - Hyperinsulinemia.
  - ◆ Mechanisms of failure.
    - Impaired folliculogenesis.
    - Increased atresia.
    - Poor oocyte quality.
    - Precocious or impaired oocyte maturation.
    - Low fertilization rates.
    - Variable implantation rates.
    - Deficient corpus luteum function.
  - ◆ Strategies to explore.
    1. Treatment of hyperinsulinemia.
    2. Supplemental use of dexamethasone is to reduce androgens.
    3. Supplemental use of GnRH agonists is to eliminate endogenous LH.
    4. Pulsatile GnRH therapy.
    5. Use of gonadotropins.

- ♦ Initial evaluation of failures.
  - Ensure that hyperprolactinemia and/or galactor-rhea have not been overlooked.
  - Evaluate the quality of the cervical mucus; if it is poor, add inseminations.
  - If no success is seen after 6 months, proceed to other options.
- ♦ Treatment of hyperinsulinemia.
  - The best therapy is weight loss.
    - At least a 5% reduction of initial weight is ideal.
    - The resumption of ovulation frequently occurs if weight loss is at least 4 to 15 kg.
    - The goal of weight loss is a body mass index (BMI) <27; even a small weight loss will have a beneficial effect.
  - Assuming that all overweight anovulatory women with PCOS are hyperinsulinemic is reasonable. The evaluation is as follows:
    - Check fasting glucose and insulin; a ratio of glucose to insulin of <4.5 is consistent with insulin resistance.
    - Check with 2-hour glucose tolerance test (75 g).
      ◇ Normal: <140 mg/dL.
      ◇ Impaired: 140 to 199 mg/dL.
      ◇ Non–insulin-dependent diabetes mellitus >200 mg/dL.
  - If the patient fails to respond to the medications described below within 2 months, then restart clomiphene at the lowest dose.
  - Metformin.
    - Improves insulin sensitivity.
    - Decreases hepatic glucose production.
    - Reduces hyperinsulinemia, basal and stimulated LH levels, and free testosterone (T) in overweight women with PCOS.
    - Increased rate of spontaneous ovulation; also improved responsiveness to clomiphene.
    - The effect may be from weight loss or from metformin itself; lean PCOS patients demonstrate reduced hyperandrogenism.
    - Lactic acidemia = a rare complication of therapy; evaluate renal chemistries of patients before administration.
- ♦ Supplemental use of dexamethasone.
  - Dexamethasone, 0.5 mg qHS, will blunt the nighttime adrenocorticotropic hormone (ACTH) peak.
  - Its use is more successful in patients with elevated dehydroepiandrosterone sulfate (DHEAS) levels.
  - Maintain treatment with dexamethasone until pregnancy occurs.
  - Restart clomiphene at 50 mg after a few weeks on dexamethasone.
  - Normal DHEAS levels do not preclude successful result following dexamethasone treatment.

- ♦ Pretreatment suppression.
  - • Six-month course of oral contraceptive pills (OCPs), followed by clomiphene.
  - • Similar rationale to the use of GnRH agonist.
    - ■ Could reduce the miscarriage rate.
    - ■ Not proven in clinical practice.
- ♦ Bromocriptine.
  - • Dopamine agonist.
  - • Directly inhibits prolactin secretion.
  - • Increases ovarian responsiveness.
    - ■ Even in patients with normal prolactin levels and no galactorrhea.
    - ■ Possibly as a result of increased sensitivity to clomiphene; LH secretion is decreased.
  - • Side effects—gastrointestinal and cardiovascular.
    - ■ Nausea and/or diarrhea.
    - ■ Dizziness.
    - ■ Headache.
    - ■ Fatigue.
  - • Dosage.
    - ■ Start with 2.5 mg qHS.
    - ■ Slowly increase the dose as needed.
    - ■ Consider intravaginal administration.
  - • Administer daily for 2 months.
  - • If no response, restart clomiphene at the lowest dose.
  - • Use of bromocriptine.
    - ■ Its use is indicated in the presence of galactorrhea or hyperprolactinemia; other use is controversial.
    - ■ Elevated prolactin levels suppress pulsatile GnRH secretion.
    - ■ The presence of galactorrhea suggests either a difference between biologic and immunologic hormones or undetected subtle elevations in prolactin.
  - • Bromocriptine for euprolactinemic women.
    - ■ Ovulation induction with bromocriptine is occasionally successful in women with normal prolactin and the absence of galactorrhea.
      - ◊ Possible elevated nocturnal peaks.
      - ◊ Possible suppression of LH.
    - ■ Administer as above for 2 months; if no response, restart clomiphene at 50 mg.
    - ■ Bromocriptine has **no** benefit in ovulatory women with unexplained infertility.
- ♦ Cabergoline.
  - • Dose: 0.5 to 3 mg/week (or 2 × 1 week).
  - • Low rate of side effects.
  - • Limited experience in pregnancy.
- IV. Induction of Ovulation with Human Gonadotropins
  - ♦ Gonadotropins have been available for over 30 years; the heavy protein content of urinary preparation required intramuscular (IM) injection.

♦ Newer, highly purified preparations and recombinant FSH can be injected subcutaneously.

Preparation	Trade Names
Human menopausal gonadotropins	Pergonal, Humegon, Menogon, Repronex
Purified urinary FSH	Metrodin, Normegon, Orgafol
Highly purified urinary FSH	Fertinex or Metrodin HP
Recombinant FSH	Puregon, Gonal-F, Follistim
hCG	Pregnyl, Profasi, APL
Recombinant hCG	Ovidrel
Recombinant LH	LHadi

♦ Patient selection.
  • Absolute requirement: ovarian competence.
  • Perform thorough infertility evaluation.
    ■ Rule out tubal and/or uterine pathology.
    ■ Check semen analysis.
    ■ Document anovulation; see workup for amenorrhea and/or galactorrhea.
♦ Use of Gonadotropins.
  • Patient education is crucial.
  • Optimal results are dependent on the clinician, not the drug preparation; consider LH-containing product in patients with LH <3 IU/L.
  • Seven to 14 days of continuous treatment is needed.
    ■ Start with one ampule per day × 7 days.
    ■ If the patient does not respond, increase to a higher dose.
  • PCOS patients require careful handling.
    ■ They have a greater risk of multiples and ovarian hyperstimulation syndrome (OHSS).
    ■ Consider adjuvant use of insulin-sensitizing agents.
  • Trigger ovulation with 10,000 U hCG; the patient should have daily intercourse on the day of hCG administration and for the next 2 days.
♦ Estrogen monitoring.
  • Allows individualization of dosage.
    ■ A level of 1,000 to 1,500 pg/mL is optimal.
    ■ A level of 1,500 to 2,000 pg/mL increases the risk of OHSS.
    ■ Levels of >2,000 pg/mL lead to a high risk of OHSS; consider cycle cancellation.
  • The risk of OHSS is 5% in conception and 1% in nonconception cycles.
♦ Ultrasound monitoring.
  • The dominant follicle is apparent by day 8 to 10.
  • Maximal mean diameter is usually 20 to 25 mm (range 14 to 28 mm) in normal cycles; in 5% to 11%, two dominants develop.
  • Rapid growth is observed during last 24 hours prior to ovulation; mittelschmerz = rapid growth *not* ovulation.

- Clomiphene follicles mature at 18 to 20 mm.
- Gonadotropin follicles mature at 15 to 18 mm.
- Ultrasound monitoring does not eliminate the risk of multiples or OHSS; a large number of small follicles (>11) should preclude hCG use.
- The greatest chance of pregnancy is seen with an endometrium >9 to 10 mm.
- With the presence of a baseline cyst on sonogram, delay treatment or use OCPs or GnRH agonist.
- ◆ Addition of clomiphene.
  - Allows a 50% reduction of gonadotropin dose.
  - Same risk of multiples and OHSS.
  - Not helpful in hypothalamic amenorrhea patients.
- ◆ Pulsatile GnRH.
  - Reproduces the pulsatile pattern of gonadotropin.
  - Administer intravenously (IV) or subcutaneously, 6 to 9 U every 90 minutes.
  - Complicated method to induce ovulation.
- ◆ Results with gonadotropin therapy.
  - It is associated with a cumulative conception rate of 90% in hypothalamic amenorrhea patients and a 23% rate of miscarriage.
  - No increased risk of congenital malformations has been observed.
  - An increased risk of ectopic pregnancy exists.
  - hCG concentration falls to <50 to 100 IU/L on day 14 after injection.
  - Use progesterone supplementation in cases of GnRH agonist.
  - Multiple pregnancy rate is between 10% and 40%.
    - Mainly dizygotic twinning.
    - Increased monozygotic twinning rate (3×).
    - Multifetal reduction (spontaneous reduction, 5%).
      - ◇ Perform transvaginally at 8 to 9 weeks.
      - ◇ Perform transabdominally at 11 to 12 weeks.
      - ◇ The procedure-related pregnancy loss rate is 10%.

V. The Ovarian Hyperstimulation Syndrome
- ◆ Can be life-threatening.
- ◆ Mild cases.
  - Ovarian enlargement.
  - Abdominal distention.
  - Weight gain.
- ◆ Moderate and severe causes.
  - Ascites.
  - Pleural effusion.
  - Electrolyte imbalance.
  - Hypovolemia with hypotension and oliguria.
- ◆ Impressive incidence of occurrence.
- ◆ Severe OHSS in 1% to 2%.
- ◆ Two-thirds of cases seen in conception cycles.
- ◆ Follicular aspiration in *in vitro* fertilization (IVF) possibly somewhat protective.

- ◆ Luteal phase hCG = a risk factor; use progesterone instead if estradiol is >2,500 pg/mL or if >15 follicles are seen.
- ◆ PCOS patients are at highest risk.
- ◆ Pathophysiology.
  - • A massive third space fluid shift occurs.
  - • Resulting hypovolemia leads to circulatory problems.
  - • The genesis of ascites is unclear.
    - ■ Possibly a local estrogen effect.
    - ■ Maybe from vascular endothelial growth factor (VEGF); severity correlates with circulating levels of VEGF.
    - ■ Perhaps due to the ovarian renin–angiotensin system; large amounts of angiotensin II in ascites fluid.
  - • Hypovolemia leads to hemoconcentration.
    - ■ Increased coagulability.
    - ■ Decreased renal perfusion (oliguria and low sodium excretion).
      - ◇ Hyperkalemic acidosis.
      - ◇ Increased blood urea nitrogen (BUN).
    - ■ Elevation in aldosterone, plasma renin, and antidiuretic hormone (ADH).
- ◆ Treatment.
  - • Conservative and empiric.
  - • Hospitalize with the following:
    - ■ Weight gain >10 lb.
    - ■ Excessive pain.
    - ■ Hemoconcentration.
      - ◇ Hematocrit >50%.
      - ◇ White blood cell count >25,000.
    - ■ Oliguria.
    - ■ Dyspnea.
    - ■ Postural hypotension.
  - • Management in hospital.
    - ■ Put on bed rest.
    - ■ Check daily weights.
    - ■ Monitor strictly intake/outputs.
    - ■ Take frequent vital signs.
    - ■ Conduct serial evaluation of the following:
      - ◇ Hematocrit.
      - ◇ BUN/creatinine and electrolytes.
      - ◇ Total protein.
      - ◇ Coagulation studies.
    - ■ Correct hypovolemia.
      - ◇ Consider the use of plasma expanders and human albumin.
      - ◇ Diuretics are not helpful.
    - ■ Consider anticoagulant therapy.
    - ■ Life-threatening acute respiratory distress syndrome can occur.
    - ■ Abdominal paracentesis can relieve severe pulmonary compromise.

- ♦ Key point—resolution occurs with time.
  - Seven days in the absence of pregnancy.
  - Ten to 20 days in the pregnant patient.
VI. Predicting Gonadotropin Failure
- ♦ Incipient ovarian failure patients have elevated levels of FSH.
  - Decreased levels of inhibin B in the follicular phase.
  - Decreased luteal levels of inhibin A.
  - Overall, probably the result of a diminished follicular pool.
  - Correlates with ovarian volume.
- ♦ Testing the ovarian reserve.
  - Day 3 FSH >10 IU/L is abnormal.
  - Day 3 FSH >25 IU/L or an age of >44 years is independently associated with a chance of success close to zero.
  - Elevated day 3 estradiol is also predictive of poor outcome; this reflects early recruitment due to increased FSH levels.
- ♦ Clomiphene citrate challenge test.
  - Bioassay of FSH response.
  - Clomiphene, 100 mg on cycle days 5 to 9; FSH, days 3 and 10.
  - Exaggerated response >26 IU/L associated with a poor prospect for pregnancy; 85% show a poor response to ovarian stimulation.
  - Abnormal tests increase with age.
    - Less than 30 years old—3%.
    - More than 39 years old—26%.
    - Unexplained infertility—38%.
  - Screening recommendations.
    - All infertile women at age 30.
    - Women of any age with unexplained infertility.
    - Women who respond poorly to stimulation.
    - May not be helpful in women >40.
  - Failure of a response to gonadotropins despite normal screening hormones places patients at high risk of rapid progression to ovarian failure.
VII. GnRH Agonist and Gonadotropin Combined Treatment
- ♦ This converts normogonadotropic anovulators to hypogonadotropic hypogonadal state.
  - May improve the response.
  - Decreases the miscarriage rate.
  - Diminishes the risk of OHSS.
- ♦ The initial response is a "flare."
  - Begin in the luteal phase.
  - Consider the use of progestational agent for 10 days (begin the GnRH agonist after 3 days).
- ♦ Progesterone supplementation or luteal phase hCG is required (increases OHSS risk).
  - hCG, 2,000 IU at 3 days and 6 days after ovulation.
  - Progesterone vaginal suppositories, 25 mg per vagina (PV) BID.
  - Oral micronized progesterone, 300 mg QD.

- Progesterone, 50 mg IM QD.
- Vaginal progesterone gel, 90 mg of 8% gel QD.

VIII. GnRH Antagonists
- Competitive inhibitor of GnRH.
- Prevents LH surge.

IX. Growth Hormone
- Could growth hormone stimulation of insulin-like growth factor I (IGF-I) facilitate ovulation induction?
- The results suggest improvements in a small percentage of poor responders; its utility is limited by the following:
  - Cost.
  - The level of the standard dose.
  - Patient selection.

X. Ovulation Induction with GnRH
- Advantages.
  - Simple to use.
  - Minimal monitoring.
  - Low risk of OHSS.
- Administer via a programmable minipump.
- Most effective in hypothalamic amenorrhea.
  - Can also be used in PCOS.
  - An alternative for hyperprolactinemic patients unable to tolerate bromocriptine.
- IV or subcutaneous administration.
  - IV leads to better absorption.
  - Use heparin 1,000 U/mL.
- Dosage.
  - IV 5 mg/bolus every 90 minutes.
  - Subcutaneous 20 mg/bolus every 90 minutes.
- Following ovulation with hCG, stop the pump; continue hCG every 3 days.
- Pregnancy rate.
  - Twenty percent to 30% per cycle.
  - Eighty percent after six cycles.
  - Ninety-three percent after 12 cycles.
- Lower success and higher miscarriage rates observed in obese women with PCOS.

XI. Ovarian Surgical Procedures
- 1935—Stein and Leventhal described 7 cases.
- They developed wedge resection as a treatment when they observed that patients began ovulating after ovarian biopsy.
- They removed 50% to 75% of each ovary.
- The physiologic basis for the resumption of ovulation is based on the following:
  - Sustained reduction in testosterone.
    - The success is proportional to the volume removed.
    - An oophorectomy can also be effective.
  - Reduction in inhibin levels.
- A risk of postoperative adhesion formation is observed.
- The modern version is performed by laparoscopy.
  - Less adhesion formation.

- • Good alternative in the patient who is unable or unwilling to explore assisted reproductive options.

XII. Superovulation and Intrauterine Insemination (IUI) for Unexplained Infertility
   ♦ Inferior to IVF but lower cost.
   ♦ Treats subtle hormonal abnormalities in women with unexplained infertility.
   ♦ Cumulative pregnancy rate of 40% after six cycles.
   ♦ IUI alone not helpful.
   ♦ IUI plus superovulation better than superovulation alone.

Pregnancy Rate per Cycle

No treatment	1.3% to 4.1%
IUI	3.8%
Clomiphene	5.6%
Clomiphene plus IUI	8.3%
Gonadotropins	7.7%
Gonadotropins plus IUI	17.1%
IVF	20.7%

XIII. Fertility Drugs and Ovarian Cancer
   ♦ Two early flawed studies suggested an increased risk.
   ♦ Several recent larger epidemiologic studies have been reassuring.
   ♦ The best evidence does not indicate an increased risk of ovarian cancer with <12 months of clomiphene or with gonadotropin treatment.

Assisted Reproduction

I. Introduction: Assisted Reproductive Technology (ART)
- ◆ Techniques involving the direct retrieval of oocytes from the ovary.
  - *In vitro* fertilization (IVF)—extraction of oocytes, fertilization in the laboratory, and transcervical transfer of embryos into the uterus.
  - Gamete intrafallopian transfer (GIFT)—the placement of oocytes and sperm into the fallopian tube.
  - Zygote intrafallopian transfer (ZIFT)—the placement of fertilized oocytes into the fallopian tube.
  - Tubal embryo transfer—the placement of cleaving embryos into the fallopian tube.
  - Peritoneal oocyte and sperm transfer—the placement of oocytes and sperm into the peritoneal cavity.
- ◆ In addition, techniques of sperm retrieval and sperm injection are now part of the ART armamentarium:
  - Intracytoplasmic sperm injection of a single spermatozoon (ICSI).
  - Testicular sperm extraction (TESE).
  - Microsurgical epididymal sperm aspiration (MESA).

II. Patient Selection
- ◆ IVF was initially used only with tubal disease but has now been expanded to wide range of causes of infertility.
- ◆ Tubal disease—IVF is treatment of choice for severe distal disease, proximal obstruction (6 months after cannulation), and failure to conceive in 2 years after surgery.
- ◆ Large hydrosalpinges can reduce the pregnancy rate; their removal is recommended prior to IVF.
- ◆ Screening tests.
  - Human immunodeficiency virus type 1 (HIV-1) and type 2 (HIV-2).
  - Human T-lymphotrophic virus type 1.
  - Hepatitis B or C.
  - Chlamydia, syphilis, gonorrhea, and cytomegalovirus.
- ◆ Age-related decline in success is observed.
- ◆ Day 3 follicle-stimulating hormone (FSH) levels are predictive of success.

III. Stimulation Protocol
- ◆ Overview.
  - Nonstimulated cycle delivery rate per retrieval is 6%.
  - Stimulated cycles were introduced to improve success.
  - Gonadotropin-releasing hormone (GnRH) agonists were introduced in the late 1980s.

- Down-regulation prevents premature ovulation (previously seen in 15% of IVF cases).
- Increased doses of gonadotropins are needed.
- This allows for flexibility of scheduling.
- Follicular phase use can increase response in poor responders; follow the "flare" protocol.
- Stimulation is usually started in luteal phase with one of the following drugs:
  ◇ Leuprolide (Lupron), 0.5 mg/day.
  ◇ Nafarelin (Synarel), nasal spray BID.
- Gonadotropins.
  - The usual starting dose is 225 to 300 IU/day.
  - New preparations can be injected subcutaneously; recombinant FSH preparations may result in slightly improved pregnancy rates.
  - The cancellation rate is usually 10% to 15%.
- Options for poor responders include the following:
  1. Increase the dose or change the mix of gonadotropins—usually unsuccessful.
  2. Use a microdose flare protocol.
  3. Lower the dose of GnRH agonist.
  4. Omit the GnRH agonist; use a GnRH antagonist.
  5. Consider the addition of growth hormone.

IV. Monitoring Response
- The goal is an estradiol level of 200 pg/mL per large (>14-mm) follicle.
- Schedule retrieval 34 to 39 hours after human chorionic gonadotropin (hCG) insertion.
- Follicle size criteria depend on each program and can vary between ultrasound machines.
- Estradiol assays are also variable.
- Elevated levels of progesterone may not interfere with pregnancy.
- The risk of hyperstimulation is significant if >25 follicles are seen or if estradiol is >4,000 pg/mL.
  - Options.
    - Cancellation.
    - Cryopreserving all embryos.
    - Coasting; give hCG once the estradiol drops below 3,000 pg/mL.
  - Pattern of the endometrium.
    - Thickness >8 mm.
    - Trilaminar pattern preferred.

V. Oocyte Retrieval
- Perform under intravenous analgesia or light anesthesia.
- Monitor by pulse oximeter.
- Usually one puncture per ovary is needed to allow sequential aspiration.

VI. Oocyte Culture
- Oocytes are identified under a microscope.
- Insemination by 4 to 6 hours after retrieval is preferred.
- The sperm are prepared usually with swim-up: 50,000 to 100,000 sperm/oocyte.

♦ Coculture is unlikely to be helpful.

VII. Fertilization
- ♦ Cumulus cells are removed the day following insemination.
- ♦ About 65% to 80% of mature oocytes will fertilize. Roughly 6% contain three pronuclei, indicating polyspermia.
- ♦ Fertilization failure can be a surprising outcome.
  - • Three cycles are needed to diagnose this accurately as a recurring problem.
  - • However, this approach is not practical so ICSI is usually recommended.
- ♦ Supernumery embryos can be cryopreserved; two-thirds survive the freeze/thaw process.

VIII. Embryo Transfer
- ♦ The transfer is most commonly performed 72 to 80 hours after retrieval with embryos at the 8- to 10-cell stage.
- ♦ The multiple pregnancy rate is 35%.
- ♦ The guidelines for the number of embryos to transfer are based on the age of the woman.
- ♦ Luteal phase supplementation is common.
- ♦ The presence of cardiac activity 5 weeks after embryo transfer is reassuring.
  - • Women <30 years of age → near 0% spontaneous abortion (SAB) rate.
  - • Women 31 to 35 years of age → 4% SAB rate.
  - • Women >40 years of age → 20% SAB rate.
  - • A history of recurrent pregnancy loss → 25% SAB rate.
- ♦ The benefit of assisted hatching is controversial.

IX. IVF Results
- ♦ Delivery rates should be presented as the success rates.
- ♦ Society of Assisted Reproductive Technology Data—1995
  - • Deliveries per retrieval.
    - ▪ IVF—22%.
    - ▪ GIFT—27%.
    - ▪ ZIFT—27.9%.
    - ▪ Women <35 years—27%.
    - ▪ Women >39 years—10%.
    - ▪ Donor ova—36%.
  - • Three percent of the resulting pregnancies are ectopic.
  - • The heterotropic rate is 1 in 30,000 spontaneous pregnancies and 1 in 1,000 IVF pregnancies.
  - • The miscarriage rate is 20%, which is similar to the rate in the infertile population.
  - • No increase in congenital malformations is observed.
  - • The multiple pregnancy rate is 35%.
    - ▪ Twins—30%.
    - ▪ Triplets—5%.
    - ▪ Higher order—0.6%.

- The chance for success drops after three failed cycles; 50% of women <35 have a live birth within six cycles of treatment.

X. Male Infertility and IVF
  ♦ Early experience demonstrated low fertilization rates.
  ♦ A variety of minimally effective modifications has been attempted.
  ♦ Micromanipulation.
    - The results with ICSI have surpassed all expectations.
    - Nonejaculated sperm can be utilized; same success occurs with even immotile sperm.
    - ICSI is also indicated for antisperm antibodies.
    - *Rescue* ICSI after failed fertilization has limited success.
  ♦ Transmission of genetic abnormalities.
    - Five percent to 7% of infertile males carry chromosomal abnormalities.
      ▪ High prevalence of Y chromosome submicroscopic deletions in azoospermia (7% to 10% in oligospermia).
      ▪ Three specific regions on Yq: AZFa, AZFb, and AZFc.
    - Ten percent of sperm carry an extra chromosome.
    - ICSI pregnancies demonstrate a 0.84% incidence of sex chromosomic abnormalities, which is higher than in spontaneous pregnancies.
    - Consider a genetic screening prior to ICSI.
      ▪ Klinefelter syndrome.
      ▪ Luteinizing hormone (LH) β subunit mutation.
      ▪ FSH receptor mutation.
    - Congenital absence of the vas deferens.
      ▪ This is seen in 1% to 2% of infertile males.
      ▪ Most of them have two cystic fibrosis mutations.
      ▪ Screen the female partner to determine the risk to the fetus.
  ♦ Long-term outcomes.
    - Questions exist about whether delayed mental development is more common in ICSI children.
    - However, other studies are reassuring regarding mental development of these children.

XI. Other Techniques
  ♦ GIFT.
    - The replacement of gametes into fallopian tube following transvaginal oocyte collection.
    - Success rates higher than with IVF; may be the result of patient selection.
    - Slightly higher ectopic rate (4.2% versus 2.6%).
    - Similar multiple rate.
  ♦ ZIFT—fallopian tube placement following *in vitro* fertilization.

XII. Ovum Donation
  ♦ A technique of proven value.

        ♦ Ideal donor <22 years of age.

        ♦ Delivery rates of 40% to 50% per cycle can be achieved.

XIII.   Preimplantation Genetic Diagnosis

        ♦ Three possible approaches are as follows:

           1.   Polar body biopsy.

           2.   Trophoblast biopsy.

           3.   Blastomere biopsy.

        ♦ Diseases to be evaluated for include the following:

           • Cystic fibrosis.

           • Duchenne muscular dystrophy.

           • Sickle cell anemia.

           • Hemophilia.

           • Tay–Sachs disease.

           • Lesch–Nyhan syndrome.

        ♦ This specialized tool is available at only a few centers.

32

Ectopic Pregnancy

I. Introduction
- Modern management of ectopic pregnancy is one of medicine's success stories.
  - Ectopic pregnancy was first described in the 11th century.
  - Previously a universally fatal event.
- Its association with pelvic inflammation was stressed by mid-19th century.
- Surgical treatment had high mortality.
  - Only 5 of 30 women survived abdominal operations in the first 80 years of the 1800s.
  - The survival rate in nontreated patients was better—one in three.
- Modern surgical management was ushered in by Robert Lawson Tait in London in 1883—ligation of the broad ligament and ruptured tube.
- Rapid drop in mortality rate from between 200 to 400 in 10,000 cases to 3.4 in 10,000 cases by 1992; however, the overall ectopic rate increased to 19.7 per 1,000 pregnancies.
- Management prior to rupture in 80% of cases is possible due to human chorionic gonadotropin (hCG) assay, sonography, and laparoscopy.

II. Etiology and Clinical Presentation
- Ectopic pregnancy still remains the second leading cause of maternal mortality in the United States and the leading cause of first trimester pregnancy-related deaths.
- Ectopic pregnancy is the great masquerader.
  - The frequency of clinical symptoms and signs is hard to assess.
  - Differential diagnosis.
    - Normal intrauterine pregnancy.
    - Ruptured ovarian cyst.
    - Bleeding corpus luteum.
    - Spontaneous miscarriage.
    - Salpingitis.
    - Appendicitis.
    - Adnexal torsion.
    - Endometriosis.
    - Diverticulitis.
  - Relevant risk factors.
    - Prior tubal surgery.
    - Use of assisted reproductive technology (ART) procedures.
    - Diethylstilbestrol exposure.
    - Previous pelvic inflammatory disease (PID).
    - Vaginal douching.
    - Method of contraception.
    - Cigarette smoking.
    - None → most patients.

- ◆ Previous PID.
  - A history of salpingitis results in a 4× increase in risk as a result of damage to the endosalpinx.
  - The risk increases with each episode of PID.
  - Circulating chlamydia antibodies are associated with a 2× increase in ectopic pregnancy.
- ◆ Prior tubal surgery.
  - The risk is increased by previous fertility surgery but is not increased by abdominal or pelvic surgery that does not involve the tubes.
  - Increased risk is seen after prior conservative surgery for an ectopic pregnancy.
  - Ectopic pregnancies occur after tubal ligations.
    - More frequent with interval sterilization by bipolar.
    - Usually occur >2 years after sterilization.
    - Probably represents fistula formation that leads to fertilization in the distal segment of the tube.
    - The overall rate of ectopic pregnancy is 80% less than in nonsterilized women, but relative risk is 3.7× that of women on oral contraceptive pills and 2.8× that of women using barrier contraception.
    - One-third of pregnancies after tubal sterilization are ectopic (Table 32.1).
- ◆ Use of ART.
  - Heterotopic pregnancy rate is increased.
  - Rate of 1 in 30,000 spontaneous pregnancies.
  - Rate of 1 in 100 ART pregnancies; probably from retrograde embryo migration following embryo transfer.
- ◆ Method of contraception.
  - The risk is reduced with all methods except the progesterone-containing intrauterine device (IUD).
  - IUD myths.
    - Previous IUD use does not increase the risk of ectopic pregnancy.

Table 32.1. Estimated relative risk of ectopic pregnancy

Risk Factor	Relative Risk
Tubal surgery	20.0
Previous ectopic	10.0
Previous salpingitis	4.0
Assisted reproduction	4.0
Age <25	3.0
Previous pelvic infection	3.0
Infertility	2.5
Cigarette smoking	2.5
Vaginal douching	2.5

Table 32.2.   Ectopic pregnancy rates per 1,000 woman-years

All U.S. women	1.50
Non–contraceptive users	3.00
Copper T 380 IUD	0.20
Progesterone IUD	6.80
Levonorgestrel IUD	0.20
Norplant	0.28

Abbreviation: IUD, intrauterine device.

- - Current use of the copper IUD does not increase the risk.
  - IUD facts.
    - IUD users are 50% less likely to have an ectopic pregnancy.
      - ◇ But, if an IUD user becomes pregnant, then the pregnancy is more likely to be ectopic.
      - ◇ Three percent to 4% of IUD pregnancies are ectopic.
    - TCu-380A IUD users are 90% less likely than noncontraceptors to have an ectopic pregnancy.
      - ◇ The risk does not increase with the duration of use.
      - ◇ Only one ectopic pregnancy per 8,000 woman-years of experience has been reported (Table 32.2).
  - ◆ Ectopic sites.
    - Almost all are in the tube.
    - The mortality rate for abdominal pregnancies is 17× greater than for the overall ectopic rate (Table 32.3).
- III. Methods of Early Diagnosis
  - ◆ The best way to diagnose an ectopic pregnancy is to be highly suspicious and to use the appropriate diagnostic tools—β-hCG measurement and sonography.
  - ◆ Quantitative measurement of hCG.
    - Level is ~ 100 IU/L at the time of missed menses.

Table 32.3.   Sites of ectopic implantation

Fallopian tube	
Ampullar segment	80%
Isthmic segment	12%
Fimbrial end	5%
Cornual and interstitial	2%
Abdominal	1.4%
Ovarian	0.2%
Cervical	0.2%

- The minimum level is 50,000 to 100,000 IU/L at 8 to 10 weeks of gestation.
- The modern assay measures the serum level of β-hCG.
  - Largest β subunit at 145 amino acids; unique 24–amino acid carboxyl terminal tail.
  - Detection level <5 IU/L—should yield no false-negative results except in extremely rare circumstances.
- A doubling rate of 48 hours in normal pregnancies was described in 1981.
  - This well-recognized pattern is seen during the first 6 weeks.
  - The rate of increase is linear from 2 to 4 weeks after ovulation.
    - ◇ Some ectopics can demonstrate a normal rise.
    - ◇ Some normal pregnancies (10%) will demonstrate an abnormal rise.
- ◆ The clinical usefulness of β-hCG measurement is as follows:
  1. Assessment of viability of pregnancy.
  2. Correlation with ultrasonography—should see intrauterine sac when titer >1,000 IU/L.
  3. Assessment of treatment results.
- ◆ Vaginal ultrasonography.
  - Identification of the gestational sac is very helpful.
    - Sonolucent center with thick echogenic rim (decidual reaction around the chorionic sac).
    - Yolk sac visualized within sac at 5 weeks; cardiac activity at 5.5 to 6 weeks of gestation.
  - Discriminatory zone of 1,000 to 1,500 IU/L usually occurs 1 week after missed menses.
  - One must also consider the possibility of a heterotopic pregnancy.
  - Color and pulsed Doppler increase the sensitivity.
    - A pseudosac is seen in 10% of ectopic pregnancies.
    - Doppler can also aid in the identification of an ectopic pregnancy in the adnexa; ultrasound should detect ectopics >2 cm.
- ◆ The progesterone level.
  - A wide overlap between normal and ectopic pregnancy is found.
  - The concentration is usually lower in ectopic pregnancies.
    - A value >25 ng/mL is associated with normal pregnancy 98% of the time.
    - A value <5 ng/mL represents nonviable pregnancy regardless of location.
  - Most patients present with progesterone between 1 and 10 ng/mL.
- ◆ Uterine curettage.
  - This is helpful with progesterone <5 ng/mL and nonrising hCG titer <1,000 IU/L.

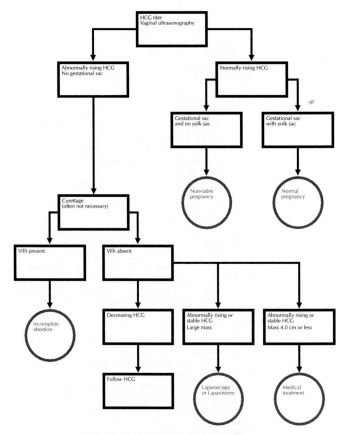

Figure 32.1.   Algorithm for diagnosis of an ectopic pregnancy.

- • Floating tissue in saline will not always identify chorionic villi.
- ♦ Culdocentesis is no longer very helpful in making the diagnosis (Fig. 32.1).
- IV. Treatment
  - ♦ Expectant management.
    - • Includes the monitoring of clinical symptoms, hCG titers, and ultrasound findings.
    - • Twenty-five percent of women can be managed expectantly; good outcomes are observed in 70%.
      - ■ The best results are in patients with hCG levels <2,000 IU/L.
      - ■ Long-term outcome is similar to active treatment interventions.
    - • **Criteria for expectant management.**
      1. Falling hCG titer.

2. Ectopic definitely in the tube.
3. No significant bleeding.
4. No evidence of rupture.
5. Ectopic not >4 cm.
♦ Medical treatment.
  • Methotrexate is a folic acid antagonist.
  • It interferes with DNA synthesis.
  • It was first used to treat an ectopic in 1982.
    ■ **Criteria for patient selection.**
      1. Patient is healthy, hemodynamically stable, reliable, and compliant.
      2. Ultrasonography fails to find an intrauterine pregnancy, and uterine curettage fails to obtain villi.
      3. Ectopic pregnancy measures 4 cm or less in its greatest diameter.
      4. No evidence of rupture of the ectopic pregnancy is observed.
      5. hCG titers >10,000 IU/L and fetal cardiac activity are relative contraindications. However, even patients with fetal cardiac activity have been successfully treated.
    ■ **Prior to methotrexate treatment.**
      1. Administer Rh immunoglobulin (RhoGAM) if the patient is Rh negative and >8 weeks of gestation.
      2. Obtain baseline liver and renal function tests and complete blood and platelet counts.
      3. Consider uterine curettage.
    ■ **Patient instructions.**
      The following are avoided until hCG titers are negative: alcohol use, sexual intercourse, and the use of folic acid–containing vitamins.
  • Multiple-dose method.
    ■ Seventy percent to 90% are successful.
    ■ Failures are more common with hCG >5,000 IU/L; the presence of fetal cardiac activity is a contraindication.
    ■ Side effects are observed in 4%.
    ■ The incidence of nonresponders or tubal rupture is 3% to 4%.
    ■ The onset of abdominal cramping 3 to 4 days after methotrexate occurs in 60%; this may require hospital observation.

Multiple-Dose Protocol

Day 1:	Baseline studies	
	Methotrexate	1.0 mg/kg intramuscularly (IM)
Day 2:	Citrovorum factor	0.1 mg/kg IM
Day 3:	Methotrexate	1.0 mg/kg IM
Day 4:	Citrovorum factor	0.1 mg/kg IM
	hCG titer	

Day 5:	Methotrexate	1.0 mg/kg IM
	hCG titer	
Day 6:	Citrovorum factor	0.1 mg/kg IM
	hCG titer	
Day 7:	Methotrexate	1.0 mg/kg IM
	hCG titer	
Day 8:	Citrovorum factor	0.1 mg/kg IM
	hCG titer	
	Complete blood and platelet counts	
	Renal and liver function tests	
Weekly:	hCG titer until negative	

- Outcome.
  - Twenty percent of patients require only a single dose.
  - Twenty percent require four doses.
  - Fertility following treatment is similar to that after laparoscopic surgery.
  - Four percent of patients require surgical therapy.
- Single-dose method.
  - Results with single dose are excellent even with cardiac activity present.
  - hCG titers keep rising for 3 days but decline by day 7.
  - Full resolution is seen in 3 to 6 weeks.
  - Repeat dosing is suggested if <15% decline is observed by day 7; this is necessary in 8% of patients.

  Single-dose protocol

Day 1:	Baseline studies	
	Methotrexate	50 mg/m^2 IM
Day 4:	hCG titer	
Day 7:	hCG titer	
	Complete blood and platelet counts	
	Liver and renal function tests	
Weekly:	hCG titer until negative	

- Important precautions.
  - Medical treatment requires compulsive compliance.
  - An ectopic pregnancy can exist in the absence of detectable hCG.
  - A satisfying decline does not guarantee against rupture.
  - The average time to hCG resolution is 4 weeks.
  - The risk of rupture is 10% with hCG <1,000 IU/L.
- Special indications—methotrexate therapy is helpful in locations where surgical therapy carries significant risk.
  - Cervix.
  - Ovary.
  - Cornua.

♦ Salpingocentesis.
  • Efficacy, safety, and long-term impact on fertility are uncertain.
  • Local treatment offers no benefit over systemic treatment.
♦ Surgical treatment.
  • Conservative surgery is more common now with earlier diagnosis.
    ■ Linear salpingostomy is the procedure of choice for ampullary ectopies.
    ■ Segmental resection is better for isthmic ectopies.
  • Milking of the ectopic out of the fimbriated end is associated with a high-risk of persistent ectopic pregnancy.
  • Salpingectomy may be a better option in the patient with tubal disease. Other indications for salpingectomy are as follows:
    ■ Child-bearing completed.
    ■ Second ectopic that has occurred in that tube.
    ■ Uncontrolled bleeding.
    ■ Severely damaged tube.
  • The surgical therapy chosen is less important in determining future fertility than is the cause of the ectopic pregnancy.

  Results with Laparoscopic Surgery

Subsequent intrauterine pregnancy	70%
Subsequent tubal patency	84%
Subsequent ectopic pregnancy	12%
Persistent trophoblast	15%

♦ Treatment of persistent trophoblastic tissue.
  • The risk of a persistent ectopic is from 5% to 15%.
    ■ Can be associated with hemorrhage and tubal rupture.
    ■ Weekly hCG measurements are necessary following conservative surgery.
  • The use of methotrexate is preferable to reoperation; consider prophylactic methotrexate (1 mg/kg) at the time of conservative surgery or a single dose (50 mg/m^2) at the time of diagnosis of persistent trophoblastic tissue.
♦ Rh sensitization—consider the use of Rh immunoglobulin in ectopic pregnancies of >8 weeks of gestation.
♦ Fertility after ectopic pregnancy.
  • Fifteen percent chance of an ectopic pregnancy in the next pregnancy.
  • The chance of a recurrent ectopic increases tenfold after two ectopics; consider *in vitro* fertilization in this setting.

Subject Index

Note: Numbers followed by an *f* indicate figures; those followed by a *t* indicate tables.